W9-ART-861

gorgeous!

Other Books by Jorj Morgan

The Complete Idiot's Guide to Good Fat, Good Carb Meals

Fresh Traditions: Classic Dishes for a Contemporary Lifestyle

At Home Entertaining: The Art of Hosting a Party with Style and Panache

At Home in the Kitchen: The Art of Preparing the Foods You Love to Eat

gorgeous!

The Sum of All Your Glorious Parts

A LIFESTYLE ENHANCEMENT GUIDE

Jorj Morgan

With Dr. Harry Moon and Mary Ellen Clark

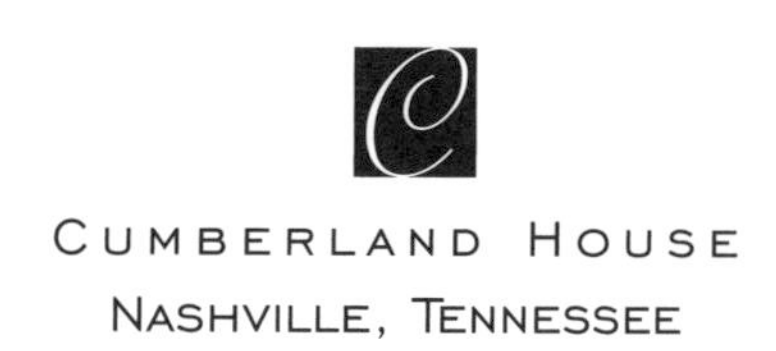

CUMBERLAND HOUSE
NASHVILLE, TENNESSEE

Gorgeous!
Published by Cumberland House Publishing, Inc.
431 Harding Industrial Drive
Nashville, TN 37211

Copyright © 2007 by Jorj Morgan

All rights reserved. No part of this book may be reproduced or transmitted in any form or by any means, electronic or mechanical, including photocopying and recording, or by any information storage and retrieval system, without permission in writing from the publisher, except for brief quotations in critical reviews or articles.

Text design: Lisa Taylor

Library of Congress Cataloging-in-Publication Data

Morgan, Jorj, 1953–
Gorgeous! : the sum of your glorious parts / by Jorj Morgan, with Dr. Harry Moon and Mary Ellen Clark.
p. cm.
Includes index.
ISBN-13: 978-1-58182-572-5 (hardcover)
ISBN-10: 1-58182-572-2 (hardcover)
1. Cookery (Natural foods) 2. Beauty, Personal. I. Moon, Harry. II. Clark, Mary Ellen. III. Title.
TX741.M65 2007
641.5'63—dc22

2006036522

Printed in Canada
1 2 3 4 5 6 7 — 11 10 09 08 07

For Mallory Marie Morgan
From your great grandmothers, your grandmothers, and your mother.
You have been given all of the tools that you will need in life.
It is up to you to go forward and make that life a most GORGEOUS one—
Not just for you, but for everyone that you touch.
We will be there for you—forever. . . .

CONTENTS

ACKNOWLEDGMENTS

I was fortunate enough to meet Jennifer Russon while working on another book. She signed on as my assistant and immediately started referring to me as Miranda (the character from the book *The Devil Wears Prada*; I still don't understand why—I think I'm such a sweeter boss . . .). Anyway, this project was on a back burner when she came to work with me. Jennifer loved it so much that she kept prodding me to get it out there. She left my employ so that she and hubby, Ryan, could give birth to the perfect son, Max. All along she kept nudging me about *Gorgeous*. When it came time to put the book together, my first call was to Jen, busy mother and all. Her research, drafting, and overall comments have been an enormous part of this book. She is an author in her own right—and I hope you will look for her writings in the future. I know I will! Thank you, Jen.

To my wonderful family for supporting me in everything that I do, merrily offering advice along the way, I say thank you and "who loves you the most bunches . . . *me*!" My everlasting love belongs to GAM, Treysers and Kimber, Chris and Jon.

To all my GORGEOUS gal pals, (you know who you are—especially Doreenie and Cindy)—you continue to inspire me and bring me not only companionship in all things but also a heck of a lot of *fun* along the way! Thank you.

To Ron, Julie, Lisa, Stacie, Tracy, and everyone at Cumberland—your faith in me is such a loving gift. Thank you for your support, your confidence, and your assistance. You continue to make my dreams come true. (Go Dolphins!)

The recipes in this book have all been thoroughly tested by a group of volunteers, many of whom have tested recipes for my previous books and really have the process down pat! They cook for hubbies, children, friends, and coworkers, soliciting opinions and offering feedback along the way. This book is one thousand percent better because of them. Thank you to this GORGEOUS group of gals:

Sharon Murrah lives in Fort Lauderdale, Florida, and seriously enjoys being at home cooking and entertaining her family and friends. She's also a devoted supporter of Saint Anthony's School and an active fundraiser for Charity Guild.

Gerri Seinberg resides in Boynton Beach, Florida. She is a registered dietitian and worked in supermarket purchasing and management for twenty-five years. She is currently a food appliance specialist focusing on recipe and appliance testing and development. How lucky were we to have Gerri onboard as a volunteer tester!

Louise Proffer is another Fort Lauderdale resident, although she tested many of the recipes from her home in Tahoe. Her hubby of twenty-five years, Paul, offered many suggestions along the way. Together, they have worked side by side at Chuck's Steak House for thirty-two years.

My oldest and dear friend, Mary Dwors, came on board as a tester for this book and jumped in with both feet. She tested for hubby Bob and daughters Sara and Liz and survived—even though she is still in need of a soup tureen!

Speaking of old and dear friends, Linda O'Bryon and daughter Jennifer were *big* helpers for this project, testing amid full-time jobs and wedding plans.

Maureen Rotella, Patty Echarte, and Lydia LaRocca tested separately and together, offering successes to their families and quietly commenting on those things that "just might need a bit of improvement." Maureen is the owner of a fine stationery store in Fort Lauderdale, and Patty is a recent empty-nester currently filling her time in real estate. Lydia works for her good friend's office—as long as she has Friday's off to cook!

Reliable and steady testers include Mel Sirois of Bethesda, Maryland. She is a fitness instructor and personal trainer, who loves running and has done several marathons. Mel is also a recreational baker and chef. Lisa Juneau is from Bridge City, Texas. She is the wife of "the best husband in the world" and a charter consultant with Taste of Home Entertaining. Kate Patch lives in Cabin John, Maryland. She is a legal secretary by day and mom to a grade-schooler and three adult stepchildren by evening. Baking is her favorite hobby, to the delight of her friends, family, and colleagues. Thanks, Kate, for all of the help on the dessert sections! Amy Kendall and her entire family tested a lot of recipes. She is from Franklin, Tennessee, is a biochemist and describes herself as a "supermom and aspiring chef."

Margaret Donkerbrook describes herself as a pampered wife and Greg's mom. She spoils her boys with food and love. She's a friend of Trey's from Arlington, Virginia. Another of Trey's pals and a fabulous tester is Mary Ellen Lemm (also known as "MEL") from Plano, Texas. She is a paralegal by trade but a baker at heart! Sandra Shu (soon to be Sandra Nanney) lives in Alexandria, Virginia. She's had a busy year with work, planning a wedding, and waiting for her new home to be finished. But she managed to find the time to be one of our most thorough testers.

Rachel Zollinger of Moon Township, Pennsylvania, has been inspired by her mother, preparing family meals and recipe collecting since the age of ten. She is a Pampered Chef consultant. If not cooking or reading recipes, she prefers to spend leisure time working in her garden. Gail Jordan lives in Raleigh, North Carolina, with her tremendous husband Dean, soon-to-be-fifteen-and-performer-of-all-things-musical-theater daughter, Carly, and eight-year-old-baseball-and-NASCAR-loving son, Adam, who are all eager tasters. Gail freelances in public relations and is a published essayist. P.J. Forbes is a marketing consultant from Virginia Beach, Virginia. She concentrates on gourmet food products and cookbook consulting. She enjoys cooking so much she made sure her new motor home had a full kitchen! P.J. has been a contributor to all of my cookbooks.

Sherry and Jon Hine, dear friends from Deland, Florida, are owners of Legacy Ferns and recent homeowners in North Carolina. Marilyn Moles-Carlisle resides in Fort Lauderdale, Florida, and is a practicing small-animal veterinarian, as well as a mother of two active, hungry boys and wife to Stephen. Lori Schrader Bachar is from Ankeny, Iowa. She is a program planner for a women's commission, wife, mother, daughter, and community volunteer.

Liz Bray is the owner of Leave It to Liz, a personal chef service in Benton, Arkansas. She taught kindergarten for twenty-one years and then studied with the USPCA. She has a wonderful, supportive husband of thirty-seven years (high school sweethearts, married right after graduation) and is the grandmother to Scarlett and her upcoming baby sister.

Other testers include Diana Shelton, Lisa Leyser of Cheverly, D.C., Anne Vitort, Ann T. Natunewicz, and Lucy Weber.

Whether testing one recipe or fifty-plus recipes like Sharon and Gerri, these *gorgeous* gals have made the dishes in this book truly easy and delicious.

gorgeous!

INTRODUCTION

Dear Fair Reader,

We believe every woman is beautiful. Do you? If you picked up this book, chances are you may not agree. And that's a problem. Our culture and the dizzying media blitz it has become convinces us that beauty is a one-size-fits-all concept, thereby labeling everything else too fat, too thin, too old, too *something*. We will debunk this outrageous myth by redefining beauty as a state of health and mind.

Even if you believe true beauty has little to do with airbrushed supermodels, American culture has more than likely taken its toll on your self-esteem, wearing you down and making you feel about as sexy as a garden slug. If you're looking to revitalize, energize, and reprioritize, this book is for you!

The beauty we will teach you how to go after celebrates uniqueness, femininity, and diversity. These things are Mother Nature's stamp on what makes us original. Notice that in a garden of breathtaking flowers, there are plenty of different varieties. It's the same with us human beings.

This is not a diet book but rather a lifestyle enhancement guide that shows smart, on-the-go women how to pamper and nurture themselves from the inside out. *Gorgeous* is crammed with information that explains the relationship between food and health. We have oodles of delicious recipes that prove *good* food is *fundamental* to living richly. Elevating the quality of our food and taking the time to enjoy it with family and friends is what this book is all about and why it will improve your life.

We talk about a lot more than just food. Starving yourself to lose weight, slathering on tons of concealing makeup, or working out so infrequently that you hurt yourself when you finally hit the gym is not being truthful to what your body needs, wants, or deserves. It's impossible to *look* good if you don't *feel* good. The presence or absence of beauty is a commentary on the quality of your overall health. If you're eating processed foods, routinely visiting fast-food restaurants, riding a stress rollercoaster every other day, and not exercising regularly, your skin, hair, eyes—*every part of you*—are going to suffer. We want you to learn how to isolate each body part, learn just what it needs to function at its best, and reinvent yourself from "head to toe."

We have prepared for you a lifestyle guide to dodge those misleading beauty bullets and help you maneuver around the demands of our increasingly fast-paced culture. We will show you other walks of life by daring to spin the globe! We remind you, our reader, that psychological well-being, personal hygiene, good nutrition, and regular exercise are the uncomplicated elixir for beauty that's at every woman's (soon-to-be-manicured, if we have anything to say about it!) fingertips. We posit that the quest for beauty is not really a quest at all but an invitation to enjoy life to its fullest while eating fresh, nutritious food.

These lifestyle changes are not difficult, and you will begin to notice the results almost overnight. Once you adopt the *Gorgeous* lifestyle, it will become part of your everyday routine. Living healthily will have you smiling for all seasons. So start today. Take stock of your health, your well-being, your appearance. Choose one thing you want to improve—your hair, your physical strength, your ability to sleep soundly, your sexual satisfaction. Begin with that chapter in this book and make the changes necessary to begin your journey toward a healthy and more satisfying lifestyle. We've made it unbelievably easy, deliciously appetizing, and amazingly luxurious.

We're here to help you improve and arrange each of your glorious parts into one *gorgeous* you!

—Jorj Morgan and Dr. Harry Moon
www.GorgeousLifestyleGuide.com

PART ONE

garden of the soul: cultivating mind & body

Your Body is a Sum of Its Parts

When you gaze into the mirror, do you see a tubby tummy, a big backside, dull hair, or a wrinkle that you swear wasn't there the last time you looked? If so, you're not alone. Most of us concentrate on the one or two parts of our bodies that we are less pleased with rather than the many parts that are doing just fine. The truth is we must begin to understand our bodies as well-designed structures. Each part of that structure has a function. When that function connects with the rest of our parts, the resulting form is a gorgeous design. It is incumbent upon each of us to nurture our bodies—each and every part—with excellent food, consistent exercise, and stress-relieving relaxation in order to obtain overall sublime gorgeousness.

I've always thought of beauty as subjective—what is attractive to one person may not raise so much as an eyebrow for somebody else. But *gorgeous* is different. Gorgeous is outstanding—it's mystical, it's universal. To feel and look gorgeous, we must consider what gorgeous is and what it is not. Media trendsetters suggest that it is airbrushed supermodels staring back at us from glossy magazine covers, stick-thin actresses in our movie blockbusters, or well-endowed college coeds recruited for Centerfold of the Year. Should these be taken as realistic representations of what strong, non-fictional women are all about? Trying to attain the impossible, in the frantic rat race the world has become today, are we guilty of neglecting our physical and emotional well-being, forgetting that these are intricately linked and dependent upon each other? The answer, sadly, is yes. The fact is we should strive for beauty simply because it's healthy, not because we mistakenly believe that with beauty comes a time-limited, A-list membership in the "Just Another Pretty Face Club." In a culture that prides itself on extreme makeovers, it is my pleasure to help you with *your* "big reveal"—one that, in contrast, lasts a lifetime and comes from a fresh, healthy, no-punches-pulled way of living. Now, *that's* gorgeous!

CHAPTER 1

gorgeous from the inside out

Creating an Individual Path to Sublime Wellness & Beauty

We've all heard the cliché "tough row to hoe;" it's an apt description when we are facing the daily challenges of living healthfully in our ever-changing, fast-paced world. A commitment to healthy, relaxed living amounts to more than just surface changes; it means a woman can be beautiful both inside *and* out. But how does a contemporary woman meet societal pressures, deadlines at work, and family obligations while still finding time to honor her body through sound diet and fitness, keeping her individuality in tact along the way?

Who are *gorgeous* women? They can be identified as those who haven't "let themselves go"—the ones who block out chatter in the frenetic contemporary life we all share and hear only a song of healing powers and sunny, regenerative living. They enjoy an exercise regime tailored for their individual lifestyle and food that's as healthy as it is pretty on the plate. Gorgeous women are the ones who take time to smell the roses, which haven't changed even today—"the roses" are and always have been fresh food, satisfying love, lust for life, and quality time spent with our families and friends. To be gorgeous, you must embrace these "tools of the well-tended."

When it comes to eating, I encourage you to make a point of living large, but only figuratively! Focus on innovation, not deprivation. Set a goal of preparing delicious recipes by eliminating the unhealthy stuff. Do this and watch the true definition of gorgeous begin to light you from the inside out. Gorgeous is your ability to feel terrific in the body you have, your desire to nurture, rather than change, what you were born and blessed with. Gorgeous is your inner contentment reflected in your outer appearance. Gorgeous is developed and embraced in every culture, in every part of the world. Being gorgeous comes from within and it starts with a healthy, well-balanced you.

Super-sizing of the 50 States

We are FAT. We are overweight because we eat out more than we eat at home. We eat alone or in front of the television. We eat junk food, fast food, processed food, and we eat too much of it. According to a poll conducted in the fall of 2005 by CBS News, a random sampling of 936 American adults revealed that, due to the demands of time or the desire to please their hungry kids, people with children are more likely than those without to eat fast food for dinner at least once a week. Still more disconcerting is research from the Produce for Better Health Foundation (PBH) which says that in those meals eaten at home, fruit and vegetable consumption is sorely lacking. Just 13 percent of American families eat the recommended minimum of five daily servings of fruits and veggies, versus 22 percent of singles, 27 percent of empty nesters, and 39 percent of the elderly. This is a poor showing for all groups concerned, especially today's families! Back when Father really did "know best," he would have told you that these statistics are associated with the country's ongoing battle with heart disease, cancer, and diabetes. Is there anything less gorgeous than that?

Striking a balance is key. Shine a detective's light on your eating habits. What's your daily intake, and, in terms of output, how much physical activity do you get from sun up to sundown? It all boils down to simple mathematics. If we keep the same level of intake (food) but our output (exercise) goes down, the end result means that we start to gain weight. So if you maintain the same level in terms of your intake and you increase your physical activity—your output—then you're more likely to lose weight. The key is finding the right balance, which is different for everyone.

What's worse than us being a society of overweight couch potatoes? It is the poor dietary habits we are instilling in our children. We're raising a nation of FAT, unhealthy kids. A growing number of overweight teens are causing the percentage of obese Americans to skyrocket; data from the National Health and Nutrition Examination Survey shows that 15 percent of kids aged six to nineteen have been, you might say, "super sized," and that, by and large (no pun intended), is a premature death sentence for our young people. Obesity is linked to a laundry list—a very dirty laundry list—of diseases: hypertension, coronary heart disease, type-2 diabetes, stroke, gallbladder disease, osteoarthritis, sleep apnea, respiratory problems, a variety of cancers, asthma, reproductive hormone abnormalities, lower back pain . . . just to name a few. Whether you are talking about your child or your grandchild, is this really what you want for the next generation? In the face of these hideous diseases, shouldn't we embrace gorgeous instead? Well, the research is in: the hope of our children growing into healthy, gorgeous adults lies in families rediscovering the nice "sit-down" dinners we associate with the

Leave It to Beaver era. Researchers from the University of Minnesota found that children ages eleven to eighteen who ate meals with their families consumed higher amounts of fruits, vegetables, grains, and nutrient-dense foods than those who ate separately. Furthermore, the *Journal of the American Dietetic Association* says that adolescents who consumed at least seven family meals per week had lower intakes of snack foods.

Beyond the bulge, there's an issue with our collective American pocketbooks as well: poor nutrition leads to staggering health-care costs for the entire nation! According to studies run by the United States government, if 88 million Americans aged 15 and up increased their physical activity and consumed less saturated fat and more calcium and fiber, national healthcare costs would go down as much as 76.6 billion dollars!

One of my favorite quotes is by Hippocrates, who said, "Let food be your medicine." While I don't advocate four-star meals as a cure for a broken leg, I *do* believe cooking fresh food and eating meals with those we love put us on the fast track to a happy heart. A happy heart is a healthy heart. Hippocrates didn't say that—that's all me—but it still sounds pretty good.

Hear Me ROAR

I am woman, hear me roar, and kudos to us for keeping that roar when our culture often gives cause to whimper. But at what price? We celebrate our equality doing double duty, holding down career jobs while parenting *and* keeping house. The U.S. Department of Labor says that 99 out of every 100 women in the U.S. will work for pay at some time in their lives. In 1950, only one-third of the U.S. labor force was female; by the year 2003 that proportion was approaching one-half (46 percent). By 2010, women are projected to account for 48 percent of the total American labor force.

For many of us busy working moms, this means burning the candle at both ends and then some, taking care of everyone around us and putting ourselves at the bottom of the list. In order to fit in all of the activities, meetings, and housework that seem to stretch into infinity, we take shortcuts. Shortcuts may seem like the answer to our prayers, but in the long run we become so focused on saving time that we lose the inherent value of the task at hand.

Here's an example of a *bad* shortcut. You are late arriving home from work, so you open a box of macaroni with a package of cheese sauce, top it with prepackaged breadcrumbs, and serve it to your unsuspecting brood. Processed foods are bad. Check out the sodium and fat content in the breadcrumbs alone to see what I mean. Likewise, just adding fresh ingredients to processed food does not a nutritious meal make. For example, browning ground beef and adding that to a can of beef soup does not produce "homemade" beef stew! I see "recipes" targeted at busy working mothers that do nothing more than manipulate processed food products. A recipe for Crab Bisque from a popular cookbook author includes in the ingredient list "1 can restaurant-style crab bisque" and "canned (not fresh) crab and parsley." The end result is supposed to be the best crab bisque ever made. Hello people! This is *not* cooking. This is combining sodium-laden, additive-filled ingredients in order to create a meal that you have little or no interaction with. Just what are we putting into our bodies?

Here's an example of a *good* shortcut. You make a meal plan and organize your grocery shopping so that one day a week you visit the grocery store for the majority of your purchases. You shop for fresh ingredients and avoid processed, prepackaged foods. When you return home, you prep as much food as you can to shorten meal preparation during the week. You wash, dry, and package lettuces into bags, and you peel carrots and slice for easy after-school snacks. This is a great expenditure of your time on your "shopping day" and an excellent shortcut to incorporate into your busy week.

As you explore your path to gorgeous, I encourage you to rediscover the joy of a leisurely dinner among family and friends. The fact is *everyone* needs quality time—even if it's just one hour—to decompress and find out what loved ones are up to. Working nutritious meals into the family's schedule is simply a matter of the two P's: pitchin' in and prioritizing! Every member of your household can be recruited for dinner prep or clean up. I know, I know . . . you're already anticipating the resistance from your husband, kids, or whoever it is that shares your roof. I believe that if you make mealtime a "fun-time," everyone will want to join in. My thirty years of family experience is a testament to this fact.

Before microwave ovens, fast food, and the extracurricular activities these conveniences enabled, the Classic Family Dinner was a no-brainer, but bring in a new line of modern conveniences and pretty soon there's no excuse to miss your son's soccer game, husband's business dinner, or night out with the gal pals. Because we can fit quick meals into a jam-packed schedule, we tend to do too much! The reality is that overscheduling engagements reduces the possibility of quiet dinners at home. I'm all in favor of finding a way to fit in nutrition *and* a kickin' social life, but in order to make this happen you must realize that the path to optimal health is paved with balance. Finding the balance among family meals, quality time to yourself, and a healthful meal plan is entirely possible—it's also essential for being gorgeous.

The Path to Gorgeous

If you want to be gorgeous, you *must* take control of your eating habits. You must carve out time to cook good, healthy meals with natural ingredients. *Just say no* to eating at fast-food drive-through restaurants. You will have to shop for fresh food. You will have to get in touch with your food. You will also have to learn where your food comes from and keep up with the ever-changing science of which foods are good for you and which ones aren't. You will have to prepare (or at least share in the preparation of) family meals. By "family" meals, I mean those for your unique and extended family, whether it be relatives or your group of closest friends. To be gorgeous you must view food with an eye toward socializing. Gorgeous people never dine alone.

Best Dressed in the Eye of the Beholder

Gorgeous begins on the inside and radiates to your outward appearance. However, how we enhance our natural beauty is another aspect for consideration. I know and you know (we all share a collective groan and eye roll on this one) that an American criterion for what constitutes gorgeous includes the category of "best-dressed" and is hinged upon the appeal of the celebrity du jour. In our rush to emulate the latest look, we often run the risk of abandoning classic good taste in personal appearance.

When I look around the workplace on casual Friday, I am dismayed to see articles of clothing that are distinctly out of place in an office environment. Pieces ranging from a "hello, cleavage!" bustier to a microscopic, cowgirl-chic miniskirt appear on all sizes and shapes—and, at the risk of sounding catty, I *cringe* at the way these items are put together and yet are still considered business-appropriate attire. Let's face it: not even Britney could pull off this look in an office! What's worse is that in our politically correct environ, it's woe to the manager or employer who utters a negative observation about a coworker's outfit. We sacrifice our two cents' worth in order to stave off lawsuits. Perhaps this lack of feedback is affecting our collective idea of what constitutes "well-groomed."

I will be the first one to admit that when time runs short, often I'm prevented from changing out of my morning "workout duds" before a round of errands, where I no doubt run across an acquaintance crossing my harried path. Usually, I reach for a pair of oversized sunglasses and a baseball cap and make like Angelina avoiding the paparazzi. However, I know women who actually live 24/7 in these clothes. When did we stay-at-home gals decide that a sweatshirt and baggy jeans constituted clothing? While I applaud those informed consumers who are not sucked in by the billion-dollar fashion and cosmetic industries, I do question a disdain for good grooming. How about just a little mascara and a bit of lip gloss? Putting on a dab of makeup does not have to be a political statement.

I believe there is a health benefit to striving to look your best and dressing in an appropriate manner. According to the National Institute of Mental Health (NIMH), women suffer from depression about twice as often as men; that's got to be at least a fraction of the reason why "the beauty business"—hairstylists, nail salons, makeup counters, and skin solutions—seems catered to us! Countless pieces of NIMH literature document a neglect of personal appearance as a symptom of depression, but could attending to your appearance actually be a *treatment*? For the layperson, it seems "sprucing up" *does* positively affect your mood and counterattack depression; otherwise, hospitals wouldn't encourage their patients to use makeup and wigs.

Gorgeous dictates that you take the time to enhance your appearance. My grandma had a sweet habit of stopping her daily chores in the late afternoon. She would draw a bath, apply her makeup, don an outfit, and greet my grandfather at the door on his return from work. (By the way, they shared supper every evening in the dining room—not the kitchen, where he later would retire to listen to the ballgame.)

I'm one of those work-at-home moms who, if I don't have an appointment, could stay at my desk all day long in my pj's without anyone ever knowing (happily, I don't have web cam). But I have long made it a practice to be dressed, with makeup and hair done, in time for afternoon carpool; even when my boys began to drive, I made a point of sprucing up before their return from school. Always, always (and this may be the most important time to shine!), I'm dressed to greet my husband when he comes home in the evening. My family would be the first to say that I'm a happy, healthy, and well-maintained woman; your family's seal of approval, by the way, satisfies the criteria for gorgeous!

Gorgeous includes good grooming, not only for your overall appearance but for your well-being. Let's face it, when you look good you feel good. You will revel in the appreciative glances of others. Who doesn't like an occasional catcall or whistle? After all, they can't help themselves 'cause you're just too beautiful!

Acting Your Age

When I find myself tempted by the latest anti-aging creams, I try to remember that aging is actually a good thing. Not only does it beat the alternative, it brings wisdom and confidence. We need only take a peek at other societies to see that older members are revered, *not* reviled. For example, in Japan, taking care of all the members of the family is the primary role for a woman. This includes the elderly, who are not shipped out to nursing homes and assisted-living centers but are instead placed at the head of the family table.

We American women are defined by demographics, mixed and remixed so that companies can convince us that we *need* this or that beauty aide. The billion-dollar anti-aging market is the perfect example. Gather the products available on department store shelves and you'll soon decipher the following disconcerting message: old equals unattractive. I'm sure you share in my personal observation that there's a product out there for every single body part—no doubt aimed at preventing, deterring, or disguising the fact that we all get old. Sure you can fight wrinkles, cover gray hair, whiten your teeth, and remove age spots from your hands, but you can't stop the birthdays from coming! Finding the balance between self-improvement and aging gracefully is a key component in discovering a more fit, focused, and gorgeous you.

Having compared notes with my peers, I realize that some are lucky and wise enough to feel, and therefore look, better and younger than their stubborn female counterparts who are so hung up on being "over the hill" that they never find that transcendent, glowing, age-appropriate ideal. Some women have yet to embrace getting older with healthy and realistic solutions in what I like to call an "aging gracefully arsenal." There is a fine balance between making good use of synthetic beauty aids and maintaining a healthful lifestyle. One does not substitute for the other. The goal is to be a healthy, vital woman—one who achieves such a state by staying true to her best interests, which is to say she avoids falling prey to advertising hype, which tends to restrict beauty to twenty-something beanpoles.

The Gorgeous Mantra

Health comes first. It will always be the predecessor to gorgeous; one can't really be had without the other. Good health is supported by living a lifestyle that includes eating fabulous, natural foods; balancing your daily activities; enhancing your personal appearance with makeup and form-flattering clothes; and accepting that you *can* age gracefully.

CHAPTER 2

truth in beauty

Let's Hear It for the Old Wives

Every person walking the earth comes with his or her own repertoire of old wives' tales; a lot of them concern how you look. You know how they typically go: "Eat this and such and such will happen." "Do this or that and the pain will go away," et cetera, et cetera, et cetera. Is there good science behind some of these myths—and which ones are truly just tales? Actually, there is *some* truth to certain wives' tales, especially the ones that vouch for "this or that" food creating beauty. Investigating the roots of these tales wipes out superstition about those little things you've always worried about but have been too embarrassed to ask others about. So what are you waiting for? Investigate! A healthy dose of sound knowledge is necessary for your path to gorgeous.

For example, how about the idea that cellulite is owed strictly to the consumption of soda. This wives' tale goes that the sodium in soda causes fat cells to swell, resulting in the thigh and buttock dimpling we're all too familiar with. Wrong! Your genes, overeating, and inactivity cause cellulite; massaging the area with a collagen-infused lotion can help, but only a procedure performed by a qualified cosmetic surgeon can vanquish cellulite.

Speaking of oiling up the legs, there's another old wives' tale—and thank God it's not true—that if you put oil on your skin, hair will grow there. Some of the biggest wives' tale whoppers involve hair—like half-baked theories concerning which natural remedies will get rid of your (existing) split ends. While a protein-rich diet can stop splits before they start, once they happen, they have to be cut; sorry, folks, but a split end never stops being a split end.

So we've covered hair and body fat. Does the Old Wives' Tale Club have anything to say about your face? Before soap was formulated with synthetic surfactants, the wives were right: a bar of soap *was* too harsh to be used for facial cleansing. Today's milder soaps have moisturizers added, so wash away, my friends.

The one tale that has been handed down from generation to generation that can definitely be placed in the "truth" column is "you are what you eat." I suggest that if you choose wisely, what you eat will make you gorgeous!

Adopt a Health Mantra: Fresh Is Best

You can't improve your body without first enlisting your mind. For the purposes of eating to be gorgeous, our "fresh is best" mantra is nothing more than a positive statement that focuses you on moving toward your goal. For instance, don't berate yourself for putting a bottled salad dressing on your bowl of freshly tossed greens; pat yourself on the back instead—at least you skipped fast food! Congratulate yourself with this mantra: "Each day, I'm getting healthier."

Antioxidants and Your Cells

Cells are the crux of all life. A poor diet wreaks havoc on your cells and diminishes physical functioning, creating health conditions and diseases. Your DNA is stored within your cells in the nucleus and the mitochondria, and a cell has many ways to keep itself safe. However, research has shown that improper nutrition—that is, nutrition low in antioxidants and other important **phytonutrients**—and environmental exposure to toxins (like pesticides) can cause your DNA to become damaged. That's when mutations form and opportunistic diseases, like cancer, can move in. The average adult has around 30 trillion cells in his or her body, and every day thousands of new cells are replicated from old ones. New cells are made to replace the old cells that become worn-out or damaged. The nutrients in your food provide raw materials for the creation of these new cells. Your cells need a full spectrum of vitamins, especially the B-vitamins, to support energy production and keep free radicals at bay. Your cells *crave* healthy fats (like the omega-3 fatty acids) and a good source of proteins to support healthy, protective membranes. Additionally, your cells need a high intake of antioxidants, like the vitamin E family compounds found in the germ of whole grains, the vitamin C in citrus, and the **carotenoids** from vegetables to protect your DNA. Phytonutrients can also act as antioxidants and help protect your cells and DNA from free radicals; these include **anthocyanidins** from fruits like grapes and strawberries and **catechins** found in green tea and fruits, especially grapes.

Five a Day

So how do you integrate antioxidants into your daily diet? Accept the "Five-a-Day Challenge," which cancer-fighting organizations and the American Heart Association encourage all of us—the young and the old—to do. The challenge requires you to eat at least five servings a day of fresh fruits and vegetables. Not only will such a goal *assuredly* make us look better, it'll maintain healthy cells and antioxidant levels, help keep us hydrated, and protect our vital organs. What do five servings look like on a plate? There are many delicious ways to achieve it, and the following is just one example: Visualize 1 cup of dark, leafy **greens**, ½ cup of **red** tomatoes, ½ cup of **yellow** peppers, 6 oz. **orange** juice, and ½ cup of **blue**berries. Imagine that, and you not only have "5-a-day," you have a rainbow of beautiful food!

Dig that Rainbow

Indulge for a minute and think of yourself as you would a baby—one who is just beginning to be nurtured by solid foods. Pediatricians urge parents to feed their children "a rainbow" every day so that all the nutritive bases are covered. The same should go for adults. Visualizing a rainbow of foods containing essential vitamins may seem juvenile, but it works—by eating just one or two things from each color in the spectrum, you assure yourself a gorgeous radiance.

In the White Beam: Peel a banana for vitamins C, B_6, magnesium, and manganese. One large banana contains 15 percent of the recommended daily allowance of fiber. A serving of raw cauliflower provides almost 20 percent of the daily recommendation of vitamin C and is high in fiber and folate. Onions and garlic boost calcium intake and lower cholesterol levels and blood pressure. The much maligned potato is an excellent source of vitamin C, potassium, vitamin B_6, niacin, and thiamin.

In the Yellow & Orange Beams: Most of us associate foods of this color with beta-carotene, one of the earliest identified antioxidants. We think of carrots as the only beta-carotene–rich food, but you can also find beta-carotene in oranges, apricots, squash, and other orange fruits and vegetables. Yellow fruits such as pineapple and papaya contain large amounts of both vitamin C and vitamin A and strengthen your immune system. One half cup of pineapple delivers almost half the daily recommendation of manganese yet weighs in at only 40 calories. Think yellow bell peppers for vitamin C; a one-half cup serving provides 300 percent the daily recommendation. One baked sweet potato provides phosphorus, vitamin E, thiamin, iron, copper, magnesium, pantothenic acid, potassium, vitamin B6, manganese, vitamin C, and vitamin A. WOW!

In the Green Beam: Avocados are high in fiber, folate, potassium, pantothenic acid, vitamin C, and vitamin B6. Honeydew melons, green peas, spinach, and collards supply important carotenoids that reduce the risk of cataracts and macular degeneration. Also included in the green group of vegetables are broccoli, Brussels sprouts, and cabbage, which are, like cauliflower, cruciferous vegetables and contain powerful carcinogen blockers.

In the Red Beam: Add tomatoes to your diet to provide lycopene, an antioxidant associated with a lower risk of cardiovascular disease. You can also get lycopene plus vitamins A and C from watermelon and pink grapefruit. The skin of a red apple is packed with two very powerful phytochemicals called epicatechin and procyanidin. Apples are also rich in pectin, a fiber that has a high capacity to absorb water and improve regularity.

In the Purple & Blue Beams: Eat purple grapes for quercetin in your diet. Quercetin has been identified as an important phytochemical in the prevention of blood clots. Blueberries, plums, purple cabbage, eggplant, and purple onion provide another phytochemical group called anthocyanins; these antioxidant phytochemicals have been linked with preserved memory and better brain function during the aging process.

Sign up for a Free Facelift Three Times a Week!

A steady diet of protein-enriched antioxidants is a first-class ticket to healthier skin; brighter, smoother complexions, and fewer wrinkles. Dark leafy greens, like methi, spinach, and amaranth are full of antioxidants. Plus, they're a great source of iron—an essential tool in fighting the war on dark circles under your eyes. Greens also contain zinc, another foe of the evil Wrinkle! Salad alone as the answer for great skin seems a bleak and boring antidote, so why not layer your greens with taste enhancers that produce the same age-defiant results, like berries. Blueberries, cranberries and strawberries are a terrific source of antioxidants known as polyphenols. Blueberries contain particularly powerful antioxidants, improving balance *and* short-term memory! The antioxidants and vitamin C in most fruits help your body reconstruct its collagen, the scaffolding that keeps skin from drooping. This fruit and leaf info is all well and good, but what if you have to have your meat? If you want to stay/be a spring chicken, look no further than the sea. Fatty fish is teaming with face-friendly omega-3 fatty acids. Also found in mackerel and shark, essential fatty acids battle collagen-damaging free radicals and help smooth out fine lines. Dermatologists recommend eating fish three times a week. If you can't stand seafood, a fish-oil supplement offers similar benefits.

Vitamin Roll Call

Because so many essential vitamins are lost in trips to the loo and in sweat, they must be replaced daily. The water-soluble vitamins are vitamin C and the many B-complex vitamins, including thiamin (B_1), riboflavin (B_2), niacin (B_3), pyridoxine (B_6), folacin (folic acid), cyanocobalamin (B_{12}), biotin, and pantothenic acid. Fat-soluble vitamins—A (retinol), D (calciferol), E (d-alpha-tocopherol), and K (menaquinone)—are transported by the fats in the bloodstream. Because the body stores fat much more readily than water, vitamins A, E, and K can be looked upon as the gravy in your daily nutrient quota.

So What Are the Quotas?

Let's start with **vitamin B**. Nutritionists advise you to get at least 400 micrograms of it a day, as it helps maintain the health of the nerves, skin, eyes, hair, liver, and mouth, as well as healthy muscle tone in the gastrointestinal tract and proper brain function. Next is **vitamin C**, the recommended daily intake is at least 35 milligrams. Vitamin C is crucial in building and maintaining collagen, which are fibers connecting tendons, ligaments, bones, and cartilage. Vitamin C heals wounds and bruises; keeps the immune system healthy; maintains healthy bones, teeth, gums, red blood cells, and blood vessels; and repairs bone fractures. Satisfy your body's thirst for **vitamin D** at between 5 and 10 micrograms a day. Vitamin D is called the sunlight vitamin because the body produces it when the sun's ultraviolet B (UVB) rays strike the skin. It is the only vitamin the body manufactures naturally and is technically considered a hormone. Essential for building strong bones and teeth, vitamin D also helps to strengthen the immune system and may prevent some types of cancer. As for **vitamin E**, get at least 15 milligrams a day if you want to boost new cell growth and keep your skin moist and youthful; you are well on your way to regaining your baby face by eating a half cup of soy a day, at least three times a week.

There Are Actually Two "F's" in Fantastic!

Want to feel fantastic? Remember the two F's: **f**olic acid and **f**iber! Ladies, get at least 400 micrograms of folic acid a day. Folic acid promotes cell division and growth, helps prevent several kinds of cancer, and is highly recommended when it comes to getting or being pregnant. Another important nutrient—for so many reasons—is fiber. Get at least 25 grams of it a day! Much like a natural appetite suppressant, fiber stops hunger immediately, keeping you content for up to several hours after you've eaten. But the true draw of fiber in your diet—as everyone knows—is keeping regular.

Good Carbs and Good Fats for a Gorgeous Complexion

Balancing the good carbs with the good fats encourages you to go ahead and eat (lord knows, ruling everything out would be a major pain). It's important to realize that some fats and carbohydrates are far from bad. In fact, some of the good ones can make you pretty. When you think fatty food, perhaps the first image that comes to mind is French fries. Ever wonder why they wreak havoc with your complexion? Many will wager the wrong guess. It may not be the *fat* in French fries that causes pimples but the simple carbohydrates in potatoes that spike insulin levels and create a ripe playing field for acne.

If you want facial skin that's clear as a bell, replace all simple carbohydrates (you can pick them out because they're chalky white in color) with complex ones, like whole wheat bread, Semolina pasta, and brown rice. Eat a lot of fish, too. Salmon, mackerel, and tuna are rich in essential fatty acids, like omega-3 and omega-6, which counteract the blocking of pores that in our youth are pimples and in our later years become wrinkles. If you don't like fish, stamp out pimples and crow's feet by grazing on almonds, hazelnuts, and flaxseed, also chock-full of fatty acids. You'll need at least 20 grams of fatty acids a day—an obligation to counteracting old skin that can be fulfilled by simply adding an avocado, nuts, or two tablespoons of olive oil to your salad.

Oil & Water

All this talk about oil, *tsk, tsk,* and we haven't moved on to water yet?! H_20 is as important to splash around in as it is to ingest. Without water, the prognosis is very, very bleak. Imagine a balloon filled with water—taut and firm to the touch. Allow some of the water out and the balloon shrinks; the rubber may even shrivel. Deprive a skin cell of water and similar things happen. Without an adequate supply of water, your cells cannot clear waste products, which stack up in the cells and blood; drink up to eight glasses of water per day to avoid this problem and enhance your appearance, but stop short of water intoxication. When too much water enters the body's cells, the tissues swell with the excess fluid. As sodium concentration drops, a condition known as "hyponatremia" results. The good news is that water intoxication is unlikely for most of us. The kidneys of a healthy adult can process fifteen liters of water a day. That's *a lot* of water! Just remember, if you are going to drink water in excess, do so over a long period of time instead of downing an enormous volume all at once. And here's another thought: water is abundant in fruits and veggies—another reason to follow that five-a-day rule.

What about the Hair?

Skin maintenance is one thing, but what about your hair? What keeps hair shining and richly textured? The answer is protein, and you'll need around 60 grams of it a day. You can accomplish that by enjoying, sometime during the day, the following examples: 2

tablespoons of peanut butter (8 grams protein), 2 cups low-fat milk (16 grams protein), 4 slivers of Cheddar cheese (14 grams protein), and 3 ounces chicken breast (11 grams protein). (*Isn't it fun to think of what you can eat, rather than what you can't?)* Always think of ways to include more protein! It's the only substance that provides your body with the amino acids it needs to repair and rebuild muscles. Protein also provides the necessary components to keep your immune system healthy; make hormones, enzymes, skin, hair, nails, and organs, and oxygenate the blood. Protein from animal sources, such as meat and milk, is called *complete* because it contains all nine of the essential amino acids. Most vegetable protein is considered incomplete because it lacks one or more of the essential amino acids. Vegetarians need not worry. Even if you can't get all the amino acids from, say, peanuts alone, you can have peanut butter on whole grain bread. Other protein-heavy veggies include legumes.

What Happens to Women Who Don't Get Enough Calcium?

Believe you me, it's not like the answer to this question is a lump of coal in your stocking. We should be so lucky. If you're not getting enough calcium, your body will take it right out of your skeleton, thinning your bone density and leading to osteoporosis. The Hunchback of Notre Dame is a great character in literature, but who wants to look like him? Male or female, you should strive to get at least 1,000 mg of calcium a day Just 8 ounces of milk puts a 300 mg dent in your 1,000-mg-a-day quota. The same amount of low-fat yogurt (8 oz.) will see you 400 mg more. Throw in a snack of any fresh cheese, and you've officially been good to your bones! And why not? It's probable that calcium reduces fracture rates by at least 10 percent! As you age, minerals in your bones are lost. Bones may get thinner and break more easily. Protect your bones by expanding your horizons past the obligatory dairy—add calcium-rich greens, broccoli, sardines, dried beans and peas, and tofu to your diet. But don't stop there! Starting each morning with calcium-fortified orange juice that includes vitamin D helps with the absorption of calcium. Vitamin D is found lots of places, including your cereal. Your body can make its own vitamin D when your skin is exposed to the sunshine, so drag your bones for some much-deserved R&R out in a lawn chair some day soon (just remember not to overdo it and to slather on the sunscreen).

An All-Women's Restaurant

Wouldn't it be great if women's restaurants went up all over the country to cater to our specific needs? Since that's not going to happen, you'll just have to treat your grocery store like an all-women's drive-thru and put goddess-friendly items in the cart.

Wouldn't it be wonderful if there was an aisle for women experiencing the negative effects of PMS? A diet low in salt, fat, and caffeine but high in fiber helps immensely. Vitamins B_6 and E, gamma-linolenic acid (GLA), calcium and magnesium have all been recommended for "that time of the month." GLA is an Omega-6 fatty acid found in plant fats; you can pick up a batch from almost any food store in the form of evening primrose oil or black currant. If you prefer not to take these as a nutritional supplement, you can have your "girl power"–replenishing GLA in a lovely cup of tea.

Middle of the Roaders

What if you're uncomfortably sandwiched between your childbearing years and change of life? Some researchers believe that high-fat diets are especially harmful to women during perimenopause. Why? Because a high-fat diet fuels estrogen production, thereby encouraging dramatic hormonal fluctuations that produce the hallmarks of menopause, like mood swings and hot flashes. Sticking with a well-balanced, low-fat diet *(please remember to enjoy healthy fats!)* can help smooth out the decline in your body's production of estrogen. The good news is that women are never completely without estrogen since adrenal glands and body fat continue to produce low levels after menopause. Also key in maintaining your health—especially now—is getting plenty of calcium, since nearing or completing the change of life takes a toll on bone density.

Falling off the Wagon

Even if you've started practicing a healthy lifestyle that works, you'll find that being around less-conscientious people, traveling on vacation, or special circumstances may tempt you to stray from your everyday routine. How do you live with those pound-packing couple of days or weeks? I suggest that if you choose a philosophy that governs the type of food you eat—whether it's in the heat of the moment or over the long haul—your choice of foods becomes automatic. The more often you make healthy food choices, the more your body will crave healthful foods. So the sooner you make up your mind to strive for a vitamin-filled, veggie-rich, protein-packed diet plan, the sooner you'll transform yourself into a more gorgeous you!

The direct correlation between nutrition and how we look is rooted in history. As we have evolved, so have our food choices. The opportunity to select healthful foods leads to a multitude of good alternatives. Explore all of your options with one thing in mind—*balance*. This is the path to gorgeous.

CHAPTER 3

gorgeous revitalizing spa secrets

Downtime Valued

For some people, the word *revitalize* conjures up images of girls scrubbing their faces with exfoliate washes or slathering on a miracle cream that, supposedly, makes pores sing. However, as far as Webster's and the real world are concerned, "revitalization" means bringing someone into activity and prominence. Furthermore, it's about having one's strength and energy restored. Revitalization presents a number of roads on the path to gorgeous.

A paramount criterion in getting that healthy glow and groove on is setting aside, or at least for petitioning, downtime. I propose the idea of "downtime" with hesitancy because I know how hard we work for our families. The obstacles standing in the way of idealized fitness and nutrition in a hoppin' twenty-first century are daunting to say the least. Take the office. Its work can be done via cell phone and laptop, from any vacation destination, or even (gasp, shudder!) a bathroom if it's close enough to an internet connection. We lucky Americans enjoy every conceivable form of communication 24/7, leaving little motivation and lots of distraction when it comes to "the how and when" of finding time to eat right, exercise, and relax in our competitive "sink or swim" madness.

Enter the booming day spa business. You can find one on almost every corner. There are hair salons, nail salons, tanning salons, and massages centers that offer a menu of choices. With limited time allotted to pampering, you must spend the time at the spa wisely.

The Spa Factor

How do our American "day spas" stack up among spas in other cultures? A globally celebrated tradition, spa treatments have been around at least since the ancient Romans.

Preserving your healthy, glowing skin through exfoliation and hydration is a fact of life the Romans were well in tune with when they discovered the first hot mineral springs in a small Belgian village called Spa. Originally popular among soldiers with aching muscles, the Romans perfected a pastime you could say was "springing" up all over the world. They made the lure of the spa—rest, relaxation, and solace—available to everyone. In fact, any free person in Rome could afford to visit the Roman baths, which were surrounded by theaters, food markets, libraries, and the all-important gymnasium.

Bathing Traditions

Today's spa experience is rooted in ancient traditions. The experience began by entering the dressing room (today known as a locker room) adjacent to large gymnasiums like those found at the modern-day local YMCAs. In ancient Rome, the public baths spanned several blocks and were called "thermae." The fee for women was twice as much as the fee for men, and separate bathing times for the two genders were strictly enforced: women bathed before the sunset and men after. Bathers entered the caldarium, a hot room filled with steam and sunken pools of hot water. Visits to the hotroom were followed by a trip to the fridgidarium, a cold environment that closed pores rendered open by the hot room.

When it comes to spas, the world over has adopted a "when in Rome" philosophy and tried to emulate the practices of the ancient Romans, coupling exercise with skin treatments and massages. Still and all, the Romans' approach isn't the only game in town.

Global Appeal

Unlike Americans, Europeans think of their spas not as a vacation retreat but rather a place of healing. Americans are usually healthy when they visit spas and the professional treatments they receive are less invasive and shorter in length. Spa treatments in the USA average half an hour, whereas in Europe they typically are longer and more expansive. It's interesting to compare what is perhaps the shortest spa ritual to the longest one. Consider the "lulur" ritual from the Indonesia region of Java in which princesses about to be married enjoy 40 days (!) of flower baths made from **turmeri**, rice, **fenugreek** (for lymphatic clearing), **gingerroot** (circulation), **jasmine** (aphrodisiac), **cempaka** (Indonesian flower), and a flower called "**ylang-ylang**," meaning "queen of the flowers." (Ylang-ylang stimulates lymph flow, reduces swelling, and acts as a Spanish fly!) After this lulur scrub is applied, yogurt is massaged into the skin and a long bath follows. Spas around the world have adopted delicious Indonesian decadences like the lulur in various packages and offerings—just ask the receptionist if there's "a Javanese lulur body treatment" and go straight to heaven!

Spin the Globe Some More!

Here's what you can find when you take a look at what other cultures do in the name of healthy, glowing skin.

- In India, **henna** is used to take away excess body heat and to help diminish and heal rashes. **Brahmi** is taken internally to rejuvenate brain cells and improve skin's elasticity.
- In Europe, the flower du jour is **chamomile**; nobility put crushed petals in their baths. In the South Pacific, it's **coconut oil** that sweetens the soul.
- The Mediterranean revere their **olive oil,** and Native Americans relied so much on mud baths and mineral springs that it drew the Spanish explorer Ponce de Leon to the Tumucuan Indians' wet beauty source, or what later came to be known as the Fountain of Youth.
- In Japan, hot **mineral springs** bubble up and kiss the spa-goer's skin.
- In Bali, rich **volcanic mud** is applied after you have been steam cleansed in a herbal sauna.
- Thailand is famous for its natural **white mud** that enhances skin texture.
- In Israel, the mineral-rich mud of the **Dead Sea**—flowing from the deepest sea in the world—rejuvenates your body with its high content of magnesium, potassium, and calcium.

Taking a Kur

"Taking a kur" is an age-old European tradition. It refers to a series of treatments begun in a spa and carried on at home over a period of ten days. But what if you want to take your "kur" with the professionals? This book suggests ways to bring the health-spa mentality to your front door, invite it in, and let it stay with you for a lifetime, but that doesn't mean a person committed to divine dining experiences and health-focused relaxation wouldn't enjoy learning all they can before picking out just the right destination spa. Prices for this total "immersion" experience generally include all meals and regular exercise classes. Here are the some of the top destination spas in the United States:

(1) and (2) **Canyon Ranch**, with locations in Tucson, Arizona, and Lennox, Massachusetts, is the ultimate "wellness spa" with an excellent medical staff.

(3) If money is no object and you're a sucker for the view from the foot of the Santa Catalina Mountains, **The Golden Door** in Escondido might be right for you; it's is a

Catalina Mountains, **The Golden Door** in Escondido might be right for you; it's is a women-only spa that serves no more than 40 guests at a time.

(4) **Miraval Life in Balance** in Catalina, Arizona, allows alcohol and also encourages creative expression through artwork and journaling.

(5) **Mii Amo** in Sedona, Arizona, borders a national forest two hours from Phoenix.

(6) **Lake Austin Spa Resort** in Austin, Texas.

(7) **Red Mountain Spa** in Ivins, Utah, is known for being more economical than the other "Top 10 Spas." It offers breathtaking Southwestern scenery and features a hiking program and outstanding outdoors guides.

(8) **Green Valley Spa** in St. George, Utah.

(9) **Cal-A-Vie** in Vista, California. This weight-loss spa is north of San Diego and has 24 guest cottages. It has both coed and women-only weeks throughout the year.

(10) **The Greenhouse** in Arlington, Texas, is a women-only weight-loss spa that has been around since the sixties. Serving only 39 guests at a time, it offers programmed activities and a "Fat Flush" program.

She's Got the Whole World in Her Tub

If you're going to stay devoted to an antioxidant-rich, omega-3-enhanced diet—the very one that's keeping your skin so supple—why not continue to reward it with the ultimate in luxuriant baths? Wouldn't it be great to "take 5" in a health spa and know a thing or two about the oils prescribed—where they come from and which indigenous people were among the first to use them?

West African Oil Bath is something your epidermal layer will sing (and demand encores) for! Mothers in Senegal and Mali rub their newborn babies with shea butter (the French inhabitants of Africa, who are also fond of shea butter, call it "karite") to form their children's features and ensure they have strong limbs. Then they use the shea butter on themselves. Shea butter is also great for your hair—it promotes growth. Spend at least 10 minutes rubbing shea butter on any and every willing body part before you go to bed. (Significant others love to help!) The babes of West Africa guarantee you'll wake up smiling.

Africa is not the only continent to have discovered the multiple benefits of a beautifying and relaxing oil bath; India knows how to do it too! They use "gingelly oil"(sesame seed oil). This is a region where oil baths are taken, regularly and famously, to keep skin soft and silky. You can follow the same **Religion of Radiant Skin** by rubbing ½ cup sesame oil all over your body. Massage your body completely to rub all the oil in. After you've done this, relax as you've never relaxed before in (or on!) a towel-draped sanctuary. In thirty minutes, draw yourself a warm bath and get into it with your most cherished loofah sponge. Scrub yourself while you soak and remove the remnants of the oil. When you emerge from the bath, you'll feel positively reborn—alive and vibrant enough to take a tiger ride into an Indian dynasty. **Sandalwood baths** from this region will treat you just as well. Close your eyes and think of the scent of woodchips in a hand-carved sandalwood chest. You can achieve the same sensual aroma with just a few discretionary drops (no less than 2 and no more than 5) of the combination of essential sandalwood, amber, sesame, and patchouli oils. Let the elixir sit overnight and bathe in it the following day.

The notes for well-worshipped skin don't begin and end in Asia. The Caribbean is renowned for its spicy (literally!) **Grenada bath**, in which cinnamon, clove, and bay leaves anoint you in the water. Boil the following ingredients, put them into a small bottle, and let them steep for a week: ¼ cup sesame oil; 2 sticks cinnamon; 6 whole cloves; large bay leaf, crumbled; 1 dash nutmeg. When ready to use, strain the spices out with a mesh strainer and pour the oil into your dream bath.

Whether you explore all of the posh (and not so posh) spas of the world or you draw a bay-oil-enhanced warm bath, scheduling downtime into your busy routine is mandatory for your road to a relaxed, revitalized, and more gorgeous you.

CHAPTER 4

mastering your glam kitchen

National surveys suggest that as many as two-thirds of American families do not eat together on a regular basis. The *Archives of Family Medicine, Parenting Magazine,* and Harvard studies are just a few of the "last word" sources on the enormous benefits family dinners provide for every member of the nuclear unit. I further suggest that a family dinner is not one that is spent outside the home. Take a look at your eating habits. Are you eating out more often than not? Have you stopped to add up the amount of money it costs you per outing? Is eating out really a convenience? I question whether rounding up everyone to get in the car, driving to a restaurant, then waiting for a table, the meal, and the check actually saves you more time than it would take you to cook a meal at home. Don't you find it difficult to discuss personal family issues in front of a server and busboy?

I've made it pretty clear that if you want to reach your highest gorgeous potential, you are going to have to learn to eat *well.* (An added benefit is that your family is coming along for the ride.) Begin with home cooking and rely on your growing expertise when making your dining-out decisions. Whether you are a career gal or a stay-at-home mom (or a combination of both), you have probably already mastered the most important skill you will need to begin your glam kitchen—*organization*. The more you organize your time and your kitchen, the easier you will find it to become a successful cook.

The Gorgeous Lifestyle Plan

Begin with a weekly meal plan. If you create a meal plan on the weekend, you won't have to wonder what you are serving your family on Wednesday night. Knowing that your meal is planned, that the ingredients are prepped and ready to go, and that your family has had some input into what everyone is going to eat eliminates the need to dash through the drive-thru restaurant on the way home from work or stop off at the grocery store for frozen entrées.

Begin by choosing a dinner meal for each day of the week. Ask the family for their food preferences or start with family-favorite meals. Plan to cook extra for kids' lunchboxes and your brown bag fare. Schedule breakfast options as well. Once your meal plan is set, make a shopping list of the ingredients you will need. Check your pantry and cross out those items on your list that you already have. Choose a shopping day that allows enough time for you to shop, prep, and put away the food for the week.

On your shopping day, stick to your list. Fight the impulse to add processed foods that *don't* fit into your gorgeous lifestyle plan. Instead, investigate new fresh ingredients that are specially featured. Anyone for jicama? You can fit these into your meals at any time.

When you return from the store, prep those ingredients that you will use during the week. For example, if turkey meatballs are on the menu mid-week, prepare them on Saturday, store them in an airtight container in the freezer, and thaw them the morning you will cook them. When you return home, all you have left to do is bake the meatballs and place them into your homemade marinara sauce.

As you work your way through your meals, you will develop a feel for how much you want to prepare on the weekends and how much time you can allot to food prep during the week. I find that chopping and slicing actually relaxes me after a long day. One of my favorite things to do is get into the kitchen to prepare a fresh and fabulous meal. So I find that my prep day is usually about washing and storing fresh veggies rather than precooking ingredients for weekly meals. But as you develop your meal plan and begin cooking more meals at home, you will find your balance point between weekend prep and preparing weekday meals.

You will discover that a huge time-saver is cooking more than the amount of food you need for one meal. In the old days this was called leftovers. In reality, five-star restaurants are run on this same premise. The chef purchases the best-quality lamb shanks offered for the best possible price. He slowly braises the shanks to perfection and offers diners his lamb shank special that evening. The next day, he reinvents the "left-over" lamb into braised lamb ravioli! You can do the same thing in your weekly meal plan. Roast two chickens for Sunday's supper, reserving one for a chicken casserole, chicken fajitas, chicken pot pie, or a simple yet succulent chicken salad. The cooking time is the same, and the benefit is that you have two (or three) meals instead of one.

The Glam Pantry

It's so much easier to cook when your fridge and pantry have the ingredients that you need to prepare the meal. It's also a whole lot easier to eat a healthful, well-balanced diet if the ingredients that you choose from are wholesome and nourishing. Let's face it, an apple is a better snack choice than a packaged cookie. Celery and carrot sticks are a better choice than potato chips. Whole grain bread is a better fiber choice that white bread made with processed flour. Olive oil is a better fat choice than butter or margarine when sautéing.

It's really simple: if you don't buy the chips, you won't find yourself eating them. This doesn't mean you can never eat another chip. But picture yourself at a friend's house for the big game. She places an appy of caramelized onion dip served with crudités and a basketful of chips! Just imagine how good those chips will taste, how rewarded you will feel, when you indulge in several, knowing that they are a *treat*—not a daily deterrent to your gorgeous lifestyle path.

Read Nutrition Labels

As you navigate the grocery store aisles, your best bet is to choose whole foods in their most natural state. However, when you must purchase items that contain nutritional information on the packaging, *be sure to read the nutrition labels.* In order to know what is actually in the food you are purchasing, look beyond food industry's clever marketing and packaging and examine the facts instead.

Rule #1—If the ingredient list is long and you cannot pronounce the words, don't purchase it.

Rule #2—Avoid those packaged foods that include high fructose corn syrup in the ingredient list. This man-made sugar is not easily digested by our bodies. Excess sugar should be avoided as well. The ingredients are listed in order of quantity. If your can of diced tomatoes lists sugar before tomatoes, look for a different product.

Rule #3—Look at the sodium content in the foods you choose. Most prepared foods are very high in sodium—even that deli-roasted chicken (many are injected with seasonings that contain high amounts of sodium). This applies to deli meats as well. Canned veggies have more sodium than frozen veggies. I like to control the seasonings in my food, so I try to choose those products with the least amount of sodium.

Rule #4—White enriched flour has been processed so that most of the nutrients have been taken out, with just a few returned. When possible, choose whole grain flour; use unbleached white flour in limited quantities. Remember, a gorgeous lifestyle plan is about balance. In certain instances, using white flour will be a better choice for taste—

not necessarily nutrition. I believe that you should satisfy your cookie craving with a delicious cookie prepared with flour, butter, and sugar. One or two home-baked cookies is a far better choice than a box of packaged cookies.

Rule #5—There are good fats and they should be incorporated into your diet, but there are very, very bad fats that are hidden in convenience foods. Avoid saturated fats and hydrogenated oils. These processed ingredients are not easily digested and remain in the body as—fat. Substitute with good fat like olive oil or canola oil in cooking rather than butter or margarine. That said, a bit of butter used sparingly to enhance a sauce is acceptable in a balanced meal plan.

Rule #6—Choose reduced-fat dairy products such as milk, cheese, and sour cream. These products reduce some of the fat but maintain taste and texture. Fat-free products, on the other hand, often manipulate the ingredients, compromising the overall quality of the food.

Read labels to choose the ingredients that best work for your gorgeous lifestyle plan. Start today. Get rid of those not-so-good-for-you items on your shelf and in your fridge and stock them instead with healthful choices. Here is a guideline:

Oils, Vinegar, and Wines

- Use vegetable, canola, or olive oil for sautéing, frying, and baking. When you sauté with a small amount of olive oil, be aware of its higher smoking point. Burning the oil will detract from its healthy benefit.
- Use good-quality olive oil when making salad dressings or tossing into a spur-of-the-moment pasta sauce. Experiment with flavorful olive oils for variety.
- Vegetable oil spray is excellent for use in preparing baking pans, casserole dishes, and sauté and grill pans so that the food does not stick. A beneficial side effect is the reduction in the amount of fat used in preparing the dish. Choose one without added ingredients. You can purchase a kitchen gadget called a quickmist oil sprayer that will allow you to diffuse your favorite oil in a spray-like bottle.
- Sesame oil is not used as often as the other oils mentioned above but is nice to have on hand when adding an oriental flavor to marinades and sautéed vegetables.
- Vinegar comes in many flavors. I keep a bottle of red wine vinegar in the pantry. I keep a large bottle of balsamic vinegar near the stove as it adds a deeply rich, tangy, sweet flavor to foods while cooking. Tarragon, raspberry, champagne, and rice wine vinegars are on my pantry shelf because they are basically interchangeable when preparing a salad dressing or creating a marinade.
- Good-quality white and red wines are used in many sauces. You do not need to purchase the most expensive wines; however, the wine must taste good. My rule of

thumb for purchasing a wine that will be used in a sauce is *if the wine is good enough to drink, then it is good enough to use in my sauce!* A wine that has turned to vinegar will make the sauce taste bitter. Sherry is bottled either dry or sweet and is sometimes called "cocktail sherry." Cooking sherry is found with cooking wines in the grocery store. I prefer to use an inexpensive bottle of dry sherry when flavoring soups.

Canned Goods

• Chicken and beef broth can be purchased in canned, boxed, or soup base form. Homemade stocks are the most desirable when making soups and sauces; however, keep a canned alternative on hand for those times when homemade stock is not available. Choose a product that meets the sodium requirements in your diet. I prefer a low-sodium broth so that I can control the seasonings of the finished meal. Fat-free, organic, and vegetable broths are also readily available.

• Chopped tomatoes also come in varying sizes of cans or boxes. I prefer to use a chopped plum tomato product rather than a stewed or pureed product. This product also gives you the luxury of creating a fresh dish like salsa or a crostini topping. Tomato paste comes in various-sized cans. I keep several small cans on hand because most recipes call for only a small amount when flavoring or thickening a sauce.

• Canned beans are a staple in my pantry because the beans can be used in many ways. They are a great addition when mixed with brown rice, perfect when rinsed and tossed into a salsa, and flavorful when sautéed with onions and puréed into a smooth, thick sauce. Read the nutritional labels to pick the best product available.

• Canned veggies like corn and peas are in my pantry; however, I prefer the lower sodium content of frozen veggies.

• Tuna and salmon can be used for everything from sandwich fillers to ingredients for dips and spreads. I keep several of each on the shelf. I prefer tuna packed in oil because it's richer in flavor and the oil is the good-for-you kind.

• Black olives, whether sliced or whole, act as a great last-minute garnish for a party platter, a colorful addition to a tossed salad, and a robust ingredient in a lemon and wine sauce.

Jars and Such

• A jar of sun-dried tomatoes packed in olive oil is the most expensive way to purchase this product, but it is a must in your pantry. A less expensive alternative is to buy packaged dried tomatoes and reconstitute them in warm water or olive oil as needed. I love the jar option because the tomatoes are tender and you can use the flavored olive oil in pasta sauce or to top a homemade pizza.

• Capers are small, salty berries that usually require rinsing before use. They are excellent in white wine and lemon sauces over fish and chicken.

• I keep jars of natural marinara and pizza sauce in the pantry. If you choose one without added salt or sugar, these products can be acceptable shortcuts for your weekly supper.

• Roasted red peppers are precooked, sliced, bottled in liquid, and presented in a jar. I love to roast my own peppers; however, jarred peppers are a good substitute in a pinch.

Condiments

• Mustard, mayonnaise, and ketchup are used for all the usual reasons. I try to use a reduced-fat mayonnaise when possible, and I also watch the sugar and salt content in my ketchup.

• Barbecue sauce is convenient to have on hand when time does not permit making your own. Again, read the labels to choose one with the least amount of added salt and sugar.

• Hot pepper sauce, although best known for its addition to tasty chicken wings, is also used to flavor soups and sauces and to spice up salsa.

• Worcestershire sauce is used in salad dressings and marinades.

• Chili sauce and chutney have very different tastes but can be used similarly. For a quick appetizer, pour the chutney over a spreadable sharp or Swiss cheese product and serve with crackers. The same is true for chili sauce served over goat cheese or cream cheese.

• Salsa from the jar is great for chip dipping. It is also well used in flavoring chicken and fish or topping vegetables like cold asparagus. Again, look at the sodium and sugar content of the brand you select.

• Soy sauce is an oriental flavoring used mostly in marinades and oriental vinaigrettes. Experiment with the tastes of light and dark soy sauce.

Pasta, Rice, & Dried Bread Products

• Pasta in its dried form comes in dozens of shapes and sizes and has a very long shelf life. I keep at least two boxes on hand at all times. A flat noodle (such as linguini or vermicelli) and a tube shape (like penne or ziti) allow me to match the pasta to the sauce I have prepared. I choose a whole wheat, semolina flour, or vegetable-flavored (like spinach or tomato) product.

• Rice comes in natural and processed varieties. Stay away from the premixed packages. As a staple, I keep one box of yellow rice and one box of brown rice on hand. A real treat to keep in the pantry is Arborio rice that can be made into risotto.

• I do stock crackers for accompaniments to quick dips and spreads. Read the label to make sure you choose a product without trans fats.

• Breadcrumbs and cornflake crumbs can be used together for crusty coatings when baking chicken or separately when topping a casserole. I keep a box of both on hand. (Actually, I prefer to make my own breadcrumbs from whole wheat bread and season them with the spices I keep on hand, but when time dictates, having boxes of these products in your pantry helps!)

• I keep an assortment of dried beans and lentils in the pantry, as they are filled with nutrition-packed stuff and can be turned into soups and stews in your slow cooker while you are out of the house.

Baking Needs

• I choose to purchase *unbleached* flour for baked goods. I use it in conjunction with whole wheat flour. I also keep bread flour on hand.

• Oats are a wonderful addition to cookies, breads, and cobbler toppings. On their own, oats work well for weekday breakfast. Pass on the instant version and instead choose old-fashioned rolled oats or steel-cut oats.

• Cornmeal has a long shelf life and is necessary when making corn muffins.

• Granulated (referred to as natural sugar in the recipes), powdered (also known as confectioners' sugar), or brown sugar is required in most baking recipes. Keep a box of each on hand, knowing that you can sometimes interchange them if you run out of one or the other. I prefer a natural cane sugar for my granulated sugar product.

• Cocoa powder is an unsweetened cooking ingredient and not a hot chocolate drink. A tin will last for a long time in the pantry.

• Honey and molasses are used in many baking recipes. Molasses comes in dark and light forms, and although they can be interchanged, it is better to follow the specifics of the recipe.

• Unsweetened chocolate squares, semisweet chocolate, and white chocolate are used in many different forms when baking cookies, cakes, and breads. Although the shelf life of chocolate is not quite as long as some other staples, I keep all kinds on hand because I tend to use chocolate a bit more often than some other ingredients.

• Nut pieces are used in toppings, cookies, and snack cakes. Depending on your preference, keep one or two packages of chopped walnuts, pecans, or almonds in the pantry.

• Cornstarch is used to thicken and smooth sauces or gravy.

• Baking powder and baking soda are two very different ingredients that are often used in the same recipe. Keep a tin of baking powder and a box of baking soda on hand, making sure that you do not mix them up!

• Yeast comes prepackaged in rapid rising or standard forms. I prefer the jar version for allowing accurate measurements when using the bread machine.

• Sweetened condensed milk and evaporated milk are used in some recipes. I prefer to keep a can on hand rather than to run out to the store for the few times that I need either evaporated or sweetened condensed milk.

• Pure vanilla extract is kept in my pantry rather than with the spices because it is used much more in baking than in cooking. I buy a large bottle of good quality vanilla and store it well sealed.

Spices

• Salt and pepper are a must and are used to your individual taste in most recipes. I choose freshly ground pepper and coarse salt. Keep both on hand as well as ground white pepper. Specialty sea salts are really fun to play around with, and since you are choosing fresh, natural food in place of processed, sodium-filled products, you can take advantage of these when cooking.

• Dried basil, oregano, tarragon, dill, and cilantro are used to season soups and stews. I prefer to use fresh herbs, but many times the dried version will work as a good substitution. Use a lesser amount of dried herbs than fresh in recipes.

• Old Bay Seasoning is a specialty spice that I like to use for chicken and fish. One tin will last a very long time.

• Bay leaves are whole dried leaves used to season soups and stews and should be removed from the dish before serving.

• Chili powder adds a uniquely rich and spicy flavor to many dishes. Keep plenty on hand as you will use more of this than you think.

• Dried red pepper flakes are a hot spice and should be used sparingly.

• Ground ginger, ground cinnamon, and ground nutmeg are spices that are frequently used in baking. However, ginger and cinnamon are sometimes called for in sauces.

• Nutmeg flavors a creamy white sauce called béchamel.

• Chinese five spice and Herbes de Provence are spice blends used in ethnic dishes. Feel free to experiment with each to punch up the flavors of your everyday dishes.

• Lemon and lime juice are found in concentrated form, packaged in bottles or frozen in cans. Although fresh is best, either of these alternatives will work well in a pinch.

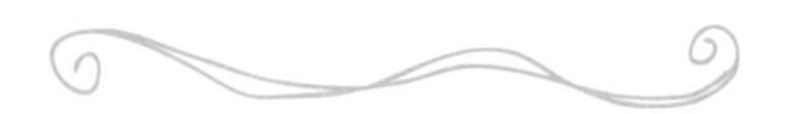

The Refrigerator Basics

Dairy Staples

• Milk, butter, and eggs will be a weekly addition to your shopping list. Remember to check the freshness dates on each. I prefer reduced-fat milk, unsalted butter, and extra large eggs.

• Read the labels on cream, fat-free cream, and non-dairy cream to determine which one works within your lifestyle plan. Again, I prefer a reduced-fat product.

• Sour cream and cream cheese are staples when making quick appetizers and are often used in sauces and baking. Again, check the labels for fat-free, reduced-fat, and soy substitutes in these products.

• Grated Parmesan cheese and many other cheeses will keep for several weeks in the refrigerator. Crumbled cheeses like Gorgonzola, blue, and Feta are great additions to a fresh, tossed salad. Goat cheese is terrific, especially when combined with sun-dried tomatoes. Packaged (shredded) sharp and mozzarella cheeses are excellent to cook with in casseroles. I choose a reduced-fat cheese when baking and a whole cheese product for salad toppers and cheeseboards.

• Jars of prepared horseradish and chopped garlic are used in sauces and when cooking. Both will keep for a long time in the refrigerator. I prefer fresh garlic (then again, I love to chop—it relieves stress), but I use the time-saving jarred version for big parties.

Your Glam Shopping List

Make your life a little easier when making your shopping list. Divide the items on your list as you will find them in the market. Your list might look something like this:

Check your pantry: List staple items such as mayonnaise and check this portion of the list against those products on your shelf.

Herbs/spices/flavorings: List items like hot pepper sauce, bay leaves, ground cinnamon. These too should be checked against your pantry.

Dairy: List items such as cream cheese and milk. Remember to check labels to determine whether you prefer a reduced-fat or fat-free product.

Produce: From now on, fruits and vegetables will take up the majority of your shopping cart. List here all of the items you will need to make sure you have plenty of variety to choose from as you aim for "5-a-day."

Meat/fish/poultry: Watch for specials in this category in order to stretch your grocery dollar. Choose skirt steak in place of flank steak or take advantage of a family pack of chicken breasts. You can always set aside some for next week.

Specialty shop: Use this category when you are looking for ingredients from ethnic shops like the Italian or Chinese market. Include that fresh loaf of whole grain bread from the bakery and the fresh catch from your fishmonger here.

Kitchen equipment: Be sure you have all of the equipment needed to prepare the upcoming week's dishes. If you need a microplane grater to zest your lemon, make a note of it in this section.

Notes: List other errands you need to do on shopping day (like searching for the perfect bottle of Pinot Noir) in this section.

Your Glam Kitchen Made So Very Easy

Hair a little dull, mood a little cranky? The chapters in this book are designed to let you focus on those areas that you feel need a *little extra* attention. Jump ahead to Chapter 16 and you will find examples of weekly lifestyle guides that incorporate all of the good things necessary to get you started on your road to stronger bones, glowing skin, and sounder sleep.

If you are looking at the larger picture, open up your laptop and visit *www.GorgeousLifestyleGuide.com*. There you can choose from the 52 weekly lifestyle plans found in chapter 16. Simply click on a plan to print your meal plan, a complete grocery list, and prep tips to help you on shopping day. We'll even throw in a couple of relaxation and exercise tips to help you balance your life. Could it be any easier?

You are well on your way to a *gorgeous* you!

PART TWO

how she became lovely: a tale of each part working toward one beautiful whole

A comprehensive, all-engrossing beauty regimen cannot be achieved by honoring one or even a few body parts. Nothing should be neglected. Each chapter in this section focuses on a specific area of the body (skin, hair, eyes, teeth, bones, toes, hands, tummies and butts) and offers the information needed to meld science with lifestyle. Begin with a glowing complexion while you work forward to a more gorgeous you.

CHAPTER 5

the richly detailed story behind great skin

"I'm tired of all this nonsense about beauty being only skin-deep. That's deep enough. What do you want, an adorable pancreas?" —*Jean Kerr*

Your Skin Tells the Story of Your Life

For radiant, healthy skin you can't slide by relying on a slew of foamy exfoliates from the skin-care industry. The care and treatment of your skin starts with a balanced, nutritious diet; without that, your skin, the body's largest organ, can't accomplish its primary functions, which are to (1) maintain a proper water and salt balance for your entire body, (2) cushion your delicate internal organs, and (3) serve as the first line of defense against germs that would otherwise invade your body. Throughout your lifetime, you'll look to your skin to *save your skin!* How dedicated and successful you are at taking care of yourself shows up in your face. It's up to you to decide if you wear the heavily lined look of neglect or the ageless glow that *gorgeous* skin has to offer.

Ask Dr. Moon

The doctor is in to answer your questions.

Q: Besides a glowing complexion, what is the function of our skin?

A: The skin, capable of self-regeneration, is the largest organ of the body and the only one that is constantly exposed to the external environment. In addition to providing the body with a protective barrier, it is also an important part of the body's immune system. Any damage to the skin, regardless of the nature of the disruption, can lead to infection, dehydration, and other life-threatening consequences.

Q: How do free-radicals affect the skin?

A: Free radicals are naturally occurring chemicals in our bodies; they attack and damage healthy cells. Free-radical damage is bad for the skin. Theoretically, free-radical damage can cause deterioration of the skin's support structures, decreasing elasticity and resilience.

Q: How do we fight free-radical damage?

A: The presence of antioxidants in the diet and, possibly, the topical application of antioxidants in skin-care products play a big part in slowing down free-radical damage.

Q: What are antioxidants?

A: They're food ingredients such as vitamins A, C, and E; superoxide dismutase; flavonoids; beta-carotene; glutathione; selenium; and zinc. Antioxidants are abundant in fresh herbs, nuts, and brightly colored vegetables.

Q: What does vitamin A do?

A: Vitamin A is a fat-soluble vitamin that helps you see normally in the dark and promotes the growth and health of all body cells and tissues. It also protects against infection by keeping healthy the skin and tissues in the mouth, stomach, intestines, and respiratory and uro-genital tracts. Vitamin A is found in dark orange (e.g., carrots, sweet potatoes, and winter squash) and dark green (e.g., broccoli, spinach, and kale) vegetables.

Q: What does vitamin E do?

A: It's found in nuts like hazelnuts and almonds and improves the quality of the skin and its ability to heal itself.

Q: What does vitamin C do?

A: It rebuilds collagen. Tomatoes, oranges, mangoes, and red peppers are rich in vitamin C.

Q: How many antioxidants should be consumed per day?

A: To obtain an ample supply of antioxidants for a standard 2000-calorie-per-day diet, you should consume 2 cups of fruit and 2 cups of vegetables daily.

Q: What part does water play in a healthy complexion, and how can you get more of it into your daily diet?

A: Dehydration causes the skin to lose elasticity and look like leather. Water is vital for cell regeneration all over your skin—especially your face. So drink plenty of water! Dress it up with a wedge of lime or lemon. Eat fruits and veggies, which are bursting with H_2O.

Q: What types of dietary fat help reduce the appearance of wrinkles?

A: Omega-3 fatty acids are building blocks of fat required by the skin to function properly; in addition to benefitting your skin, Omega-3 reduces inflammation throughout your body, keeps your blood from clotting excessively, and maintains the fluidity of your cell membranes. Fish with the highest omega-3 content include mackerel, fresh or canned albacore tuna, and salmon; walnuts and flax oil are other good sources.

Q: How do I choose skin-care products and programs?

A: First, develop a skin-care program that works with your schedule. Second, determine your skin type. Lastly, choose a moisturizer supplemented with vitamins A, C, and E to block pollutants, while staying conscientious of the fact that *direct sunlight is best avoided.*

Q: If I use sunscreen, will I still get a tan?

A: The higher SPFs (anything more than SPF-15) provide over 80 percent protection from the sun, so no, you won't get a deep, dark tan with that kind of protection working for your skin; notice I said "for" and not "against." The ultraviolet radiation of direct sunlight destroys and scars skin cells and makes them lose their elasticity.

Q: Is smoking bad for my complexion?

A: Yes! Stay away from tobacco smoke! Smoking causes vasoconstriction, which means the skin is starved of nutrient-bearing blood.

Q: Do French fries and chocolate cause acne?

A: Despite the myths, acne isn't caused by junk food. Studies have found no connection between acne and chocolate, chips, or pizza; however, researchers are currently investigating whether there's a link between acne and high glycemic index (GI) foods, such as white bread and potatoes.

Q: What are the similarities and differences between dermabrasion and dermaplaning, and who is a good candidate?

A: Both procedures help to "refinish" the skin's top layers through a method of controlled surgical scraping. The treatments soften the sharp edges of surface irregularities, giving the skin a smoother appearance. Dermabrasion is most often used to improve the look of facial skin left scarred by accidents or previous surgery or to smooth out fine facial wrinkles, such as those around the mouth. It's also sometimes used to remove the pre-cancerous growths called keratoses. Dermaplaning is commonly used to treat deep acne scars.

Q: Should I get a facelift?

A: The best candidate for a facelift is someone whose face and neck have begun to sag but whose skin still has some elasticity and whose bone structure is strong and well-defined. A facelift can make you look younger and fresher, and it may enhance your self-confidence in the process. But it can't give you a totally different look, nor can it restore the health and vitality of your youth. Before you decide to have surgery, think carefully about your expectations and discuss them with your surgeon.

Q: What are the different "facelift" procedures?

A: The "full facelift" traditionally includes the brow, the entire face, and the neck. Commonly, when just the term "facelift" is used, the face and neck are what is being referred to. There are also neck-only lifts, face-only lifts, and regional facelifts.

Jorj's Skin-Savvy Glam Kitchen

While we all benefit from some patented lathers and creams, skin-care products aren't relegated to the health & beauty aisle; in fact, many are edible! What our skin craves first and foremost is the right diet. Through the pleasures of *certain* scrumptious fruits and veggies, nuts and cheeses, meats and grains, a girl subtracts years from her face, while adding—no *multiplying*—compliments. It's the perfect equation. Clear some space in your kitchen for these helpings of skin-friendly glam—below are my age-defying favorites.

Cornucopia of Color

Glowing skin testifies to good health; keeping it gorgeous on the outside requires a commitment to nurturing it on a cellular level—the part no one sees. If you want to keep things below your epidermal layer humming along, start with antioxidant-rich foods. These include **red** and **yellow bell peppers**, **soy**, **broccoli**, **spinach**, **carrots**, **garlic**, cooked **tomatoes**, **apples**, **raspberries**, and fresh **oranges**—remember that the brighter the fruits and vegetables, the more antioxidants they have to offer.

H_2O: Where to Hit the Mother Load

Water may very well be your skin's dearest friend. To flush out skin-threatening toxins, seek out water-filled fruits and veggies, like **watermelon**, **grapefruit**, **peaches**, **mangoes**, **cantaloupe**, **cucumbers**, and *every kind* of **lettuce**. These are just a few of the earth's treasure trove of fruits and veggies that will hydrate you, in turn promoting elasticity of the skin and regeneration of new, healthy skin cells—H_2O also helps skin maintain a balanced pH!

Spring Chickens of the Sea

Oil-rich fish in your well-balanced diet are guaranteed to give you a youthful glow. Why? Because of their antioxidant-rich omega-3 fatty acids. Go to the nearest seafood department or fishmonger and pick up **salmon**, **halibut**, **sardines**, **trout**, **herring**, **mackerel**, fresh or canned **albacore tuna**, and **shrimp**. Don't forget to buy **clams**, light chunk **tuna**, **catfish**, **cod**, **walnut oil**, **flaxseed oil**, **canola oil**, **spinach**, **walnuts**, **hazelnuts**, **almonds**, **sesame seeds**, and, for the most delicious fun of all, **cocoa**—the ultimate antioxidant-rich dessert!

"Fresh Faced": The Chemistry Behind the Simplicity

The chemical composition of the foods you eat plays a big part in determining who has dull, patchy skin and who possesses a dewy, fresh-faced countenance. If you want to look more like the latter, aim for a diet chock-full of alpha-hydroxy acids (AHA); these help your skin slough off the layer of dead cells and regenerate healthy new ones. AHA also balances your skin's pH. Our skin surface is slightly acidic and needs to remain so for the skin's protection and overall health; seek out recipes with **milk**, **grapes**, **blackberries**, **strawberries**, and all **citrus** fruits and juices.

How to Get "A-List" Skin

To promote the growth and health of all body cells and tissues—simultaneously protecting your mouth, stomach, and other internal organs from infection—load your grocery cart with vitamin A–rich foods, such as liver, sweet potatoes, dried apricots, egg yolks, and mozzarella cheese. Vitamin C helps rebuild collagen and is abundant in broccoli, cabbage, and tomatoes. Fight free-radical damage with red grapes, plums, cherries, apricots, bananas, Granny Smith or red delicious apples, corn, and kale.

Give Us This Day Our Daily Bread

Beautiful skin may ask several things of you, but one request in particular is: Eat those bread crusts! Whole grains are rich in phytochemicals, and the crusts of those breads are rich in antioxidants. The crusts may even provide a much stronger health benefit than the rest of the bread. So choose crusty **whole grain bread** over refined white breads; the latter contains simple carbohydrates your skin won't love as much as the complex carbs in **multi-grain unrefined bread**.

Nutty Bean Fiends Are 4-Ever Young

Love those legumes! **Red beans**, **kidney beans**, and **black beans** are at the top of the heap when it comes to antioxidants. Go nuts! **Pecans**, **hazelnuts**, **peanuts**, and **almonds** in raw form and **nut butter** are a terrific source of vitamin E and phytochemical antioxidants—not to mention omega-3 fatty acids.

Lend a Bit of Spice

Go heavy on the fresh herbs—your skin and taste buds implore you to do so, and it just so happens that like so many of the more delicious foods out there, herbs, too, are an abundant source of antioxidants. According to the U.S. Department of Agriculture, of all the herbs tested, **oregano** had the highest antioxidant capacity—so the Italians are onto something! A little spice is nice; ground **cloves** and **cinnamon** are two more of your skin's favorites.

Skin-Savvy Recipes

Start Your Day

Main Plates

On the Side

Snacks & Sweets

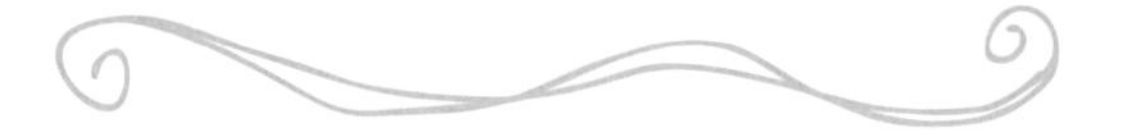

JUICED-UP FRUIT-AND-HERB BREAKFAST DRINKS

Combining fresh fruit with fresh herbs packs a double dose of antioxidants and lends a sophisticated twist to the everyday smoothie. Experiment with different combinations to keep your quick breakfast drink interesting and imaginative.

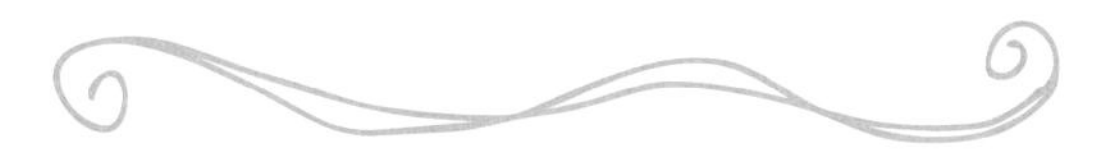

I like the PROTEIN and DAIRY that yogurt adds to the equation, but you can substitute with SOY MILK if you prefer. Also, I add a bunch of ice cubes to give a frothy result; again, you can eliminate this for a smoother, thicker drink.

Makes 2 generous servings each
Prep Time: 5 minutes

For Apple-Mint Power Drink

- 2 medium apples, peeled, cored and cut into ½-inch cubes (about 2 cups)
- 1 cup apple juice
- 1 cup reduced-fat vanilla-flavored yogurt
- 1 tablespoon chopped fresh mint leaves

For Cantaloupe-Tarragon Power Drink

- 2 cups cantaloupe, cut into 1-inch cubes
- 1 cup white grape juice
- 1 cup reduced-fat vanilla-flavored yogurt
- 1 tablespoon chopped fresh tarragon leaves

For Blueberry-Basil Power Drink

- 1 pint fresh blueberries (about 2 cups)
- 1 cup fresh grapefruit juice
- 1 cup reduced-fat vanilla-flavored yogurt
- Zest of 1 medium lemon (about 2 tablespoons)
- 1 tablespoon chopped fresh basil leaves

For each drink, combine all of the items in a blender. Add ice cubes to the top. Pulse to emulsify.

To serve the drink, pour into 2 tall glasses. Add a sprig of the fresh herb on top for garnish!

FRESH FRUIT SALAD

with Citrus Basil Dressing

Fresh fruit is brightly enhanced with a touch of sweetness and a sprinkle of fresh herbs. Use your favorite fruit combination and experiment with different fresh herbs to make this your own family-favorite dish.

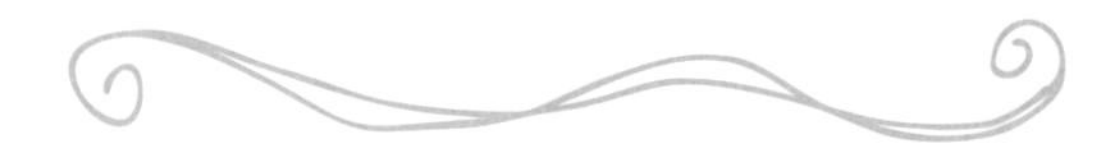

MINT makes a nice substitute for basil in this recipe. Try the different variations of mint for an even more unique flavor experience.

Makes 6 servings
Prep Time: 20 minutes

For the dressing

- 2 tablespoons chopped fresh basil leaves
- Juice of 1/2 medium orange (about 2–3 tablespoons)
- Zest of 1/2 medium orange (about 1 tablespoon)
- Juice of 1 medium lime (about 1 tablespoon)
- 1 tablespoon natural sugar

For the salad

- 2 cups honey dew melon, cut into 1-inch cubes
- 2 cups cantaloupe, cut into 1-inch cubes
- 2 cups seeded watermelon, cut into 1-inch cubes
- 2 large mangos, pitted, peeled, and diced into 1-inch cubes (about 2 cups)
- 1 pint fresh blueberries (about 2 cups)

Place all of the ingredients for the dressing into the bowl of a food processor or blender. Pulse to combine.

Combine all of the salad ingredients in a serving bowl. Pour the dressing over top and toss gently.

FRUIT AND YOGURT BREAKFAST PARFAITS

with Granola Crunch

Granola is chock-full of oats and nuts—and in many cases dried fruit. Adding ground flaxseed pumps it up to a bigger, badder breakfast food. You can purchase ground flaxseed or you can grind it yourself using a spice grinder.

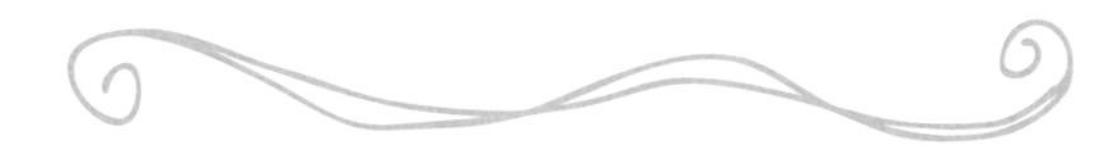

One-fourth cup whole flaxseeds will yield about 6 tablespoons ground FLAXSEED.

Makes 4 parfaits plus an extra 3 cups granola
Prep Time: 10 minutes
Cook Time: 30 minutes

For the granola

- 2 cups old fashioned rolled oats
- 1/3 cup ground flaxseed
- 1/3 cup sliced almonds
- 1/3 cup chopped pecans
- 2 teaspoons ground cinnamon
- 1/2 teaspoon ground nutmeg
- 1/3 cup apple juice
- 1/3 cup honey
- 2 tablespoons dark brown sugar
- 2 teaspoons canola oil
- 1 teaspoon vanilla extract

For the parfaits

- 1 cup fresh blueberries
- 1 cup fresh raspberries
- 1 cup strawberries, hulled and quartered
- Zest of 1 medium lemon (about 1 tablespoon)
- 2 cups plain reduced-fat yogurt

Preheat the oven to 300 degrees.

In a small bowl mix together the oats, flaxseed, almonds, pecans, cinnamon, and nutmeg. In a pot over medium heat, heat the apple juice, honey, and brown sugar until the sugar is dissolved, about 3–5 minutes. Remove the pan from the heat. Stir in the oil and vanilla. Pour the apple juice/honey mixture over the oat mixture and stir. Spread the coated mixture onto a jelly-roll pan that has been coated with vegetable oil spray. Bake for 10 minutes, stir and bake for 15–20 minutes more, or until the granola is golden brown. Cool and break into small pieces.

To serve, mix together the fruit and lemon zest in a small bowl. Divide the fruit into 4 parfait glasses (or bowls). Top the fruit with ¼ cup yogurt. Sprinkle 1–2 tablespoons granola on top of each parfait. Dig in!

On Shopping Day: Prepare granola and store in an airtight container at room temperature for up to 2 weeks.

BREAKFAST BURRITOS

With Red Pepper Salsa

Start your day with a breakfast rich in vitamin A–filled veggies and the protein found in eggs. Add a splash of spice and a splurge of creamy garnish, and you have a dish that beckons *you to breakfast.*

Make this meal in RECORD time using PREPARED SALSA as a substitute. Check the labels to make sure you are choosing a product without added salt or sugar.

Prepare the salsa by tossing together the onion, red bell pepper, tomatoes, cilantro, and basil in a small bowl. Sprinkle with lime juice and olive oil. Season with salt and pepper. Toss again and set aside.

Prepare the burritos by lightly coating each tortilla with vegetable oil spray. Stack them on a sheet of parchment paper and wrap completely. Warm them in a microwave oven on medium-high setting for 45 seconds. Set aside.

Prepare the filling by whisking together the eggs and egg whites in a medium bowl until frothy. Stir in the chili powder. Heat 1 tablespoon olive oil in a nonstick skillet over medium heat. Pour in the egg mixture. Use a spatula to continually stir the eggs until soft curds form, about 4–5 minutes. Stir in the cheese until melted, about 2–3 minutes more. Season with salt and pepper. Remove the skillet from the heat.

Assemble the burritos by unwrapping the tortillas, placing each onto a plate. Layer with spinach leaves. Divide the egg mixture among the tortillas. Roll each one by folding burrito-style. Top with 2 tablespoons Red Pepper Salsa and 1 tablespoon reduced-fat sour cream.

On Shopping Day: Prepare salsa and store in the refrigerator for up to 4 days.

Makes 4 servings
Prep Time: 10 minutes
Cook Time: 6 to 8 minutes

For the salsa

- 1 small white onion, finely diced (about 1/2 cup)
- 1 large red bell pepper, seeded and chopped (about 1 cup)
- 6 medium plum tomatoes, seeded and diced (about 3 cups)
- 1 tablespoon chopped fresh cilantro
- 1 tablespoon chopped fresh basil
- Juice of 1 medium lime (about 1 tablespoon)
- 1 tablespoon olive oil
- Salt and freshly ground pepper

For the burritos

- 4 6-inch whole wheat tortillas
- 3 large eggs
- 4 large egg whites
- 1/2 teaspoon chili powder
- 1 tablespoon olive oil
- 4 ounces reduced-fat, grated Monterey Jack cheese (about 1 cup)
- 1 cup fresh spinach leaves, washed and dried
- 1/4 cup reduced-fat sour cream

SUSHI-STYLE SALMON WRAPS

Packages of cooked and drained salmon are excellent products to store in your pantry. Canned salmon is equally good, but you will have to work a little harder draining and cleaning. Another good substitution is leftover roasted salmon. You can cook it once and eat it twice!

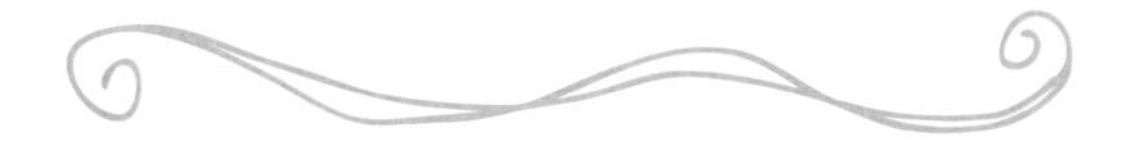

SALMON is a natural source of OMEGA-3 fatty acids. These building blocks of FAT are necessary for your skin to function optimally.

Makes 4 to 6 servings
Prep Time: 15 minutes

2 7-ounce packages drained skinless, boneless pink salmon
Juice of 1 medium lemon (about 2 tablespoons)
Zest of 1 medium lemon (about 1 tablespoon)
1 1-inch piece ginger, grated (about 1 tablespoon)
1 tablespoon light soy sauce
1 tablespoon sesame oil
1 teaspoon honey
2 cups cooked brown rice
1 8-ounce can sliced water chestnuts, drained
1 bunch (6–8) green onions, thinly sliced on the diagonal (about 1/2 cup)
2 tablespoons sesame seeds
4 10-inch whole grain tortillas
2 cups arugula leaves, washed and dried
Salt and freshly ground pepper

Place the salmon into a bowl. In a separate bowl stir together the lemon juice, zest, ginger, soy sauce, sesame oil, and honey. Pour this mixture over the salmon. Toss to combine. Stir in the rice, water chestnuts, green onions, and sesame seeds.

Lay the tortillas onto your work surface. Layer each one with arugula leaves. Divide the salmon mixture among the tortillas. Use a spatula to spread out the salmon over the leaves. Season with salt and pepper. Tuck in the sides and roll the bottom edge of the tortilla over the filling to form a cylinder. Repeat with remaining tortillas.

To serve, roll each wrap in parchment paper. Cut in half, and peel back paper to bite.

MEDITERRANEAN TUNA MELT

Behold, an update on the traditional tuna melt! Filled with veggies and vitamin-rich tuna, this sandwich is a breeze to make. Consider serving it with a bowl of Butternut Squash Soup (page 70).

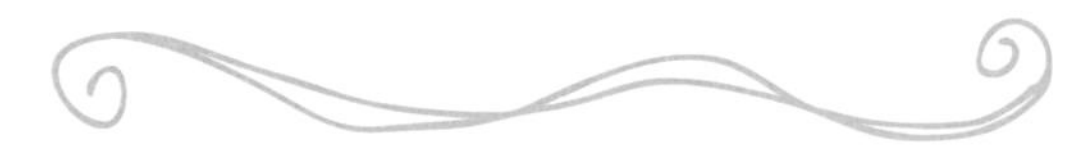

I like to use TUNA packed in OIL because of the benefits of the OMEGA-3 fatty acids and because of the flavor boost. If you choose tuna packed in water, drain first and then consider adding a tablespoon or two of good-quality OLIVE OIL to the tuna mixture.

Makes 6 servings
Prep Time: 10 minutes
Cook Time: 6 to 8 minutes

1 12-ounce can tuna, packed in oil
10–12 Nicoise (or other good-quality) large olives, pitted and chopped (about 1 cup)
1 14-ounce can artichoke hearts, drained and chopped
1 16-ounce can cannellini beans, drained
Salt and freshly ground pepper
1 16-ounce whole grain (French bread style) loaf, cut in half horizontally
2 ounces Parmesan cheese, grated (about ½ cup)

Preheat oven to 400 degrees.

In a bowl combine the tuna, olives, artichoke hearts, and cannellini beans. Season with salt and pepper.

Scoop out some of the bread in each loaf half to create a bowl. Fill each half with tuna salad. Sprinkle with Parmesan cheese. Bake until the cheese is melted and the tuna is warmed through, about 6–8 minutes.

To serve, cut each half into 3 pieces.

SWEET POTATO APPLE SALAD

With Honey, Ginger, and Mustard Dressing

Sweet potatoes, tossed with fresh fruit and flavor-filled dressing, star in this super salad—great for luncheons or for a lite veggie meal.

Makes 6 servings
Prep Time: 15 minutes
Cook Time: 10 minutes

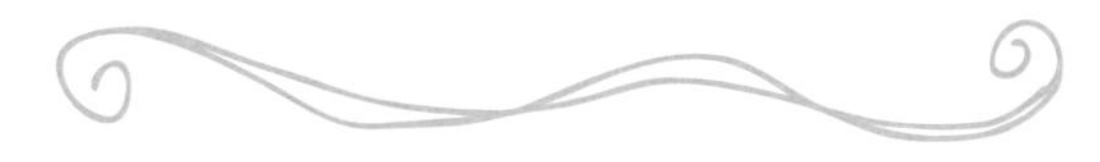

You can add a boost of FLAVOR by ROASTING the sweet potatoes with SPICES. Toss with olive oil and a combination of your favorite spices. (I like chili powder, cumin, and paprika.) Roast until golden, cool, and continue with the recipe.

For the dressing

- 1/2 cup honey
- Juice of 3 medium limes (about 1/4 cup)
- 1/4 cup olive oil
- 1 1-inch piece ginger, grated (about 1 tablespoon)
- 2 tablespoons Dijon mustard
- Salt and freshly ground pepper

For the salad

- 2 medium sweet potatoes, peeled and diced into 1-inch cubes (about 2 cups)
- 2 cups fresh pineapple, cut into 1-inch cubes
- 2 medium apples, peeled, cored, and cut into 1/2-inch cubes (about 2 cups)
- 2 medium celery ribs, diced (about 1/2 cup)
- 1 cup finely chopped walnuts
- 4 ounces mesclun lettuce mix (about 4 cups)

In a small bowl whisk together salad dressing ingredients. Season with salt and pepper.

Preheat the oven to 350 degrees. Place the potatoes onto a rimmed baking sheet that has been coated with vegetable oil spray. Cook until tender, about 8–10 minutes. Cool to room temperature. Toss together the remaining salad ingredients.

To serve, pour the dressing over the salad, toss and season with additional freshly ground pepper.

GRILLED HALIBUT

With Salsa Verde

Halibut is a fresh-tasting fish that laps up the flavors that surround it. Grilling shortcuts this whole dish, making it a quick insertion into your mid-week meal repertoire.

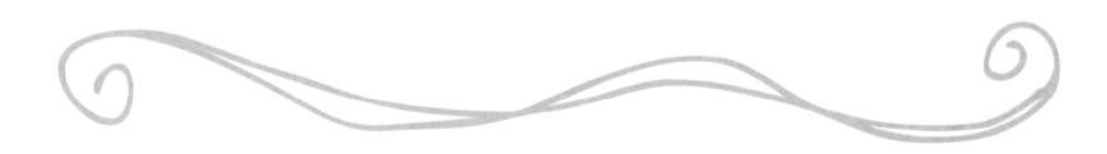

This salsa is really a cross between a PESTO and a CHIMICHURRI sauce. Feel free to make it your own by substituting with your favorite nuts and herbs. WALNUTS and pine nuts are terrific substitutes, as are mint leaves and tarragon.

Preheat the oven to 350 degrees. Spread the almonds onto a rimmed baking sheet and bake until golden, about 5–8 minutes. Cool to room temperature.

Place the almonds, herbs, garlic, and jalapeño pepper into a blender (or food processor). Season with salt and pepper. Pour in lime juice. Process until the ingredients are thoroughly chopped. With the machine running, slowly pour in the olive oil until the mixture becomes a thick paste.

Heat a grill pan over medium-high heat. Brush the fish with 1 tablespoon olive oil and season with salt and pepper. Grill, turning once, about 5 minutes per side for a 1½-inch-thick steak. Place the steaks onto a platter and keep warm. Pour the remaining 1 tablespoon olive oil into the grill pan. Grill the onion and pepper until just beginning to char, about 5 minutes.

To serve, place the grilled veggies onto a platter. Top with the grilled halibut. Drizzle with Salsa Verde.

Makes 4 servings
Prep Time: 10 minutes
Cook Time: 8 to 10 minutes

For the salsa

- 1/4 cup sliced almonds
- 1 cup fresh parsley leaves
- 1/2 cup fresh basil leaves
- 1/2 cup fresh cilantro leaves
- 4 medium garlic cloves
- 1 medium jalapeño pepper, seeded and diced (about 2 tablespoons)
- Salt and freshly ground pepper
- Juice of 1 medium lime (about 1 tablespoon)
- 3/4 cup olive oil

For the halibut and veggies

- 4 6- to 8-ounce halibut steaks
- 2 tablespoons olive oil, divided use
- 1 large red onion, sliced (about 1 cup)
- 1 large red bell pepper, seeded and thinly sliced (about 1 cup)

CHICKEN THIGHS

With Sage and Caramelized Peaches

Caramelized fruit makes a wonderful addition to a pan sauce. Fruit also contains antioxidants—so it's kinda like getting all the good stuff rolled into one dish.

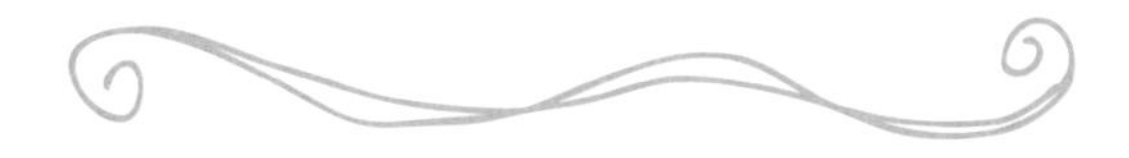

Substitute with FROZEN sliced peaches if fresh are not available, or chicken breasts if you prefer WHITE meat. It all works!

Makes 4 servings
Prep Time: 10 minutes
Cook Time: 20 minutes

- 4 boneless, skinless chicken thighs
- Salt and freshly ground pepper
- 1 tablespoon olive oil
- 2 ripe peaches, pitted and sliced into wedges
- 1 tablespoon natural sugar
- 1/2 cup red wine
- 2 sprigs sage leaves

Season the chicken thighs with salt and pepper. Heat the olive oil in a sauté pan over medium-high heat. Place the chicken into the pan. Cook, turning once until the chicken is golden, about 5–7 minutes per side. Transfer to a platter and keep warm.

Place the peach wedges into the pan. Sprinkle with sugar. Cook until the slices are tender and begin to brown. Pour in the wine. Reduce until the sauce begins to thicken. Remove the peaches from the skillet. Return the chicken thighs to the skillet. Add the sage. Cook for 5–7 minutes more or until the chicken is cooked through.

To serve, place the chicken onto a platter. Top with peaches and drizzle the pan juices over the top.

SPINACH SALAD WITH WARM CHIPOTLE CHILI VINAIGRETTE

Topped with Chicken Strips and Crisp Sweet Potato

Salads are a great way to build an easy-to-make midweek meal and include everything from left-overs to good-for-you veggies. This is just one example of the many fabulous salads you can create when you include brightly colored veggies in your meal plan.

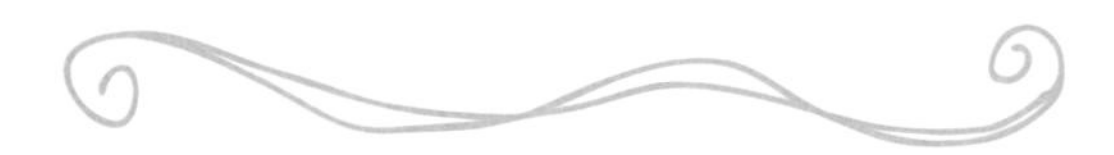

You can purchase CHIPOTLE CHILIES in a can in the ETHNIC department of your grocery store. These reconstituted peppers come packed in a rich, RED sauce and are very SPICY. If you are not as keen on spice as I am, feel free to cut the amount of chipotle in half (or even less to start with). You can always add more as you build your palate to HOT, HOT HOT!

Preheat the oven to 400 degrees. In a small bowl stir together the chili powder, cumin, salt, and pepper. Toss the potato sticks in 1 tablespoon olive oil. Sprinkle with half of the chili powder mixture. Spread the potato sticks onto a rimmed baking sheet. Roast until the sweet potato is crisp and golden, about 10–15 minutes.

Heat a sauté pan over medium-high heat. Toss the chicken strips with remaining 1 tablespoon olive oil and the remaining chili mixture. Cook until golden, about 3–5 minutes. Drain on paper towels.

Prepare the vinaigrette by placing the chipotle pepper, sun-dried tomatoes, balsamic vinegar, and brown sugar into a blender. Pulse to combine. With the machine running, slowly pour in ½ cup olive oil. Season with salt and pepper. Place this mixture into the sauté pan and warm over medium-low heat.

Place the spinach, romaine, and basil leaves into a large serving bowl. Drizzle with 2 tablespoons of the warm vinaigrette. Toss well.

To serve, place the dressed greens onto a platter or into a shallow pasta bowl. Top with sweet potato strips, chicken strips, red onion and avocado. Drizzle with additional warm vinaigrette.

Makes 4 servings
Prep Time: 20 minutes
Cook Time: 15 minutes

For the salad

- 1 teaspoon chili powder
- ½ teaspoon cumin
- ½ teaspoon kosher salt
- ½ teaspoon ground black pepper
- 1 medium sweet potato, peeled and cut into matchstick-size strips (about 1 cup)
- 2 tablespoons olive oil, divided use
- 2 4- to 5-ounce skinless boneless chicken breast cutlets, cut into thin strips
- 4 ounces fresh spinach leaves, washed, dried, and chopped (about 2 cups)
- 1 medium head romaine lettuce, washed, dried, and torn (about 6 cups)

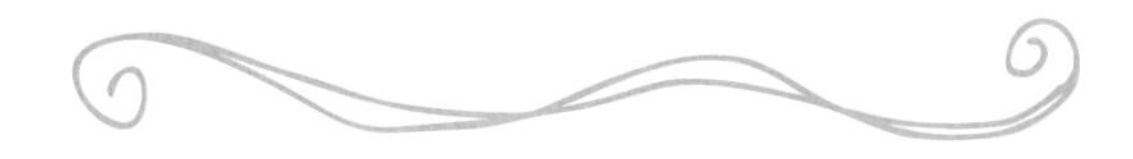

- ½ cup basil leaves
- 1 small red onion, thinly sliced
- 1 large avocado, peeled, pitted, and diced (about 1 cup)

For the vinaigrette

- 1 chipotle pepper in adobo sauce, seeded and finely diced (about 1 tablespoon)
- ¼ cup minced oil-packed sun-dried tomatoes, drained
- 2 tablespoons balsamic vinegar
- 1 tablespoon dark brown sugar
- ½ cup olive oil

OPEN-FACED CHICKEN TACOS

This meal comes together in minutes, making it an excellent midweek supper. It's full of lean protein, fresh veggies, and herbs, deeming this dish an antioxidant windfall!

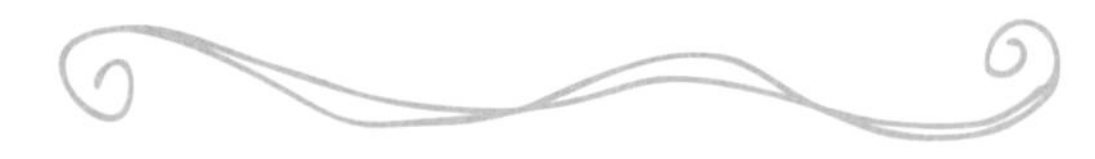

Turmeric is thought to be an anti-inflammatory spice, boosting the good-for-you aspect of this dish.

Makes 4 servings
Prep Time: 15 minutes
Cook Time: 10 to 15 minutes

2–4 tablespoons olive oil, divided use
1 large red bell pepper, seeded and cut into thin strips (about 1 cup)
1 yellow bell pepper, seeded and cut into thin strips (about 1 cup)
1 large red onion, peeled and cut into thin strips (about 1 cup)
Salt and freshly ground pepper
2 teaspoons ground cumin
1/2 teaspoon turmeric
1/2 teaspoon ground oregano
2 large (6 to 8-ounce) skinless, boneless chicken breast halves, pounded to 1/2-inch thickness, cut into strips (about 3 cups)
4 6-inch whole wheat tortillas
1 medium head Boston lettuce, washed, dried, and torn (about 2 cups)
1/2 medium plum tomato, seeded and diced (about 2 tablespoons)
2 tablespoons chopped fresh cilantro
Reduced-fat sour cream

Heat 2 tablespoons olive oil in a skillet over medium-high heat. Add the red and yellow bell peppers and onion. Season with salt and pepper. Cook until the veggies are soft and begin to turn brown. Use a slotted spoon to transfer the veggies to a platter.

In a medium bowl combine the cumin, turmeric, and oregano. Toss the chicken strips in the bowl until well-coated. Season with salt and pepper. Heat the remaining olive oil in the same skillet. Add the chicken and cook until golden, about 6–8 minutes.

Stack the tortillas and wrap in parchment paper. Warm on low in the oven or in a microwave until soft.

To serve, place 1 tortilla on each plate. Top with lettuce leaves. Place one-fourth of the onion/pepper mixture on top of the lettuce. Top with one-fourth of the chicken strips. Top with diced tomatoes, fresh cilantro, and a dollop of sour cream.

ROASTED TOMATO BASIL SOUP

With Sea Bass Center

This dramatic dish features succulent roasted sea bass, surrounded by vibrant red soup. Not only is it delicious, but you'll get raves for your inventive presentation.

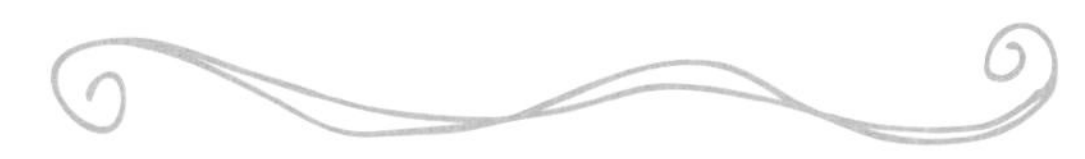

You can substitute your favorite fish in this dish. Try red snapper or mackerel, or the freshest fish your market has to offer.

Preheat the oven to 400 degrees. Place the tomatoes on a rimmed baking sheet coated with vegetable oil spray. Sprinkle with 3 tablespoons olive oil, oregano, salt, and pepper. Roast until the tomatoes are golden and beginning to caramelize, about 45 minutes to 1 hour.

Heat 2 tablespoons olive oil in a large pot over medium-high heat. Add the onion and garlic and cook until soft, about 5 minutes. Add the diced tomatoes, the roasted tomatoes, and the basil leaves (reserving some for garnish). Pour in the chicken broth. Bring the soup to a boil, reduce the heat, and simmer for 20 minutes. Use a handheld blender (or food processor) to emulsify the ingredients. Keep the soup warm.

Preheat the oven to 350 degrees. Place the sea bass into a baking dish. Top with diced onion and bell pepper. Sprinkle with 2 tablespoons olive oil and Worcestershire sauce. Season with salt and pepper. Bake until the fish is cooked through, about 15–20 minutes for 1½-inch-thick filet.

To serve, divide the fish into 4 portions. Place each portion into the center of a shallow pasta bowl. Ladle the soup around the fish. Garnish with reserved fresh basil leaves.

On Shopping Day: Prepare the roasted tomatoes and store in an airtight container in the refrigerator for up to 5 days.

Makes 4 servings
Prep Time: 30 minutes
Cook Time: 45 minutes for the tomatoes, 30 minutes for the soup and fish

For the soup

- 16 medium plum tomatoes, cut in half lengthwise (about 2½ pounds)
- 3 tablespoons olive oil
- 2 teaspoons dried oregano leaves
- Salt and freshly ground pepper
- 2 tablespoons olive oil
- 1 medium yellow onion, diced into ½-inch squares (about 1 cup)
- 3 medium garlic cloves, minced (about 1½ teaspoons)
- 1 28-ounce can diced tomatoes
- 2 cups fresh basil leaves, divided use
- 3 cups chicken stock or low-sodium chicken broth

For the sea bass

- 1 12- to 16-ounce sea bass filet
- 1 medium yellow onion, diced into ½-inch squares (about 1 cup)
- 1 medium red bell pepper, diced into ½-inch squares (about 1 cup)
- 2 tablespoons olive oil
- 1 tablespoon Worcestershire sauce

BUTTERNUT SQUASH SOUP

Flavored with Orange and Tarragon

Prepare this soup on shopping day and serve it warm, either by reheating or by simmering on low, in a slow cooker. As with most soups, the longer it simmers, the more its flavors meld. This soup is a low-maintenance dish, savory and comforting—ideal to come home to after a long, busy day.

Makes 4 servings
Prep Time: 10 minutes
Cook Time: 30 minutes

- 1 tablespoon olive oil
- 1 large yellow onion, diced into 1-inch squares (about 1 cup)
- 1 medium butternut squash, peeled and diced into 1-inch squares (about 4 cups)
- Salt and freshly ground pepper
- 1 teaspoon ground cinnamon
- 1/2 teaspoon ground cumin
- 1 quart homemade chicken stock or low-sodium chicken broth
- Juice of 1 medium orange (about 1/3 cup)
- Zest of 1/2 medium orange (about 1 tablespoon)
- 1/4 cup brandy
- 2 tablespoons chopped fresh tarragon leaves

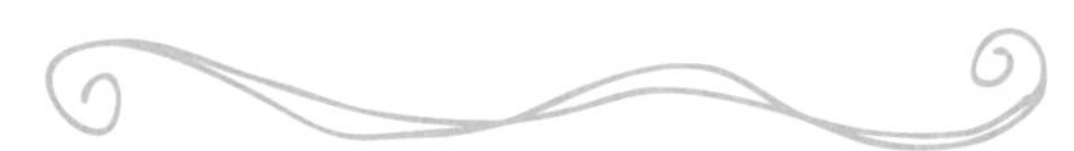

Brightly colored veggies like BUTTERNUT SQUASH and fresh herbs such as TARRAGON contain ANTIOXIDANTS that are important in fighting our bodies' inherent free radicals, which damage skin, creating wrinkles. Soups like this one are a delicious means to a GLOWING complexion.

Heat the olive oil in a large, deep pot over medium-high heat. Stir in the onion and cook until opaque, about 4–5 minutes. Stir in the butternut squash. Season with salt, pepper, cinnamon and cumin. Pour in the chicken broth. Bring to a boil. Reduce heat, cover the pot, and simmer until the squash is soft, about 15–20 minutes.

Remove the pot from the heat. Use a hand held blender (or food processor) to purée the soup until smooth. Return the pot to medium heat. Stir in the orange juice, zest, brandy and tarragon. Simmer the soup for 5 more minutes, so the flavors can blend. Taste to adjust seasonings.

STEWED TOMATOES

With Garlic and Black Beans

This antioxidant-filled side dish morphs into a complete meal by simply adding a spoonful of brown rice! The veggies store so well you can use them later in the week to fill burritos or stuff bell peppers. Voilà—two more quick meals!

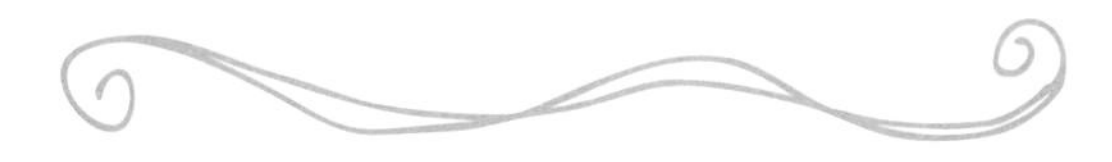

To cut BASIL LEAVES into CHIFFONADE, begin by piling leaves on top of each other. Roll them into a tight cylinder. Use a sharp knife to cut through the roll, rendering it into THIN STRIPS. Separate the thin curls and sprinkle onto the dish.

Makes 6 generous servings
Prep Time: 5 minutes
Cook Time: 30 minutes

- 1 tablespoon olive oil
- 1 large yellow onion, finely diced (about 1 cup)
- 4 medium garlic cloves, chopped (about 2 teaspoons)
- 1 28-ounce can diced tomatoes
- 1 16-ounce can black beans, drained
- Salt and freshly ground pepper
- 2 tablespoons fresh basil leaves, cut into chiffonade

Heat the olive oil in a pot over medium-high heat. Add the onion and cook until soft, about 4–5 minutes. Add the garlic and cook for 3–4 minutes more. Pour in the tomatoes. Reduce the heat and simmer for 5 minutes. Pour in the beans. Season with salt and pepper. Continue simmering until much of the liquid has been reduced and the stew is thickened, about 15–20 minutes.

To serve, spoon the stew onto a plate or into a shallow bowl. Sprinkle basil over top.

ROSEMARY ROASTED CARROT STICKS

When your complexion asks, "What's up, doc?" answer with a simple preparation of a healthful veggie.

Makes 4 servings
Prep Time: 5 minutes
Cook Time: 20 to 25 minutes

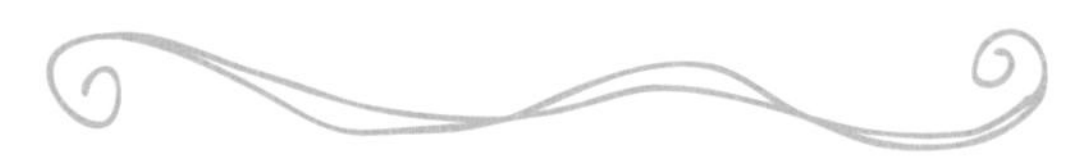

6 large carrots, peeled and cut into strips, 4-inches long and 1/2-inch thick
2 tablespoons olive oil
Salt and freshly ground pepper
Fresh rosemary sprigs

Preheat oven to 350 degrees. Toss the carrot sticks with olive oil, salt, and pepper. Place onto a baking sheet. Place rosemary springs alongside the carrot sticks. Roast until the carrots are soft and begin to turn brown, about 20–25 minutes.

To serve, discard rosemary and place carrots in a serving dish. Season carrots with salt and freshly ground pepper.

STUFFED SWEET POTATOES

With Spinach and Corn

It's not about sugar and marshmallows in this sweet potato dish. Instead, we stuff them with fresh spinach and corn for a side dish that is just about a meal in itself.

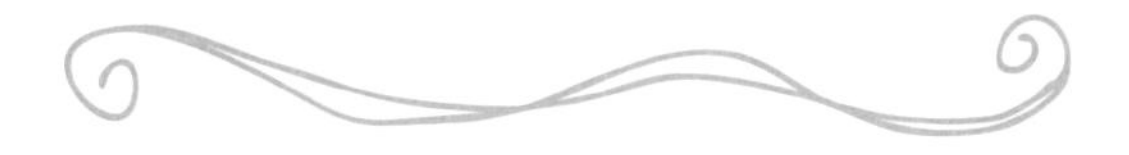

Get an extra dose of VITAMINS and FIBER in this dish by eating the OUTSIDE as well as the inside. The skin of the potato is oh-so-good-for-you, too!

Preheat the oven to 375 degrees. Use a fork to pierce the skins of the potatoes. Bake the potatoes until soft, about 40–45 minutes (depending on size).

Heat 1 tablespoon olive oil in a skillet over medium-high heat. Add the onion and garlic and cook until soft, about 5 minutes. Add the corn and spinach, cook for 5 minutes more. Season with salt and pepper.

Stand up each potato, on its small end, in a baking dish. Cut the top fourth from each potato. Remove the flesh from the inside, leaving 4 sweet potato shells. Roughly chop the flesh and stir into the spinach mixture. Stuff each potato with one-fourth of the spinach/potato mixture. Drizzle with the remaining 1 tablespoon olive oil. Reduce the heat to 350 degrees and bake for 20 minutes.

On Shopping Day: Bake the sweet potatoes, cool, and store in an airtight container for up to 1 week.

Makes 4 servings
Prep Time: 20 minutes
Cook Time: 45 minutes to roast potatoes and 20 minutes to cook the dish

4 medium sweet potatoes (about 2 pounds)
2 tablespoons olive oil, divided use
1 medium yellow onion, diced into 1/2-inch squares (about 1 cup)
2 medium cloves garlic, minced (about 1 teaspoon)
4 ears of fresh corn, kernels sliced from cob (about 2 cups) or two cups frozen corn, defrosted
6 ounces fresh spinach leaves, washed, dried, and chopped (about 4 cups)
Salt and freshly ground pepper

ROASTED FIGS

With Sweetened Orange Sauce

Roasting fruit brings out its natural sweetness. Linger over this dessert, as each bite brings a new flavor explosion.

Makes 6 servings
Prep Time: 10 minutes
Cook Time: 15 to 20 minutes

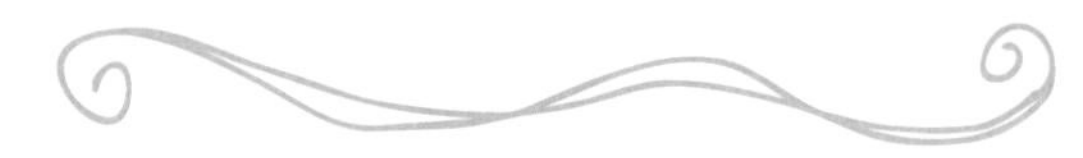

If FRESH figs are not available, you can substitute with dried figs. If the figs become too dry, double the cooking time and add additional ORANGE JUICE as the figs roast.

For the sauce

- Juice of 3 medium oranges (about 1 cup)
- Zest of ½ medium orange (about 1 tablespoon)
- 2 tablespoons honey

For the dessert

- 1 pound fresh Mission figs cut into quarters
- Reduced-fat sour cream (for garnish)
- Fresh mint leaves (for garnish)

Place the orange juice, zest, and honey into a small saucepan over medium heat. Simmer until the mixture thickens and is reduced to about ½ cup, about 10 minutes.

Preheat oven to 400 degrees. Place the figs into a baking dish. Pour the sauce over top. Roast until the figs are soft and the sauce is syrupy, about 15 minutes.

To serve, spoon the figs and the sauce into a bowl. Garnish with a dollop of sour cream and a sprig of fresh mint.

BANANA FLAXSEED BREAD

With Warm Strawberry Sauce

This recipe demonstrates how easy it is to include flaxseed in your favorite baked goods. Quick breads like this one are easily prepared on the weekend for a grab-and-go weekday snack.

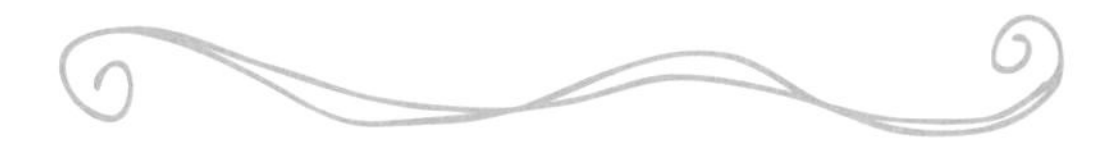

FLAXSEED is a nutritional megastar. It is the only plant source of OMEGA-3 fatty acids and the richest plant source of ANTIOXIDANTS.

Makes 12 servings
Prep Time: 20 minutes
Cook Time: 1 hour

For the banana bread

- 1½ cups unbleached all-purpose flour
- 1 cup whole wheat flour
- ½ cup ground flaxseed
- ¾ cup natural sugar
- ¼ cup dark brown sugar
- 1 tablespoon baking powder
- 1 teaspoon ground cinnamon
- ½ teaspoon salt
- ¼ teaspoon baking soda
- ¼ teaspoon ground nutmeg
- 1 cup reduced-fat vanilla yogurt
- 1 large egg, beaten
- ¼ cup canola oil
- 1 teaspoon pure vanilla extract
- 3 very ripe bananas, mashed (about 1½ cups)
- ½ cup chopped walnuts

For the sauce

- 2 cups natural sugar
- Juice of ½ medium orange (about 2–3 tablespoons)
- Zest of ½ medium orange (about 1 tablespoon)
- 2 pints strawberries, hulled and quartered (about 2 cups)
- 1 tablespoon cornstarch mixed with 2 tablespoons cold water

Preheat oven to 350 degrees. Coat a 9 x 5-inch loaf pan with vegetable oil spray.

In a large bowl whisk together the flours, flaxseed, sugars, baking powder, cinnamon, salt, baking soda, and nutmeg. In a second bowl stir together yogurt, egg, canola oil, and vanilla. Stir in the bananas.

Stir the yogurt/banana mixture into the flour mixture until just combined. Fold in the walnuts. Pour the batter into the prepared loaf pan. Bake for 1 hour or until a wooden pick inserted in the center comes out clean. Cool on a rack.

To prepare the sauce, place the sugar, orange juice, and orange zest into a small pot over medium-low heat. Stir until the sugar dissolves, about 10 minutes. Add the strawberries to the pot. Simmer over low heat until the strawberries begin to break down. Stir in the cornstarch mixture and simmer until the sauce thickens.

To serve, remove the loaf from the pan and slice into ¾-inch-thick slices. Serve with a drizzle of warm sauce.

PEACH GINGERBREAD

With Walnut Streusel

Enjoy this yummy snack cake as an easy dessert or a mid-morning pick-me-up.

Makes 9 servings
Prep Time: 10 minutes
Cook Time: 40–45 minutes

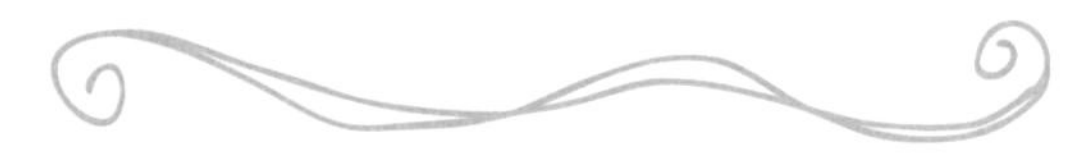

CRYSTALLIZED ginger comes in a JAR and is found in your grocery store near the specialty food items.

If fresh peaches are not available, feel free to substitute with fresh FROZEN peaches.

For the streusel

- 1/3 cup finely chopped walnuts
- 1/4 cup natural sugar
- 2 tablespoons crystallized ginger, finely chopped

For the cake

- 2 cups unbleached all-purpose flour
- 3/4 cup dark brown sugar
- 2 teaspoons ground ginger
- 2 teaspoons baking powder
- 1 teaspoon baking soda
- 1/4 teaspoon salt
- 2 ripe peaches, cut in half, pitted, and peeled
- 1/2 cup reduced-fat buttermilk
- 1/4 cup canola oil
- 2 large eggs, slightly beaten

To make the streusel, in a small bowl stir together the walnuts, sugar, and chopped ginger.

For the cake, preheat the oven to 350 degrees. Coat a 9-inch square baking pan with vegetable oil spray. In a large bowl combine the flour, brown sugar, ground ginger, baking powder, baking soda, and salt. Place the peaches into a food processor, pulse to purée. Place the peach purée into a large bowl. Stir in the buttermilk, canola oil, and eggs. Whisk in the flour mixture until smooth.

Pour half of the batter into the prepared pan. Sprinkle with half of the streusel. Pour in the remaining batter. Top with the remaining streusel. Bake until the bread springs back when touched and a tester inserted into the center comes out clean, about 40–45 minutes. Remove from the oven and cool.

To serve, cut the cake into 9 (3-inch) squares.

OVEN-ROASTED FRUIT

With Vanilla Yogurt Sorbet

This deliciously satisfying dessert comes together in no time. You control the amount of sugar, or substitute with honey for a distinctive flavor.

Makes 6 to 8 servings
Prep Time: 10 minutes
Cook Time: 30 minutes

For the sorbet

- 2 extra-large egg whites
- 1/3 cup honey
- 2 cups reduced-fat vanilla flavored yogurt

For the fruit

- 2 ripe peaches, pitted and quartered
- 2 ripe plums, pitted and quartered
- 1/4 cup natural sugar
- 1 pint fresh blueberries (about 2 cups)
- 1 pint fresh raspberries (about 2 cups)
- 2 sprigs rosemary
- 1 tablespoon olive oil

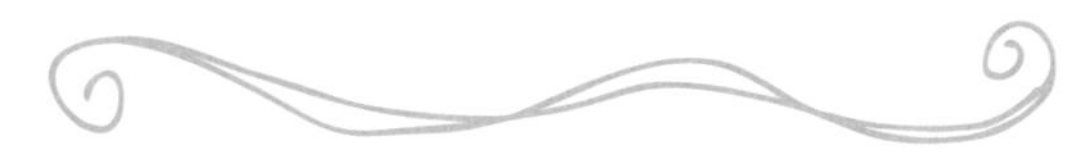

This recipe calls for UNCOOKED eggs, which have been linked to salmonella. By choosing the FRESHEST eggs you can find and making sure that they are refrigerated properly and that the shells are intact (not cracked), you reduce the risk of CONTAMINATION. If you are nonetheless concerned, simply eliminate the egg WHITES in the sorbet recipe.

Use an electric mixer to whip the egg whites until frothy. Add the honey and whip until the egg whites are stiff and shiny. Whisk the yogurt in a bowl until soft. Gently fold in the egg white mixture. Place into the bowl of an ice cream maker and freeze according to the manufacturer's directions.

Preheat the oven to 425 degrees. Place the peaches and plums into a baking dish coated with vegetable oil spray. Sprinkle with 1/4 cup sugar. Sprinkle the blueberries and raspberries on top. Place the rosemary sprigs into the fruit. Drizzle olive oil over the top. Roast until the fruit is tender and golden and the berries have released their juices, about 25–30 minutes. Remove the rosemary sprigs.

To serve, place a scoop of the sorbet into a bowl and top with warm fruit.

On Shopping Day: Prepare the sorbet, store in an airtight container in the freezer for up to 5 days.

Gorgeous Home Spa Secrets . . . Just for Your Skin

Penny-pinching has never been this much fun! Just think . . . creating dual purposes for your food—you can eat it or apply it! The best home facial takes advantage of foods most of us already have on hand: milk; olive, safflower, sesame, and flaxseed oils; certain herbs; and from your medicine cabinet, witch hazel.

Livin' Steamy

Next time you have a Southern gentleman caller at the door, tell him you're out of mint for those summer Juleps and use it, instead, as part of an invigorating facial blend! Juiced-Up Fruit-and-Herb Breakfast Drinks (pg. 57) features mint in the recipe, which can be used to make your own invigorating **Mint Facial Steam**. Just place a handful of mint leaves in a pot of water, boil, then reduce the heat and simmer for 5–10 minutes. Pull your hair back, wash your face with a gentle soap, and then do double-facial-beatification duty. Carefully transfer the pot with the warm minted water to your table or countertop. Have a few tablespoons of sesame seed oil standing by. Apply the oil to your face before you begin your facial steam; this will act as a beauty buffer. Make a tent over your head with a towel, being very careful not to get too close to the pot so you do not burn yourself. Keep your face in the sweet mint steam for about five minutes. Afterward, rinse your face with cold water and close your newly invigorated pores with an astringent, such as witch hazel. Not only will you look years younger afterward, but such a ritual preps the skin for future homemade facial masks and cleansers.

Skin Like Milk

If you have oily or combination skin, try a foaming cleanser. For dry skin, a cream or **Milky Cleanser** works best. You can make your own cleanser with a warmed mixture of 1 to 2 tablespoons buttermilk and several drops of olive oil. If you're planning to make the Peach Gingerbread with Walnut Streusel (pg. 76), you'll already have plenty of buttermilk on hand! After you've prepared a small amount of the buttermilk and olive oil facial cleanser to cover your face, use your fingers to get a gentle exfoliating scrub going, in a circular motion, all over your face. Make sure to concentrate on the areas around your nose and forehead. If you have combo skin, work harder on the areas that tend to be "greasy." Rinse your face well since traces of exfoliating scrubs have been known to dry out the face.

Home-Baked Beauty

Who knew a "home-baked" exfoliate was within arm's reach when you were readying those old-fashioned rolled oats for the Fruit and Yogurt Breakfast Parfaits with Granola Crunch (pg. 59)? Begin your **Oatmeal Peel** by mixing ½ cup dry oatmeal, 3 tablespoons almond oil, 1 tablespoon fine sea salt, and 1 tablespoon chopped fresh mint into a paste. Apply to your face, let sit for 10 to 15 minutes, and then wash off with warm water.

Busy Bee

A great facial mask for dry skin is pure and simple: Just mix together 1 teaspoon honey, 1 teaspoon aloe vera gel (you can find this at any pharmacy or health food store), and 1 vitamin E capsule (slit the capsule open and stir its liquid contents in with the other ingredients). Spread your **Honey Mask** onto your face, making sure not to get too close to your eyes. Leave on for 10–15 minutes. Gently rinse off with warm water.

Toner Secrets

To open your pores and really cleanse them, fill your sink with warm water, dip a wash-cloth, in and press it to your face. Repeat 2–3 times. Infuse the water with your favorite fragrant herbs such as chamomile, eucalyptus, and lavender. If you're looking for an excellent homemade **Natural Facial Toner**, use equal parts juice from an orange (a few recipes in chapter 5 use oranges; they get top billing in the Butternut Squash Soup Flavored with Orange and Tarragon (pg. 70) and witch hazel. Another great orange facial cleanser calls for a food processor; purée 2 tablespoons each: juice from tomato and cucumber, parsley, olive oil, carrot, and rosemary sprigs leftover from the Rosemary Roasted Carrot Sticks (pg. 72). Juice from tomatoes like those in the recipe for Stewed Tomatoes with Garlic and Black Beans (pg. 71) mixed with witch hazel also makes an au natural toner fit for Venus herself.

Eat Dessert and Get Younger . . .

The Oven-Roasted Fruit with Vanilla Yogurt Sorbet recipe (pg. 77) has everything you need to tighten up your complexion like a twenty-one-year-old's! Fruit acids make for a fabulous facial peel. Utilize puréed fruit as a mask; apply, let sit, and wash off. Two egg whites to tighten pores followed by a slather of plain yogurt and a good wash can also brighten your complexion.

Apples Conjur Loveliness

Sweet Potato Apple Salad (pg. 63) features, obviously, apples, which can be used to smooth the fine lines on your face. Press alpha-hydroxy–rich apple slices on crow's feet and laugh lines, lie back and relax, smelling the sweet, relaxing aroma of the fruit as you do so. Later on, moisturize with products that are free of retinols or acids since these will over-exfoliate your skin.

Calming Wrinkles

Stress shows on your face. If you reduce your stress level, your complexion will clear and your frown lines will calm down. Eliminate your stress issues. Start with the frustration of road rage—at least yours! Smooth worry lines while driving around town by hooking up with the latest and greatest audio book. Unabridged and dramatically read, these productions are a fabulous way to lose yourself while you are driving. Stopped in traffic?—no need to fret, just go on to the next chapter. Most current best-sellers and a whole bunch of classics are available for rent or purchase. Start a driving book club and share titles with other moms or commuters and discuss the book at your next luncheon. Check out amazon.com to find the title that is best for you. Remember, no cheating—be sure to choose the *unabridged* version.

Keep in mind that a little pampering and beautiful food equals beautiful skin (even when we're talking "topical application" rather than ingestion), and you're well on your way to a glowing and more *gorgeous* you!

CHAPTER 6

every day is a good hair day

"I'd luv to kiss ya, but I just washed my hair." —Bette Davis

Every Day Is a Good Hair Day

What would Vidal Sassoon or Paul Mitchell place on your "good hair day" menu? Delicious foods that are rich in vitamin A, copper, zinc, protein, and iron are your answer! This chapter is all about the hair—what makes it shine and grow stronger, thicker, longer, and more lustrous. We'll also dish on the not-so-comely facts responsible for unglamorous conditions, like brittle, sparse, or dull hair. Hold on to your hats . . . then get ready to toss them up and celebrate because what lies underneath that cap—at least after you've sampled these recipes—is going to be so healthy and gorgeous you can't help wanting to shake your locks out for the whole world to see.

Ask Dr. Moon

The doctor is in to answer your questions.

How thick or thin your hair is depends on heredity; its natural state (straight, wavy, or curly) lies in your DNA, but whether your hair is gorgeous or not . . . now, that's something you alone control. What you eat is more important to your hair than its shampoo, beautician, hair dryer, or curling iron. A well-balanced diet and plenty of exercise keep the body healthy and the circulatory system, which is so important to hair follicles, working at optimal levels. The following Q&A with Dr. Moon proves the point.

Q: What is the function of hair?

A: Our hair serves primarily to insulate us as well as to shield us from harmful ultraviolet radiation.

Q: When is hair loss normal?

A: Losing hair is part of a natural cycle of growth and replacement. Hair loss becomes a problem when the resting phase of hair grows longer and the regrowth (anagen) stage gets shorter.

Q: Is hair loss more prevalent in women as they age? What causes hair loss?

A: On average, your hair grows about ½ inch per month and 100 to 150 strands are lost per day. Here's how factors like age and daily stressors aggravate natural, normal hair loss: **(1) The age factor:** As women get older, they lose estrogen and retain testosterone, a condition that affects some more than others, and can, for some women, set the stage for hair loss as seen in male pattern baldness. **(2) Relax! Stress will thin your hair!** Because it raises testosterone levels, stress can be a factor in hair loss. **(3) Certain over-the-counter supplements are to blame!** DHEA has been linked to hair loss. DHEA is a dietary supplement touted as having anti-aging effects.

Q: So can I combat hair loss?

A: Treatments like Rogaine work better for women than for men. One hair-saving option is the hair transplant; many surgeons find it beneficial to use a combination of two or more types of grafts in order to achieve the best appearance. For example, smaller grafts work very well along the front of the hairline where we typically have much finer hair growing naturally. Depending on the procedures used, the entire process of a hair transplant surgery may take up to two years and involve multiple procedures. New groundbreaking gene therapy and hair follicle cloning are also are currently being explored. Making lifestyle changes may stave off hair loss. Stop stressing! Get plenty of iron, zinc, and other hair-loving vitamins, and use botanical shampoos that pack a protein punch.

Q: Does monoxidil really work?

A: There has been success with monoxidil. About two-thirds of people who have used it have reported hair growth. Monoxidil was first used in tablet form for the treatment of high blood pressure. Increased hair growth was observed as a side effect in patients taking the drug. Tests were then carried out to see if monoxidil could be applied to the scalp as a topical (liquid) preparation. Clinical trials involving thousands of people showed success.

Q: Why is iron important for strong hair?

A: Hair can't go through the natural process of shedding and replacing itself without enough iron; without iron your follicles are starved for oxygen, so get a variety of meats and/or plenty of dark green veggies in your diet!

Q: How do you encourage stronger, silkier locks?

A: With protein-rich recipes. Since hair is made of protein, a diet chock-full of it can produce stronger, silkier locks and help you avoid most hair problems. Meats, fish, beans, yogurt, tofu, and soy are where it's at!

Q: What is the value of H_2O when it comes to your hair? What are a few sample foods that are both delicious to eat and water-rich?

A: Water makes up one-fourth of the weight of a strand of hair. Moisture also makes the hair supple, so be sure to get *plenty* of fluids and eat foods that contain water. For example, a cup of watermelon contains almost a cup of water; the same for milk and cooked broccoli. A cup of yogurt is about 80 percent water; a baked potato or cooked rice about 70 percent.

Q: Can you improve the texture of dry hair?

A: Yes! Improve the texture of dry hair with foods rich in zinc. Zinc also helps with the absorption of iron. Seafood and liver are rich sources.

Q: What other things are necessary for a healthy scalp and great hair?

A: Vitamin A is good for the scalp—look to cheeses, brightly colored fruits, veggies, and liver. Foods rich in copper can affect hair pigmentation in a very gorgeous way—find it in shellfish, nuts, seeds, fresh veggies, and your local meat department.

Jorj's Good Hair Day Glam Kitchen

When we think of foods most often associated with a healthy "do," we should think of those filled with protein like that found in red meat and peanut butter. However, gorgeous hair requires more than iron and protein to thrive; the locks you've styled and stressed in so many different ways throughout the course of your life thirst too for zinc, copper, vitamin A, and plenty of water.

Beyond Steak

Iron is more than just a T-bone on a plate. While the stars of your iron-rich show are generally meats, like liver and shellfish, you can dress up the rest of the entrée with tasty accompaniments from the dark green veggie family, namely spinach, kale, broccoli, and green beans. When you make mashed potatoes, keep the skins in the mix. Doing so not only lends this popular side dish a more gourmet look but also provides extra iron. In the morning, look for your first serving of iron in any fortified cereal. That being said, your pantry *and your hair* are in crisis without whole grains! A good showing from this family of foods is a pantry that includes brown rice, whole wheat bread, wheat germ, and oatmeal.

Inspired Dishes

With the right spices and savory additions, side dishes of red beans and spinach, both good for your hair, go from "I'll pass" to "pass that right over here!" There will be no end of praise from those seated at your dinner table when the chicken and pork have been simmered in exotic sauces, the lamb is a coconut dream, and the calf's liver is served with caramelized onions so tasty you forget you're eating healthy. Ditto for zinc-laced lobster and mussels shared over that perfect bottle of wine. Be adventurous in the meats you choose; for instance it doesn't have to be a winter holiday to bake a juicy turkey! Dark turkey meat is great for the health of your hair, no matter what time of year it is.

A Fine Substitute

Everybody knows that protein-rich dishes, like cheeses and meats, are just that: *rich*—rich in flavor and in fat, but it doesn't have to be so. You can be proactive and choose lean protein, which contains the same benefits for your hair without the extra fat and calories. Look for reduced-fat mozzarella, Cheddar, pepper jack, and gouda. Put reduced-fat milk, lean corned beef, lean turkey, and lean chicken breasts in your grocery cart; entertain the notion of swordfish before baby-backed ribs; and make soups that apologize for the absence of heavy cream with dried beans. Instead of tossing your summer salads with bacon bits and bits of egg, use flaxseeds, mixed nuts, sunflower seeds, kidney beans, chickpeas, snowpeas, or plain old sweet peas.

Notes on Water & Vitamin A

You may very well be the kind of person who believes, rightfully, that water is vital for healthy organs, let alone great hair. The problem is, you're not so keen on drinking eight glasses of water a day. The good news is you don't have to seek the recommended daily intake of water in beverages alone. You can load up on life-giving H_2O in the foods you eat. Do "watery" foods like raspberries and vegetable stock–based soups, tomato sauces, and frozen fruit dessert. Get a double dose of water and vitamin A in rhubarb, pears, bell peppers, Swiss chard, and tomatoes.

Start Your Day

Main Plates

On the Side

Snacks & Sweets

CREAMY FRENCH-STYLE EGGS

Garnished with Chopped Tomatoes and Chives

These delicious eggs are cooked slowly and have a much creamier consistency than your everyday scramble. Using a touch of butter and a dollop of sour cream adds to the texture and to the flavor of the dish. I know it's a little over the top, but every once in a while. . . .

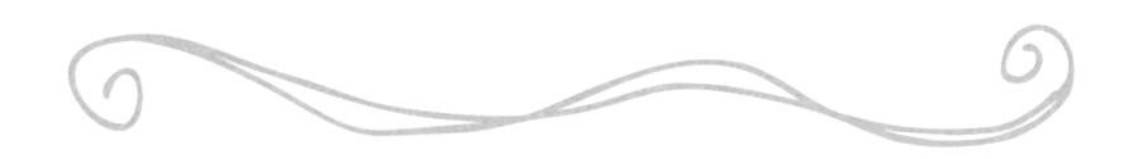

If you do not have a double boiler, you can use a BOWL placed over the SIMMERING water. You can also prepare this dish in a skillet; just make sure that you keep the heat very LOW.

Makes 2 servings
Prep Time: 3 minutes
Cook Time: 6 to 8 minutes

- 4 large eggs
- Salt and freshly ground pepper
- 1 tablespoon unsalted butter
- 1 tablespoon reduced-fat sour cream
- 2 slices whole grain bread, toasted
- 1 medium plum tomato, seeded and diced (about 2 tablespoons) (for garnish)
- 1 tablespoon chopped fresh chives (for garnish)

Pour water into the bottom of a double boiler and heat until the water barely simmers. Top with another pot making sure that the simmering water does not touch the bottom of the top pot. Crack the eggs into the top pot. Season with salt and pepper. Use a whisk to constantly stir the eggs. If the eggs begin to scramble, lower the heat. Cook until the eggs form a light film, about 5 minutes. Continue stirring the eggs. The end result will be a thick, pudding-like consistency. Remove the pot from the water and whisk in the butter and sour cream.

To serve, place 1 slice of toasted bread on each plate. Top with half of the eggs. Repeat with remaining ingredients. Garnish with chopped tomatoes and fresh chives.

EGG WHITE OMELETS

With Bell Peppers and Turkey Sausage

This healthy breakfast is filling, delicious, and so good for you that you'll crave a version of this dish every day!

Makes 4 servings
Prep Time: 10 minutes
Cook Time: 10 to 12 minutes

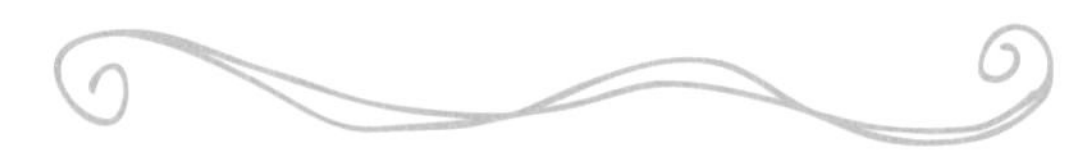

Reserve the egg yolks for another use like making your own lemon curd!

For the filling

- 1 tablespoon olive oil
- 1 small yellow onion, peeled and diced (about ½ cup)
- 1 large red bell pepper, seeded and cut into ¼-inch dice (about 1 cup)
- 1 pound ground turkey sausage
- Salt and freshly ground pepper

For the omelets

- 10 egg whites
- ½ teaspoon chili powder
- 4 ounces shredded Parmesan cheese (about 1 cup)
- 2 tablespoons chopped fresh tarragon (for garnish)

Heat the olive oil in a skillet over medium-high heat. Add the onion and bell pepper and cook until soft, about 5 minutes. Stir in the turkey sausage. Cook until browned, about 5 minutes more. Season with salt and pepper. Drain off any residual liquid. Set aside.

In a bowl whisk together the egg whites until fluffy. Season with chili powder, salt and pepper. Coat a nonstick omelet pan with vegetable oil spray. Pour one-fourth of the egg white mixture into the pan. Cook until the egg whites stand up, pushing the outer edges to the center and allowing the uncooked portion to run into the sides of the pan. Spoon one-fourth of the filling mixture onto one side of the omelet. Fold over the other half to form a semicircle. Top with one-fourth of the grated cheese. Cook until the cheese begins to melt, about 2 minutes. Use a spatula to slide the omelet to a plate. Continue with the remaining ingredients to make three more omelets.

To serve, garnish with fresh tarragon.

RASPBERRY OATMEAL MUFFINS

With Macadamia Nut Butter

These hearty muffins are worthy of the rich nut butter. What a great way to get your day going!

FROZEN berries will hold their SHAPE better in this recipe than fresh ones. You can purchase them FROZEN or grab some fresh berries and put them in the freezer for 20 minutes.

On Shopping Day: Prepare the muffins, cool, and store in an airtight container for up to 5 days. Prepare Macadamia Nut butter and store in an airtight container for up to 5 days.

Makes 12 large muffins
Prep Time: 15 minutes
Cook Time: 25 minutes

For the muffins

- 1 2/3 cups old-fashioned rolled oats
- 2/3 cup unbleached all-purpose flour, plus 2 tablespoons to toss with raspberries
- 1/2 cup whole wheat flour
- 3/4 cup brown sugar
- 1 teaspoon ground cinnamon
- 1/2 teaspoon ground nutmeg
- 1 teaspoon baking powder
- 1 teaspoon baking soda
- 1/2 teaspoon salt
- 1 1/2 cups reduced-fat buttermilk
- 1/4 cup canola oil
- 2 large eggs
- 1 teaspoon vanilla
- 2 cups frozen raspberries

For the butter

- 1 cup macadamia nuts
- 2 teaspoons canola oil
- 2 teaspoons honey
- 1/8 teaspoon ground cinnamon

Preheat the oven to 400 degrees. Place the oats into the bowl of a food processor. Pulse to grind the oats into crumbs. Pour the oat crumbs into a large bowl. Add flours, brown sugar, cinnamon, nutmeg, baking powder, baking soda, and salt into the bowl. Whisk to combine. In a separate bowl stir together the buttermilk, canola oil, eggs, and vanilla. Stir the buttermilk mixture into the flour mixture until just combined.

Toss the raspberries with 2 tablespoons flour. Gently fold into the batter. Spoon into a muffin tin with paper liners. Bake until the muffins spring back when touched and a tester inserted into the center comes out clean, about 20–25 minutes. Cool on wire racks.

Prepare the butter by placing the nuts into the bowl of a food processor. Pulse until the nuts are finely ground. Pour in the oil, honey, and cinnamon. Pulse until the mixture is puréed. Store in an airtight container for up to 1 week in the refrigerator.

To serve, split 1 muffin in half horizontally. Spread one half with a dollop of macadamia nut butter and place the top half back onto the muffin.

PECAN BANANADANA MUFFINS

Easy to make, easy to bake—kinda reminds you to let them eat cake!

Makes 12 servings
Prep Time: 15 minutes
Cook Time: 20 to 25 minutes

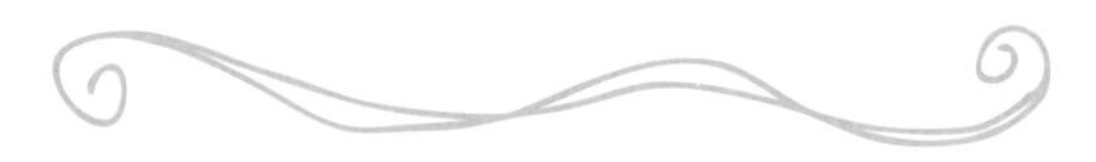

Use very RIPE bananas for very MOIST muffins.

- 1/3 cup pecans, toasted
- 1 cup unbleached all-purpose flour
- 1/3 cup whole wheat flour
- 1 1/2 teaspoons baking powder
- 1/2 teaspoon baking soda
- 1/2 teaspoon ground nutmeg
- 1/2 teaspoon salt
- 2/3 cup brown sugar
- 2 tablespoons canola oil
- 1 teaspoon vanilla extract
- 1 cup reduced-fat vanilla-flavored yogurt
- 1 large egg
- 3 very ripe bananas, mashed (about 1 1/2 cups)
- Honey

Preheat the oven to 400 degrees. Place the pecans into the bowl of a food processor. Pulse until finely ground. Place into a large bowl. Add flours, baking powder, baking soda, nutmeg, and salt. Whisk to combine.

Place the brown sugar in a medium bowl. Stir in the canola oil, vanilla extract, yogurt, and egg. Add to the flour mixture. Use a wooden spoon to just combine the ingredients. Fold in the mashed bananas. Spoon the batter into a muffin tin with paper liners. Bake until the muffins spring back when touched and a tester inserted into the center comes out clean, about 20–25 minutes. Cool on wire racks.

Serve warm with a drizzle of honey.

ROSEMARY ROASTED CHICKEN BREASTS

With Smoky Almond Sauce

A perfect make-ahead dish, this spruces up an ordinary everyday supper.

Makes 4 servings
Prep Time: 10 minutes
Cook Time: 15 to 20 minutes

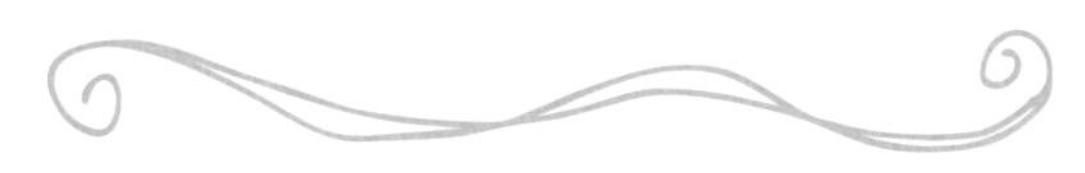

Chop the ALMONDS using a mini food processor or sharp knife on a cutting board. A ROUGH chop is all you need.

For the chicken

- 4 medium (6- to 8-ounce) skinless, boneless chicken breast halves
- 1 tablespoon chopped fresh rosemary
- Juice of 1 medium lemon (about 2 tablespoons)
- 1 tablespoon olive oil
- Salt and freshly ground pepper

For the almond sauce

- 1/2 cup reduced-fat sour cream
- 1/2 cup reduced-fat mayonnaise
- 1 tablespoon Dijon mustard
- 1 bunch (6–8) green onions, thinly sliced on the diagonal (about 1/2 cup)
- 1/2 cup smoked almonds, chopped
- 1 tablespoon chopped fresh rosemary

Preheat the oven to 400 degrees. Place the chicken breasts into a baking dish. In a medium bowl whisk together the rosemary, lemon juice, and olive oil. Brush this mixture on both sides of the chicken. Season with salt and pepper. Bake until the chicken is golden brown and still very moist in the center, about 15–20 minutes depending on thickness. Remove and cool to room temperature.

In a medium bowl whisk together the sour cream, mayonnaise, and mustard. Stir in the onions, almonds, and rosemary. Season with salt and pepper.

To serve, cut the chicken into thin slices. Top with sauce.

LAMB CHOPS

With Coconut Skillet Sauce

Bring a little bit of the islands to your dinner table with this easy-to-prepare dish.

Makes 4 servings
Prep Time: 10 minutes
Cook Time: 15 minutes

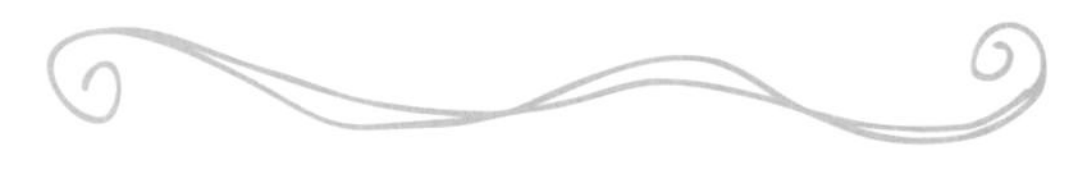

Fried PLANTAINS (pg. 100) are a great ACCOMPANIMENT to this dish.

You can substitute with lamb shoulder chops for a more budget-friendly ingredient.

For the lamb chops

- 2 tablespoons olive oil
- 2 teaspoons ground cumin
- 1/2 teaspoon red pepper flakes
- 8 4- to 5-ounce loin lamb chops, cut 1 1/2- to 2-inches thick
- Salt and freshly ground pepper

For the sauce

- 2 tablespoons tomato paste
- 1 teaspoon curry powder
- 1/2 teaspoon ground cinnamon
- 1 5-ounce can coconut milk
- Juice of 1 medium lime (about 1 tablespoon)
- Fresh coconut flakes (for garnish)

In a small bowl mix together the olive oil, cumin, and pepper flakes. Brush this mixture over the lamb chops. Season with salt and pepper.

Heat a skillet over medium-high heat. Cook the lamb chops until medium rare, about 3–4 minutes per side, turning once. Remove to a platter and keep warm.

Cook the tomato paste, curry, and cinnamon in the same skillet over medium heat for 1 minute, stirring constantly. Pour in the coconut milk. Bring the sauce to a simmer and cook until thickened, about 5 minutes. Add the lime juice. Season with salt and pepper.

To serve, pour the sauce over the lamb chops and garnish with fresh coconut flakes.

LOBSTER

In an Orange Curry Butter Sauce

I know, I know . . . there is an entire stick of butter in this dish—well, it is a butter sauce. So, if you've overdone your bad fats this week, do not include this dish in your meal plan. However, if you have been a very good girl, this dish is divine!

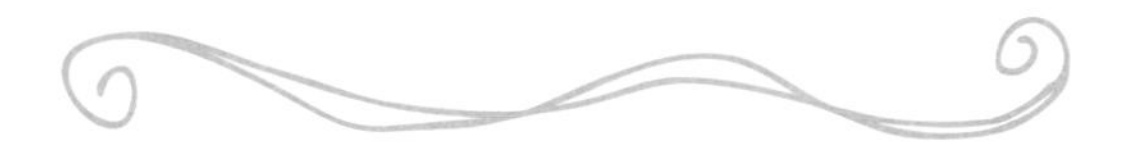

You can purchase FROZEN, cooked lobster meat and keep it in your freezer to create this elegant dish for impromptu dinner guests.

Makes 4 servings
Prep Time: 10 minutes
Cook Time: 6 to 8 minutes

- 2 pounds cooked lobster meat
- Juice of 3–4 medium oranges (about 1 cup)
- 1 tablespoon white wine vinegar
- 4 green onions, thinly sliced (about 1/4 cup)
- 1 teaspoon curry powder
- 1/2 cup unsalted butter (1 stick), cut into pieces
- Salt and freshly ground pepper
- 2 cups cooked couscous
- Fresh mint (for garnish)
- Lime zest (for garnish)

Cut the lobster meat into 1-inch pieces. Set aside. Pour the orange juice into a skillet. Add the vinegar, green onions, and curry. Cook until reduced by one-third, about 4–6 minutes. Stir in the lobster. Cook for 2 minutes more. Remove the skillet from the heat. Add the butter, a few pieces at a time, and swirl the liquid around, melting the butter into the sauce.

To serve, place the lobster and sauce over the couscous. Garnish with fresh mint and lime zest.

MUSSELS WITH BRUSSELS

In a White Wine Butter Sauce

If you like Brussels sprouts as much as I do, you'll find this combination of veggie and shellfish a natural.

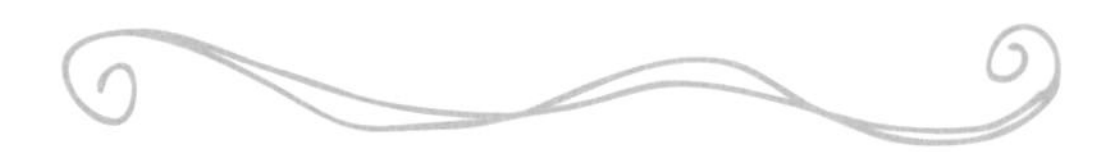

Brussels sprouts are rich in VITAMIN C. They also supply good amounts of folate (folic acid), potassium, vitamin K, and a small amount of BETA-CAROTENE.

Most MUSSELS are cultivated and shipped frozen to stores. When you do come across FRESH mussels, feel free to choose them. If a shell is partially open, pinch it back together. A fresh mussel will close its shell if prodded.

Trim the stems from each Brussels sprout. Peel away the outer leaves and cut an *X* into the bottom. Blanch the sprouts in salted boiling water until crisp-tender (insert the tip of a knife into the stem to test for doneness). Drain and place into a bowl filled with ice water to stop the cooking process. Drain and slice into halves.

Heat the olive oil in a large sauté pan (with a lid) over medium-high heat. Add the onion and cook until golden. Stir in the garlic and sun-dried tomatoes. Pour in the wine. Add the Brussels sprouts and mussels. Reduce heat to medium, cover, and cook until the mussels open, about 5 minutes.

Remove the lid and turn off the heat. Sprinkle the dish with lemon juice and season with salt and pepper. Add the butter and stir until melted. Sprinkle with fresh parsley.

To serve, divide the mussels into serving bowls. Ladle the Brussels and sauce over top. Offer warm whole grain bread for lapping up all of the good stuff.

Makes 4 appetizer servings
Prep Time: 10 minutes
Cook Time: 6 to 8 minutes

For the Brussels

1 pound Brussels sprouts (about 4 cups)
Salt

For the mussels

1 tablespoon olive oil
1 large red onion, diced into 1/4-inch cubes (about 1 cup)
4 medium cloves garlic, thinly sliced (about 2 teaspoons)
1/4 cup minced oil-packed sun-dried tomatoes, drained
1 cup white wine (you can substitute with chicken broth)
1 pound mussels, scrubbed, beards removed (discard any with open shell)
Juice of 1 medium lemon (about 2 tablespoons)
Salt and freshly ground pepper
2 tablespoons chilled butter
2 tablespoons chopped fresh parsley

GRILLED SKIRT STEAK AND VEGGIE OPEN-FACED SANDWICH

Serve this sandwich for a lazy Saturday afternoon get-together or as an easy mid-week meal. Make sure you serve with a knife and fork!

Makes 4 servings
Prep Time: 10 minutes
Cook Time: 25 minutes

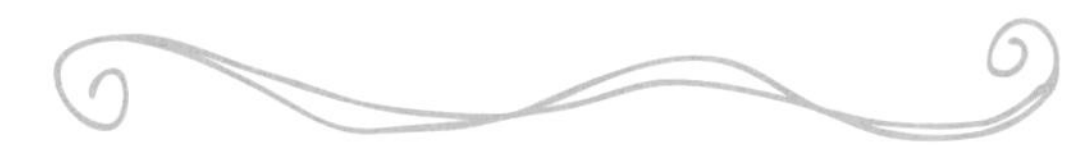

If you can't find CIABATTA bread, serve this sandwich on a hearty WHOLE GRAIN bun or sub roll.

For the skirt steak

- 1 1-pound skirt steak
- 1/4 cup olive oil
- 2 tablespoons Worcestershire sauce
- 1 tablespoon steak seasoning
- 4 large portobello mushrooms, stem and gills removed
- 1 large red onion, cut into 4 1/2-inch slices
- 2 large red bell peppers, seeded and cut into quarters
- Salt and freshly ground pepper

For the sandwich

- 1 ciabatta loaf, sliced in half horizontally
- 1/3 cup reduced-fat mayonnaise
- 1 tablespoon Dijon mustard
- 1 tablespoon prepared chili sauce
- 2 ounces mesclun lettuce mix (about 2 cups)
- 2 large tomatoes, sliced into 1/4-inch thick slices (about 8 slices)

Place the skirt steak onto your work surface between 2 sheets of parchment paper. Use a meat mallet to pound the steak to about ¼-inch thickness. Set the steak into a shallow baking dish. In a small bowl whisk together the olive oil, Worcestershire sauce, and steak seasoning. Pour the mixture over the skirt steak. Cover and marinate for at least 30 minutes or in the refrigerator overnight. Heat a grill pan over medium-high heat. Grill the skirt steak, turning once until medium-rare, about 6–8 minutes per side.

Toss the mushrooms and veggies in the remaining marinade. Season with salt and pepper. Grill the veggies, turning once, until soft and golden, about 3–5 minutes per side.

To serve, lay the ciabatta loaf onto your work surface. Cut into quarters. Stir together the mayonnaise, Dijon, and chili sauce. Spread this mixture onto the cut side of the four bread pieces. Top with lettuces leaves. Cut the steak into slices and place these on top of the lettuce. Cut the veggies into slices and place on top of the steak. Top the veggies with slices of tomato.

ROASTED PORK TENDERLOIN

With Swiss Chard

Swiss chard is filled with antioxidants, making this delicious entrée an excellent choice for your well-balanced lifestyle plan.

Makes 6 servings
Prep Time: 15 minutes
Cook Time: 20 minutes

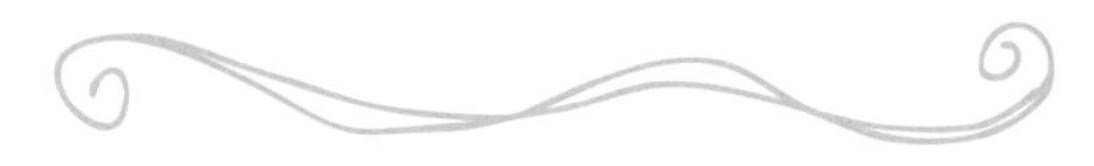

Don't stop at tenderloin; this dish would be just as good with PORK CHOPS! Look for the specials on shopping day and make a BUDGET-WISE selection.

For the pork

- 2 12- to 14-ounce pork tenderloins
- Salt and freshly ground pepper
- 1 teaspoon ground allspice
- 1 teaspoon dried thyme
- 1–2 tablespoons olive oil

For the greens

- 1 medium yellow onion, peeled and diced into ½-inch squares (about 1 cup)
- 2 medium cloves garlic, minced (about 1 teaspoon)
- 1½ pounds Swiss chard, washed, dried, stems removed, leaves torn (about 8 cups)
- 1 cup homemade chicken stock or low-sodium chicken broth
- 2 tablespoons balsamic vinegar
- 1 tablespoon Dijon mustard

Season the tenderloins with salt, pepper, allspice, and thyme. Preheat the oven to 400 degrees. Heat 1 tablespoon olive oil in a large skillet over medium-high heat. Brown the tenderloin in the skillet until all sides are golden. Place onto a rack in a baking dish. Place the baking dish in the oven and roast the tenderloins until medium-rare, about 10–15 minutes. Remove from the oven and allow to rest for 5 minutes.

Meanwhile, add the onion and garlic to the skillet. Cook until soft, about 5 minutes. Add the chard, a handful at a time, until it is wilted down. Stir in the chicken broth, balsamic vinegar, and mustard. Season with salt and pepper. Reduce heat and simmer until the liquid is evaporated, about 10 minutes.

To serve, spread the chard onto the bottom of a platter. Cut the pork tenderloins into 1½-inch diagonal slices. Arrange on top of the chard.

On Shopping Day: Clean the chard by removing the stems. Wash and dry leaves, wrap in paper towels, and place into a plastic bag. Use a fork to pierce holes in the bag for circulation. Store in the refrigerator for up to 5 days.

CALF'S LIVER

With Golden Onions

Eaten in moderation, calf's liver is a delicious and satisfying dish.

Makes 4 servings
Prep Time: 5 minutes
Cook Time: 6 to 8 minutes

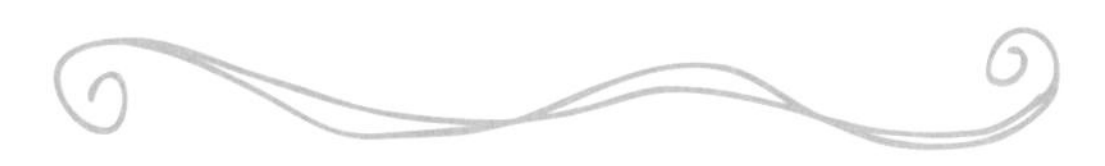

Calf's liver is an exceptionally NUTRIENT-DENSE food, a good source of PROTEIN and IRON. Although calf's liver is also high in cholesterol and saturated fat, its concentration of so many beneficial nutrients makes it an extremely HEALTHFUL food.

- 1½ pounds thinly sliced calf's liver
- Salt and freshly ground pepper
- ½ cup unbleached all-purpose flour
- ¼–½ cup olive oil
- 1 large red onion, peeled and thinly sliced (about 1 cup)

Season both sides of the calf's liver with salt and pepper. Place into a plastic bag with the flour. Shake well. Remove the dusted liver, shaking off excess.

Heat ¼ cup olive oil over medium-high heat. Place the calf's liver into the oil. Cook, turning once, until golden, about 2–3 minutes per side. Remove to a platter and keep warm.

Cook the onion in the pan. (You may add more oil if needed. Make sure that added oil is hot before you put the onion in the pan.) Cook until golden, stirring often, about 4–5 minutes.

To serve, place the calf's liver onto a platter. Top with golden onions.

PAELLA

With Chorizo, Asparagus, and Shellfish

There are a couple of steps to this dish, but it comes together faster than you might think. Prepare it on a day when comfort food is what you crave and the family is ready to swarm the table.

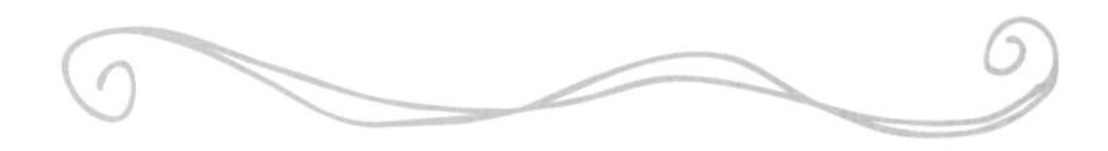

Saffron is an EXPENSIVE ingredient. If you can't find it in your grocery store, check out your specialty market or let your fingers do the clicking online. Store well and it will keep for several months.

Place the asparagus into a casserole dish with lid. Pour in 1 inch of water. Cover and microwave on high until just crisp-tender, about 3–4 minutes. Drain, plunge into cold water, drain again, and set aside.

Heat the wine in a pot (with lid) over low heat. Remove from the heat, add the chicken broth and saffron, cover, and set aside 5 minutes to steep.

Heat the olive oil in a large skillet with lid. Add the sausage and cook until golden, about 5–7 minutes. Add the onions and cook until soft, about 5 minutes. Add the garlic and tomatoes and cook for 2 minutes more. Stir in the red pepper and paprika. Season with salt and pepper. Stir in the rice.

Preheat the oven to 350 degrees. Pour the saffron-infused wine and chicken broth into the skillet. Bring to a boil and simmer for 3 minutes. Tuck the seafood into the rice mixture. Stir in the peas and toss in the asparagus. Cover and place into the oven. Cook until the rice is tender, most of the liquid is absorbed, and the shellfish have opened, about 20–25 minutes. Carefully remove from the oven. Sprinkle with lemon juice, cover, and allow to rest for 10 minutes.

To serve, transfer the paella to a large shallow dish. Garnish with fresh parsley.

Makes 6 to 8 servings
Prep Time: 30 minutes
Cook Time: 40 minutes

- 1 pound fresh thin asparagus spears, ends trimmed, cut diagonally into 1/2-inch lengths (about 2 cups)
- 1 cup dry white wine
- 5 cups homemade chicken stock or low-sodium chicken broth
- 1/2 teaspoon saffron threads
- 2 tablespoons olive oil
- 4 chorizo sausage links (about 12 ounces), cut into 1/2-inch slices
- 2 large Spanish onions, peeled and diced (about 2 cups)
- 4 medium garlic cloves, minced (about 2 teaspoons)
- 2 medium plum tomatoes, seeded and diced (about 1 cup)
- 1 roasted red pepper (drained from jar), diced
- 2 teaspoons paprika
- Salt and freshly ground pepper

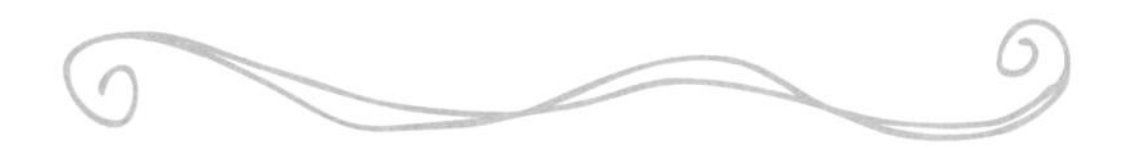

- 2 1/2 cups yellow rice
- 1 pound small clams
- 1 pound mussels, scrubbed, beards removed
- 1 pound large uncooked fresh shrimp, peeled and deveined (about 20)
- 1 10-ounce package frozen baby peas, thawed
- Juice of 1 medium lemon (about 2 tablespoons)
- Chopped fresh parsley (for garnish)

FRIED PLANTAINS

Plantains are not sweet like bananas. You must work with them a bit to soften their texture; but, oh when you do . . . . Serve them crispy and hot. Mmmmm, mmmmm—so good!

Makes 4 servings
Prep Time: 20 minutes
Cook Time: 15 minutes

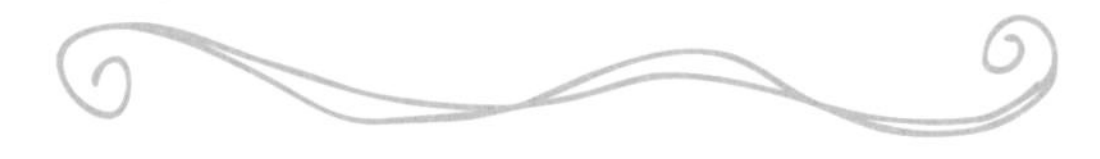

The darker the PLANTAIN, the riper it is.

- 2 ripe plantains
- Canola oil for frying
- Salt

Peel the plantains using a vegetable peeler. (Alternatively, you can peel plantains with a sharp knife, cutting the peel off in long strips.) Cut the plantains into 1-inch pieces. Heat about ½-inch canola oil in a deep skillet to 325 degrees. Place the plantains (in batches) in the skillet. Cook over medium-high heat, turning once, until golden, about 2 minutes per side. Remove the plantains to a parchment-lined baking sheet. Use a spatula to smash the plantains into circles.

Place the plantain circles into the oil again. Cook until golden brown, about 3–5 minutes per side. Drain on paper towels. Season generously with salt.

CREAMY CAULIFLOWER SOUP

With Arugula and Crispy Bacon Garnish

I'm an ardent fan of potato soup—hot, cold, or in between. This soup has the same creamy satisfaction you're used to, not to mention veggies galore and extra nutrition.

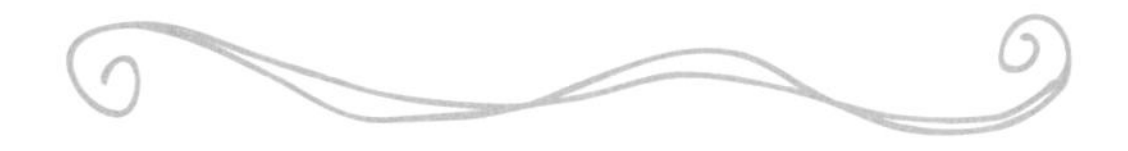

Adding HALF AND HALF to the soup gives it an extra depth of RICHNESS. You can substitute with heavy cream for an even richer dish, or you can lighten up by adding skim milk, or eliminate this step altogether. It's totally up to you!

Cook the bacon in a deep soup pot over medium-high heat until crisp. Remove the bacon with a slotted spoon and drain on paper towels. Add the leek and onion to the pot and cook until just beginning to brown. Add the cauliflower and potatoes. Pour in the chicken broth and pour in 2 cups of water. (The liquid should cover all of the vegetables.) Bring the soup to a boil, reduce the heat to medium, cover and simmer until all of the vegetables are soft and falling apart, about 15–20 minutes. During the last few minutes of simmering, add the rosemary sprigs. Season with salt and pepper.

Remove the pot from the heat. Remove the rosemary stems. Use a handheld blender (or food processor) to puree the soup until smooth. Return the pot to medium heat. Stir in the sherry, arugula, and nutmeg. Adjust seasonings. Cover and simmer over low heat for 5 minutes. Stir in the half and half.

To serve, ladle the soup into bowls. Garnish with the chopped bacon.

On Shopping Day: Prepare the cauliflower and store in a plastic bag in the refrigerator for up to 5 days.

Makes 4 cup servings, plus extra for tomorrow's desktop lunch.
Prep Time: 15 minutes
Cook Time: 30 minutes

- 6 ounces lean bacon, about 4–6 strips, chopped into pieces
- 1 leek, white part only, rinsed well and sliced
- 1 large yellow onion, peeled and thinly sliced (about 2 cups)
- 2 small heads cauliflower, or 1 large, cut into small bunches of florets
- 2 medium potatoes, peeled and cut into 1/2-inch pieces
- 1 quart homemade chicken stock or low-sodium chicken broth
- 2 cups water
- 2 sprigs rosemary
- Salt and freshly ground pepper
- 1/4 cup dry sherry
- 1 cup arugula leaves, washed, dried, and cut into very thin strips
- 1/2 teaspoon ground nutmeg
- 1/2 cup half and half

LOUISIANA-STYLE RED BEANS

You can prepare this dish in a slow cooker if you have one.

Makes 6 to 8 servings
Prep Time: 10 minutes plus soaking beans
Cook Time: 2 to 2½ hours or longer if using a slow cooker

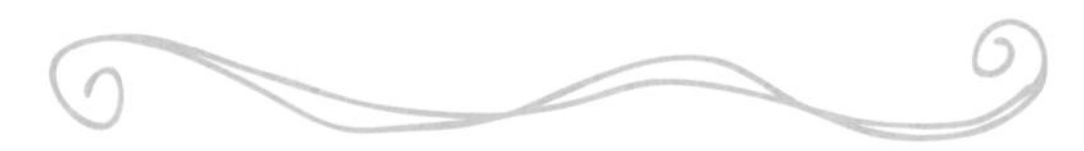

To prepare the BEANS, place them into a pot. Cover with about 1 quart water. Bring to a boil and cook 5 minutes. Turn off the heat and let the beans soak in the water for at least 1 hour. Drain and continue with the recipe.

- 1 pound red beans, washed, drained, and soaked
- 1 quart homemade chicken stock or low-sodium chicken broth
- 1 pound smoked sausage, sliced into rounds
- 1 large red onion, peeled and thinly sliced (about 1 cup)
- 2 medium celery ribs, diced (about ½ cup)
- 4 medium garlic cloves, minced (about 2 teaspoons)
- 1 dried bay leaf
- Salt and freshly ground pepper
- Cooked brown rice
- 2 tablespoons chopped fresh parsley (for garnish)

Place the beans into a deep pot. Pour in chicken broth. Stir in the sausage, onion, celery, garlic, and bay leaf. Season with salt and pepper. Bring to a boil. Reduce heat and simmer until the beans are very soft, about 2–3 hours. Add water if the liquid reduces too quickly. Use a potato masher to smash some of the beans.

To serve, ladle over brown rice and garnish with fresh parsley.

On Shopping Day: Prepare this dish while you are working in the kitchen, and it will be ready for you during the week.

TOASTED CORN

With Sautéed Spinach and Cherry Tomatoes

This simple veggie side dish is an example of how delicious it is to blend fresh ingredients with those that you have in your pantry. Season with your favorite spices or substitute with your best frozen veggies.

Makes 4 servings
Prep Time: 10 minutes
Cook Time: 10 minutes

- 1 tablespoon olive oil
- 1 10-ounce package frozen corn kernels, thawed
- 6 ounces fresh spinach leaves, washed, dried, and torn (about 4 cups)
- 1 pint ripe cherry tomatoes or mixed baby tomatoes, cut into halves
- Salt and freshly ground pepper

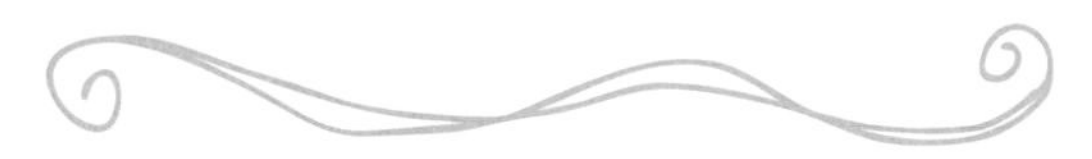

Leftover corn KERNELS from Sunday's corn on the cob will work just fine in this recipe, as will frozen, thawed corn.

Heat the olive oil in a skillet over medium heat. Add the corn and cook until the edges just begin to turn brown (watch for popping!), about 3 minutes. Add the spinach and cook until wilted, about 3–5 minutes. Stir in the tomatoes and cook until warmed through, about 3 minutes more. Season with salt and pepper.

BAKED PEARS

In Brandy Sauce

Use reduced-fat ice cream as a garnish when serving warm fruit; it'll boost flavors to the max!

Makes 4 servings
Prep Time: 10 minutes
Cook Time: 60 minutes

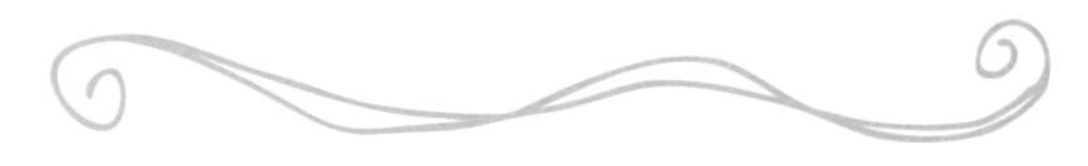

Large, ripe PEARS work best in this recipe.

- 4 large pears, peeled, cut into halves, and cored
- 1 cup brown sugar
- 2 teaspoons ground cinnamon
- 1 teaspoon ground ginger
- 1/2 teaspoon ground cloves
- 1/2 teaspoon allspice
- 1/2 teaspoon ground nutmeg
- 2 tablespoons canola oil
- 1/2 cup brandy

Preheat the oven to 400 degrees. Place the pears in a shallow baking dish. In a medium bowl mix together the brown sugar, cinnamon, ginger, cloves, allspice, and nutmeg. Pack the mixture into the center and over the top of the pears. Drizzle with canola oil. Pour the brandy into the dish, drizzling over the pears. Cover the dish with aluminum foil.

Bake for 1 hour in the preheated oven, or until pears are very soft and the sauce is slightly runny.

To serve, place each pear into a dessert bowl. Ladle the sauce over the top and garnish with a dollop of reduced-fat vanilla ice cream.

RHUBARB AND STRAWBERRY FROZEN YOGURT

With Fresh Mint

This refreshing dessert can be prepared on shopping day and served during the week. Better yet, just prepare the rhubarb on shopping day, then right before supper place all of the ingredients into the ice cream freezer and start. Everyone is sure to clean their plates in anticipation of dessert!

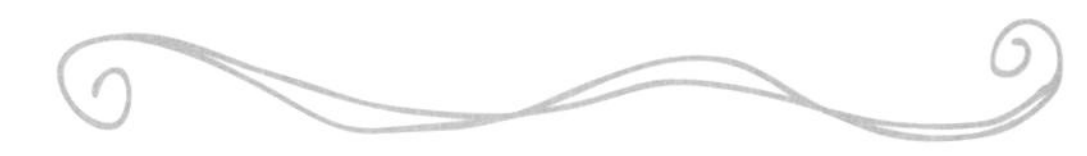

Use more or less SUGAR depending on your own PREFERENCE.

Makes 4 servings
Prep Time: 30 minutes, plus ice cream maker time

- 1 pound rhubarb, trimmed and sliced (about 2 cups)
- 2 tablespoons natural sugar
- 2 teaspoons pure vanilla extract
- 1 cup water
- 1 pint strawberries, hulled and quartered (about 2 cups)
- 1½ cups cranberry juice
- 2 tablespoons chopped fresh mint
- 1 cup reduced-fat vanilla yogurt

Place the rhubarb, sugar, vanilla, and water into a saucepan over medium-high heat. Bring to a boil. Reduce the heat and simmer until the rhubarb is very soft and the sugar is dissolved, about 20 minutes. Pour this mixture into the bowl of a food processor (or blender). Pulse to emulsify. Transfer to a bowl.

Add the strawberries, cranberry juice, and mint to the processor and pulse until smooth. Combine the strawberry mixture with the rhubarb. Chill the mixture in a refrigerator until thoroughly cool.

Stir in the yogurt. Freeze the mixture in an ice cream maker according to the manufacturer's directions. Store in an airtight container (in the freezer) for at least 4 hours (or overnight) before serving.

To serve, spoon the frozen yogurt into bowls.

On Shopping Day: Prepare the rhubarb and store in an airtight container for up to 4 days.

OATMEAL SNACK CAKE

Oats and dried cranberries make this simple cake an excellent mid-morning snack.

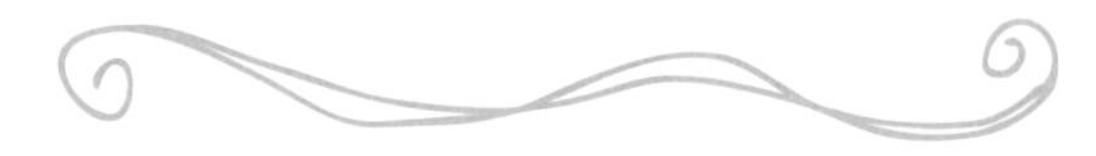

Makes 8 servings
Prep Time: 15 minutes
Cook Time: 45 to 50 minutes

- 1/2 cup old-fashioned rolled oats
- 1 cup dried cranberries
- 1 cup boiling water
- 1 1/2 cups unbleached all-purpose flour
- 1 teaspoon baking soda
- 1 teaspoon ground cinnamon
- 1/2 teaspoon salt
- 1/2 cup butter, room temperature (1 stick)
- 1 cup natural sugar
- 1/2 cup brown sugar
- 2 large eggs
- 1 teaspoon pure vanilla extract
- Reduced-fat cream cheese (for garnish)

Place the oats and the cranberries into a pan. Add 1 cup boiling water. Warm over low heat until the oats and fruit soften slightly, about 5 minutes.

Preheat the oven to 350 degrees. In a large bowl whisk together the flour, baking soda, cinnamon, and salt. In a separate large bowl use an electric mixer to combine the butter and sugars until soft and fluffy. Add the eggs one at a time. Stir in the vanilla. Add the flour mixture in 3 additions, until just combined. Stir in the oat/cranberry mixture.

Pour the batter into a 9-inch diameter round baking pan that has been coated with vegetable oil spray. Bake until the cake springs back when touched and a tester inserted into the center comes out clean, about 40–45 minutes.

To serve, cut into wedges and serve warm with a dollop of reduced-fat cream cheese for garnish.

SAUTÉED BANANAS

With Sweet Mascarpone and Walnut Crunch

This update on the classic banana split will brighten up that weekday supper.

Makes 4 servings
Prep Time: 15 minutes
Cook Time: 10 minutes

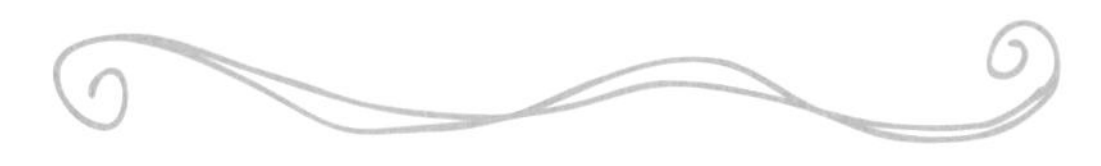

Choose a ripe, but firm, BANANA for this dish.

For the walnut crunch

- 1 tablespoon unsalted butter
- 1 cup chopped walnuts
- 2 tablespoons natural sugar
- 1/8 teaspoon salt

For sweet mascarpone

- 1/2 cup mascarpone cheese
- 1 tablespoon whipping cream
- 1 tablespoon honey
- 1 1/2-inch piece ginger, grated (about 2 teaspoons)

For the bananas

- 2 tablespoons unsalted butter
- 1/4 cup brown sugar
- 2 bananas, peeled and cut half lengthwise

Heat 1 tablespoon butter in a skillet over medium heat. Add the walnuts and stir. Sprinkle with sugar and salt. Cook until the nuts are golden and the sugar dissolves, about 5 minutes. Pour this mixture onto parchment paper and cool to room temperature.

In a medium bowl whisk together the mascarpone cheese, whipping cream, honey, and ginger until smooth.

Heat 2 more tablespoons butter in the skillet over medium heat. Stir in the brown sugar and cook until the sugar is melted. Cook the bananas in the butter sugar, turning often to coat, about 3–5 minutes.

To serve, place one banana half onto a plate or banana boat. Top with a dollop of mascarpone cheese. Drizzle extra brown sugar sauce over top. Sprinkle with walnut crunch.

On Shopping Day: Prepare the walnut crunch; cool and store in an airtight container.

Gorgeous Home Spa Secrets . . . for Great Hair Days

Like it or not, hair can "make or break" a pretty face. As we all know (and may like to forget), a girl can spend a fortune ensuring gorgeous hair, and while this may do the trick in transforming manes from mousy to magnificent, it's certainly not the only way to achieve awesome locks. Those hair-beautifying foods you've been enjoying in this chapter contain certain ingredients that can be applied directly to your the tresses, providing the final answer for not just luxurious, but *luminous*, hair.

Color Me Gorgeous

If we're not trying to "wash that man right out of our hair," then we're desperately trying to "wash away the gray." The men are easy enough, but the question is what to replace "the gray" with. Before I dish on simple pantry items that color you gorgeous, let's dispel a popular and frightening myth regarding gray hair: when you pluck just one, do a dozen more come in its place? The answer is a resounding *no*! The reassuring scientific truth of the matter is *if one gray hair is pulled, exactly one will grow back*—so pluck away! You can nip the graying process in the bud by applying some natural color enhancers; then hit the beach with a good book and a trusty tube of sunblock.

Blonde Bombshell

Brew a cup of very strong chamomile tea. Let it cool to lukewarm. Spray or comb into dry hair. Leave on twenty minutes (if possible sit in the sun). Shampoo and rinse; this gives a **Color Lift** and subtle highlights to blonde and light brown hair.

When Life Gives You Lemons

Whether you've got lemon juice on the brain because you're making the Rosemary Roasted Chicken Breasts With Smoky Almond Sauce (pg. 91) or entertaining your guests with scrumptious lemon juice–infused Mussels with Brussels in a White Wine Butter Sauce (pg. 94), this ingredient ought to be at your immediate disposal. Use a spray bottle and spritz ¼ cup lemon juice (or massage liberally) into wet hair and get some sun for 30 minutes or so. Then rinse and shampoo, being sure to note that the acidity in lemons can dry out your hair; you'll *definitely* want to moisturize it after every lemon juice application . . . and what better way than to use our au natural hair masks? Read on!

When a Brunette Needs an Extra Kick

Dark-haired beauties can create bewitching and enchanting color highlights with tea, walnuts, and coffee. Boil one cup of chopped walnuts with one cup water. Strain the liquid, cool to room temperature, and pour over your hair. Leave on for thirty minutes and rinse with freshly brewed tea or espresso (also cooled to room temperature). Leave this on for another thirty minutes and then shampoo. This will add sparkling highlights to black or brown hair.

Be "That Little Redhead . . ."

At any health food store or beauty supply shop, one can find all-natural henna for safe application at home. Using henna on gray hair presents a challenge since it has a harder time attaching to silvery hair—all due to changes in the protein base of gray hair. Just so you know, there are three major types of henna plant, as well as different plant parts, each yielding a different color. Although red is the most well known shade of henna, there is also a neutral and a black henna. Blending these three shades of henna in the right proportions can create an arresting and lovely vivid red, rich auburn, chestnut, or mahogany. Best of all, the Food and Drug Administration has given henna its nod of approval.

Shampoo the Do!

Hair gets dirty when sebum, an oily substance secreted by the skin's sebaceous glands, coats the shaft. Dead skin cells and airborne dirt stick to the sebum. Whether dry or greasy, hair should be washed as often as required to look good. How often you wash your hair will depend on your hair's texture, the weather, and your lifestyle. The best home hair-care products are easily whipped up in your own kitchen by using herbs and natural ingredients.

Invite Your Hair to a Masked Ball!

Of course, we all need to shampoo with regularity, but is there anything we can do before "the daily shampoo" that will make the blow-dried final result better than ever? Yep! **Hair Masks** that can be whipped up from everyday food items rev up your hair's softness, shine and volume.

Try this **Fruit Mask**. Get out your blender and mix a few chunks of banana, avocado and cantaloupe, with 1 tablespoon wheat germ oil and plain yogurt. For extra conditioning, squeeze in the contents of a vitamin E capsule. Massage into your hair and leave in for 15 minutes. Now, go vigorously shampoo and rinse thoroughly. Once blow-dried, your hair will look sweeter than the fruit that went into it!

We Call it "The Olive Oil"

A great conditioner for your hair—one that's enhanced Italian women's raven locks for centuries—is an **Olive Oil Hair Mask**. Mix 5 tablespoons of olive oil with 2 eggs (or use those leftover yolks from your Egg White Omelets with Bell Peppers and Turkey Sausage (pg. 88). Massage into your hair. Wrap your head with plastic wrap or use a shower cap. Leave on for 15 minutes then shampoo and rinse thoroughly.

Stop the Frizzies & Start Damage Control

For damaged hair mash a ripe banana with a few drops of almond oil. Massage into your hair. Leave in for at least 15 minutes. Rinse with soda water, then shampoo and condition. Calm frizzed out hair by mixing 1 tablespoon honey into a liter of water. Use this mixture as a rinse after you shampoo your hair.

Your Perfect Hairstyle

Match the shape of your face to the hairstyle that complements your looks. There are five different facial shapes: oval, heart, square, rectangle, and round. Almost every cut works if you have an oval-shaped face. You'll look gorgeous with a short style that brings out your eyes and balances your nose. For a heart-shaped face, choose a style that grows hair to shoulder length, fluffing out at the chin—like a sweeping pageboy. For a square-shaped face, allow your hair to grow past the shoulders with soft layers and fringy bangs that will soften your look. If your face is elongated in a rectangular fashion, choose layered hair that reaches about mid-neck with long, wispy bangs. For a round face, choose a close-cropped cut that offers more height on the top of your head without teasing.

Have a Do-Over

Just because your high school yearbook picture shows you with a better flip than Farrah Fawcett does not mean that you should wear your hair in this style *forever*. Don't be afraid to change your hairstyle and accentuate your hair color from time to time. Make an appointment every few months with a stylist and update your look. Learning a few tricks along the way can keep you—and your hairdo—looking fresh and current.

Shed a Few Inches

When the time comes for a total hair makeover (when those long locks start to bring you down), why not think about donating the clippings to boost up someone else? Check out www.locksoflove.org. Even if you don't have *luscious* locks to donate, you do have an hour or two during the week to help out a sister in need by volunteering for this organization.

CHAPTER 7

a closer look—the eyes have it!

"The face is the mirror of the mind, and eyes without speaking confess the secrets of the heart."
—Saint Jerome

We are a highly visual species, so when it comes to what constitutes good eye health and its importance in a human being's life, there should be no end to questions and answers. However, with so much healthy cooking awaiting us, we'll stick to an abridged line of questioning, requesting of Dr. Moon only the most essential Q&As. Here we make it our quest—our *vision*—to seek the best, most comprehensive answers.

Ask Dr. Moon

The doctor is in to answer your questions.

Q: How important is good eye health?

A: Once you understand the enormity of what the human eye does, you'll answer this question with one word: critical. Most of our information about the world comes to us through our eyes, and most of our cultural and intellectual heritage is stored and transmitted as words and images to which our vision gives access and meaning. Vision is a complex process involving not only the eyes but also eyelids, tear ducts, and optic nerve, as well as the electrical impulses from the eye to the brain. Taking care of our eyes for good vision involves more than just popping in to see our optometrist once a year; *that's only the beginning*. One major contributor to vision problems is a poor diet, so taking care of our eyes starts with the food choices we make every day.

Q: What foods practically guarantee that I'll maintain good vision?

A: It's plain to see that eggs are good for your eyes. That's because egg yolks contain lutein and zeaxanthin (L&Z), two antioxidants from the carotenoid family that contribute to improving eye health and protecting eyes from ultraviolet rays. L&Z help to reduce the risk of age-related macular degeneration. What's more, data from the Beaver Dam Eye Study shows that people who eat eggs every day have less risk of developing cataracts.

Q: Is there any further explanation you can give when it comes to the importance of carotenoids in one's daily diet and their relationship to eggs?

A: Carotenoids protect the retina from UV rays. These antioxidants are also found in certain leafy green vegetables, such as spinach. However, the body metabolizes the L&Z found in eggs more efficiently—yet another reason why eggs are good for your health.

Q: What nutritional support should we include in order to prevent problems and maintain the eyes' peak function?

A: Supplementing several key nutrients, such as vitamin A and beta-carotene, can be very beneficial to eye health and good vision. It is well documented that the antioxidants vitamin E and selenium, along with phytonutrients, such as lutein and other carotenoids, help preserve peak visual health. A lifelong practice of adequate supplementation, along with a good diet, helps to avoid the eye problems associated with aging and disease. Quercetin also protects the eye from sunlight and other sources of oxidation. Quercetin-rich foods may be helpful because they help neutralize the damaging effects of pollution. You can find this potent antioxidant in cabbage, grapefruit, cranberries, kale, grapes, pears, and, if you're looking for a highly concentrated dose, the skin of apples.

Q: Okay, Mr. Plastic Surgeon, what health & beauty aid products make your eyes look their best?

A: Over-the-counter wrinkle creams are helpful in erasing the fine lines that surround your eyes. Retinol is a vitamin A derivative and is the first antioxidant to be widely used in over-the-counter wrinkle creams. But you can do far more detective work when it comes to choosing the best antiaging products. Scan the ingredient information on health & beauty aids for these acids: alpha hydroxy, beta hydroxyl, and poly hydroxyl. These are all synthetic versions of acids derived from sugar-containing fruits and are a sweet, age-defiant salve to your skin. They're also exfoliates, substances that remove the upper layer of old, dead skin and stimulate the growth of smooth, evenly pigmented new skin.

Q: Are there any other chemical wonders that decrease signs of aging around the eyes?

A: Yes. Alpha-lipoic acid is an antioxidant that penetrates skin cell membranes, where it neutralizes free radicals and increases the effectiveness of other antioxidants such as vitamins C and E. It may also work as a superficial chemical peel to exfoliate dead skin and reduce the appearance of wrinkles.

Q: What if "crow's feet" don't respond to over-the-counter treatments? What surgical procedures will make a person look younger around the eyes?

A: If cutting-edge drugstore creams aren't cutting the mustard, you may want to consider injections. Botox inserted into the muscles by a surgeon will relax the wrinkles around eyes known as crow's feet. Upper eyelid blepharoplasty can make a remarkable difference in the appearance of the face, alleviating the appearance of tiredness and old age. The eyes appear fresher and more youthful, and these results may last for many years. The degree of improvement varies from patient to patient. Blepharoplasty is done to remove fat bags and excess skin around the eyes.

Q: What are the common procedures used to improve vision?

A: Sometimes surgical enhancements are necessary for improved vision. If your level of refractive error is small and you're not basing your decision on price alone, lasik might be for you.

Jorj's Eye-Catching Glam Kitchen

It's been said before and it'll be said again: you're moaning and groaning after partaking of that huge Thanksgiving spread because "your eyes were bigger than your stomach." As a visual species, *what* we see and *how* we interpret it is the reigning force behind the reality of what winds up on our plates. What *looks* good isn't always good for you. How can we make our eyes more discriminating with a nod, not to mention an *eye*, toward good health. And wouldn't it be ironic and wonderful if, as well as picking out the healthiest foods in sight, we also selected the fruits, veggies, meats, and cheeses that benefited our eyes most of all? Here are a few staples promoting what Jorj's Eye-Catching Glam Kitchen recognizes as food that's not just good but optimal for optics.

Eyes on Vitamin B!

Good eye health is synonymous with what's right for the entire body. The area around and immediately beneath the eye is just as vulnerable as its interior and will sometimes suffer from puffiness and wrinkling. Vitamin B, which promotes circulation and prevents inflammation, is always in demand for your eyes and the delicateness surrounding them. Get your vitamin B, bidding adieu to bags and circles under your eyes, by enjoying **cheeses** of the world, **milk**, **oatmeal**, **brown rice**, **brewer's yeast**, **black strap molasses**, **steak**, and **soybeans**.

The Q Word

Many of us, and wisely so, won't drive without sunglasses, fearing overexposure to the sun poses a "down the road" threat of cataracts. Quercetin, the magic Q word, protects the eye from sunlight and other sources of oxidation, and if that's not enough in terms of a glowing recommendation, quercetin neutralizes free radical damage caused by airborne pollutants we come in contact with every day. Get Q-rich from making visually appealing, tasty breakfasts, lunches, and dinners featuring **cabbage**, **grapefruit**, **cranberries**, **kale**, **grapes**, **pears**, **garlic**, **onions**, **egg yolks**, and **apples**.

Is Your Veggie Crisper Insured?

Brightly colored veggies and dark leafy greens contain vitamin A, beta-carotene, and carotenoids—all magical components in the equation that lends your eyes sun-safe pigmentation, good blood circulation, and, above all, the ability to absorb these and other eye-loving nutrients. **Acorn squash**, **carrots**, **spinach**, **sweet potatoes**, **corn**, and **collard greens** are your eyes' insurance policy against eye problems associated with old age and disease. Also in the carotenoid family are the good ol' lutein and zeaxanthin found in farm-fresh **eggs**, **romaine lettuce**, **zucchini**, **Brussels sprouts**, and garden **peas**.

Getting the Red Out

Nothing brings home the image of bloodshot eyes like cartoons of our sleep-deprived favorites, their orbs a network of angry blood vessels pried open with toothpicks. Though we true-to-life humans can't get *that bad*, we've certainly come close. What kind of healthy diet eradicates the need for eye drops? The answer is vitamin C, critical for growth and repair of tissues in all parts of your body, including healthy blood vessels at work in your eyes. Find vitamin C in **green** and **red peppers**, **tomatoes**, **broccoli**, **strawberries**, **turnip greens**, **potatoes**, **cantaloupe**, and **citrus** fruits and their sweet juices.

Magnificent

Clear eyes and skin owe their perfection to a nutritious diet, which would be incomplete without magnesium. The nutrient most beneficial to the body's circulation, magnesium benefits your heart and nervous system, bones, and stunning eyes. Magnesium-rich foods are **avocados**, **cashews**, **dark chocolate**, **Swiss chard**, **whole grains**, cooked **beans,** and **fish**.

Of Cosmetic Concern

For great skin around your eyes, load up on vitamin E found in **almonds**, **sunflower seeds**, and **vegetable** (olive!) **oils**. Further combat the ravages of free-radical damage (which leads to wrinkling) with foods containing bioflavonoids, chemical compounds that work with vitamins to promote cellular integrity. They are in **cherries**, **celery**, **parsley**, **endive**, **radishes**, **leeks**, and **red wine**.

Eye-Catching Recipes

Start Your Day

Main Plates

On the Side

Snacks & Sweets

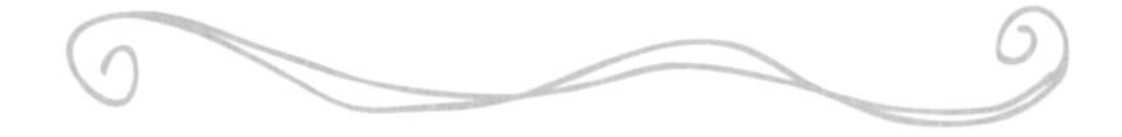

BROILED GRAPEFRUIT

With Honey Mascarpone Cream

Make your everyday breakfast fit for a queen with this simple, yet luscious, breakfast starter.

Makes 4 servings
Prep Time: 5 minutes
Cook Time: 10 minutes

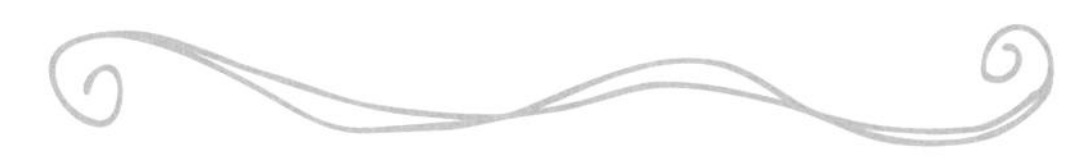

Slice a SMALL piece from the bottom of the grapefruit to make sure it sits up in the pan without wobbling.

For the grapefruit

- 2 tablespoons brown sugar
- ½ teaspoon ground ginger
- ¼ teaspoon ground cinnamon
- 1 teaspoon vanilla
- 2 large pink grapefruits

For the mascarpone cream

- 1 cup mascarpone, room temperature
- 2 tablespoons honey
- ½ teaspoon pure vanilla extract
- 2 tablespoons reduced-fat half and half
- Fresh mint leaves (for garnish)

Preheat the broiler. In a small bowl whisk together the sugar, ginger, cinnamon, and vanilla. Cut each grapefruit in half (crosswise) and run knife around each section to loosen membranes. Arrange grapefruits, cut-side up, in a baking dish or on a rimmed baking sheet that is just large enough to hold them in one layer and sprinkle with sugar mixture. Broil grapefruits about 2–3 inches from heat until sugar melts and tops begin to brown, about 8–10 minutes.

In a small bowl whisk together the mascarpone, honey, vanilla extract, and half and half until smooth.

To serve, cool the grapefruits to room temperature. Serve with a swirl of mascarpone cream and garnish with fresh mint leaves.

On Shopping Day: Prepare the mascarpone cream and store in an airtight container in the refrigerator for up to 4 days.

SCRAMBLED EGGS

With Red Grape and Avocado Salsa

Juice up the everyday scramble with a sweet and spicy salsa that's chock-full of antioxidants.

Makes 4 servings
Prep Time: 15 minutes
Cook Time: 8 minutes

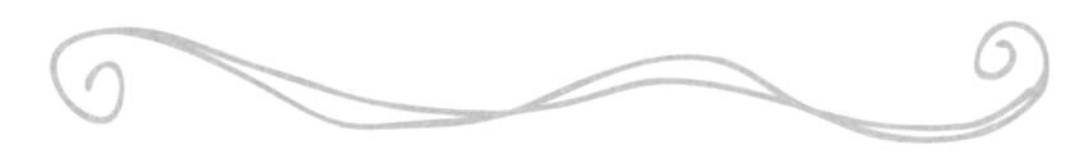

Make a DOUBLE batch of the salsa on shopping day, and use it on your weeknight CHICKEN or FISH dinner.

For the salsa

- 1 cup red seedless grapes, cut in half
- 1 large avocado, peeled, pitted, and diced (about 1 cup)
- 1 medium green bell pepper, seeded and cut into 1/4-inch dice (about 2/3 cup)
- 2 tablespoons finely diced red onion
- 1 small jalapeño pepper, seeded and diced (about 1 tablespoon)
- Juice of 1 medium lime (about 1 tablespoon)
- Juice of 1 medium orange (about 1/3 cup)
- Salt and freshly ground pepper

For the eggs

- 1 tablespoon unsalted butter
- 8 large eggs
- 2 tablespoons reduced-fat half and half

Place the grapes, avocado, bell pepper, red onion, and jalapeño pepper into a large bowl. Pour in the lime and orange juices. Season with salt and pepper. Toss and chill for at least 1 hour.

Heat the butter in a skillet over medium-high heat. Whisk together the eggs with the half and half until fluffy. Season with salt and pepper. Pour the eggs into the pan. Cook, moving the eggs from the edges to the center, until soft curds form, about 5–8 minutes.

To serve, divide the eggs onto 4 plates. Pour the salsa into a colander to drain the juice. Serve 1–2 tablespoons salsa with the eggs.

On Shopping Day: Prepare the salsa (without the avocado) and place into an air-tight container. Refrigerate for up to 4 days. Add avocado just before serving.

POACHED EGGS

In Spicy Tomato Sauce

Get your day off to a great start by waking up to this spicy dish!

Makes 4 servings
Prep Time: 10 minutes
Cook Time: 20 minutes

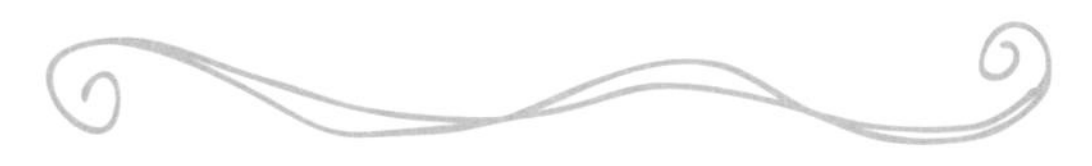

Turn this dish into a fun brunch with friends by adding SHRIMP and ASPARAGUS to the sauce as it simmers. Serve with fresh-baked tortilla chips on the side.

For the sauce

- 1 tablespoon olive oil
- 1 large red onion, peeled and thinly sliced (about 1 cup)
- 1 28-ounce can diced tomatoes
- 2 tablespoons tomato paste
- 1 teaspoon natural sugar
- 1/2 teaspoon crushed red pepper flakes
- Salt and freshly ground pepper

For the eggs

- 3 ounces thick bacon (about 4–5 strips), cut into 1/2-inch pieces
- 8 large eggs

Heat the olive oil in a skillet over medium-high heat. Add the onion and cook until soft and golden, about 5 minutes. Pour the tomatoes into the skillet. Stir in the tomato paste, sugar, and red pepper flakes. Bring to a boil. Reduce the heat and simmer the sauce until it thickens and reduces by about one-third, about 15 minutes. Season with salt and pepper. Keep warm.

Cook the bacon in a skillet over medium heat. Use a slotted spoon to transfer the bacon to paper towels to drain.

Poach the eggs in an egg poaching pan, or in a pot filled with water and a bit of vinegar.

To serve, ladle the sauce into bowls. Place 2 poached eggs in each bowl. Top with crumbled bacon.

On Shopping Day: Prepare the tomato sauce and store in an airtight container in the refrigerator for up to 4 days. Reheat before serving.

MELON BOWLS

With Strawberry Ginger Sauce

A simple combination of fruits and spice makes for a fast and healthful breakfast.

Makes 4 servings
Prep Time: 10 minutes

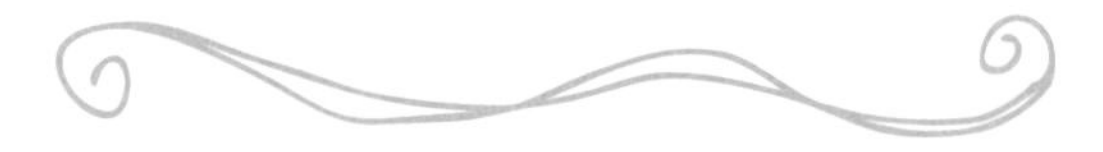

Hollowed out MELONS act as the serving bowls for this fun, fresh fruit snack.

- 1 pint strawberries, hulled (about 1 cup)
- 1 1-inch piece ginger, grated (about 1 tablespoon)
- 1 small honeydew melon, sliced in half, fruit cut into 1-inch cubes (about 2 cups)
- 1 small cantaloupe, sliced in half, fruit cut into 1-inch cubes (about 2 cups)

Place the strawberries and ginger into the bowl of a food processor. Pulse to emulsify.

Toss the melon cubes together.

To serve, hollow out the melons and cut a slice from each end so that each half sits flat on a serving plate. Divide the melon cubes among the four melon "bowls." Pour the strawberry ginger sauce over top.

On Shopping Day: Cut up the fruit and store in an airtight container and chill for up to 4 days. Cover and store the melon "bowls."

ROASTED VEGGIE BURRITOS

With Chipotle Chili Tomato Sauce

Serve this dish with rice and beans for a satisfying veggie meal.

Makes 4 servings
Prep Time: 30 minutes
Cook Time: 35 minutes

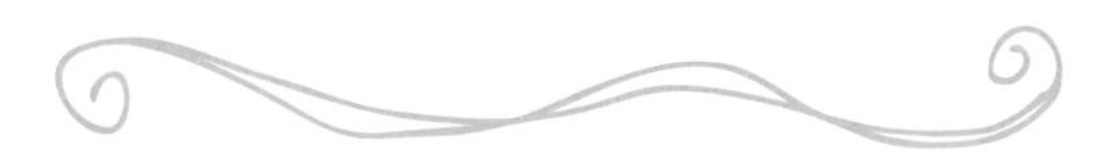

Canned CHIPOTLE chilies can be found in the ethnic section of your grocery store or in specialty markets. Be careful—this is a HOT addition to the dish. Start small—you can always add more.

For the veggies

- 4 large portobello mushrooms, stems and gills removed
- 1 large red onion, peeled and thinly sliced (about 1 cup)
- 1 medium eggplant, sliced into ½-inch-thick lengths
- 1 large green bell pepper, seeded and cut into quarters
- 1 large red bell pepper, seeded and cut into quarters
- 6 plum medium tomatoes, cut in half lengthwise (about 1 pound)
- 3 tablespoons olive oil
- 1 tablespoon ground chili powder
- 1 teaspoon ground cumin
- Salt and freshly ground pepper

For the sauce

- 1 28-ounce can diced tomatoes
- 2 tablespoons tomato paste
- 1 canned chipotle chili pepper in adobo sauce, seeded and finely diced (about 1 tablespoon)
- 1 teaspoon natural sugar

For the burritos

- 4 10-inch corn tortillas
- 4 ounces reduced-fat grated Monterey Jack cheese (about 1 cup), divided use

Preheat the oven to 375 degrees. Place the mushrooms and vegetables onto a rimmed baking sheet. Toss with olive oil, chili powder, cumin, salt, and pepper. Roast until the vegetables are soft and golden, about 15–20 minutes. Cool and slice into similar-size strips.

Place the tomatoes, tomato paste, chili pepper, and sugar into a saucepan. Simmer over medium heat until the sauce thickens and is reduced by one-third, about 15 minutes. Season with salt and pepper.

Wrap the tortillas in parchment paper. Warm in the microwave until soft. Arrange the veggies on top of the tortillas. Cover with ½ cup of the cheese. Roll up, burrito-style and lay seam-side down in a baking dish that has been coated with vegetable oil spray.

Pour the tomato sauce over the burritos. Top with remaining ½ cup cheese. Reduce oven temperature to 350 degrees. Bake the burritos until the cheese begins to melt, about 20 minutes.

On Shopping Day: Roast the veggies and cool to room temperature. Store in an airtight container in the refrigerator for up to 3 days.

CHICKEN PAPRIKASH

Served over Egg Noodles

This comfy home-style dish comes together on your stovetop in mere minutes!

Makes 6 servings
Prep Time: 10 minutes
Cook Time: 20 minutes

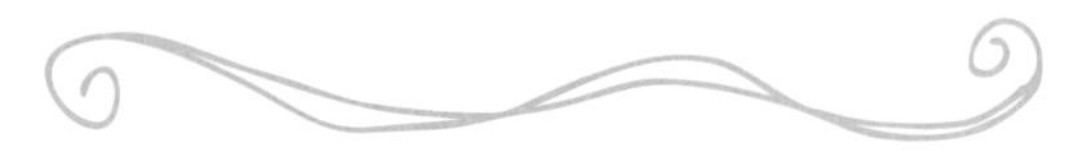

The BETTER the paprika, the BETTER this dish. Experiment with the various VARIETIES available in your grocery store or specialty markets.

* * *

For a COLORFUL presentation substitute with SPINACH FETTUCCINI or WHOLE WHEAT SPAGHETTI in place of the egg noodles.

- 1 tablespoon olive oil
- 2 large (8-ounce) skinless, boneless chicken breast halves, cut into 1-inch strips (about 3 cups)
- 2 tablespoons unbleached all-purpose flour
- Salt and freshly ground pepper
- 12 ounces egg noodles
- 1 medium yellow onion, peeled and diced into ½-inch squares (about 1 cup)
- 1 large red bell pepper, seeded and thinly sliced (about 1 cup)
- 3 medium garlic cloves, minced (about 1½ teaspoons)
- 1 14.5-ounce can diced tomatoes
- ½ cup reduced-fat half and half
- 2 tablespoons tomato paste
- 1 tablespoon paprika
- Chopped fresh parsley (for garnish)

Heat the oil in a large skillet over medium-high heat. Toss the chicken with flour and season with salt and pepper. Cook the chicken in the oil until golden. Remove with a slotted spoon to a platter.

Bring a pot of water to a boil over high heat. Season generously with salt. Cook noodles according to package directions.

Add the onion, bell pepper, and garlic to the skillet. Cook until soft, about 3–5 minutes. Pour the tomatoes into the skillet. Place the chicken back into the skillet. Pour in the half and half. Stir in the tomato paste and paprika. Reduce the heat, cover, and simmer until the chicken is cooked through and the sauce thickens, about 5 minutes more.

To serve, ladle the chicken and sauce over egg noodles. Garnish with fresh parsley.

STIR-FRY CHICKEN AND BROCCOLI

With Chopped Peanuts

Nothing beats stir fry for a quick and healthy midweek meal. This one is reminiscent of Kung Pao Chicken—but who cares what it's called as long as it's this good!

Makes 4 servings
Prep Time: 20 minutes
Cook Time: 20 minutes

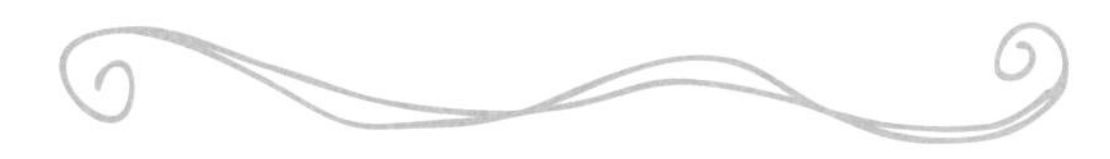

BLANCHING veggies to use in your stir fry speeds up the cooking process and guarantees a CRISP-TENDER result. Place the veggie into rapidly boiling, salted water. Cook until the color deepens but the veggie is still crisp. Remove the veggie with a slotted spoon to a bowl filled with ICE WATER; this will halt the cooking process. Drain and store, or continue with the recipe.

- 2 tablespoons olive oil, divided use
- 1 1-inch piece ginger, grated (about 1 tablespoon)
- 1/2 teaspoon crushed red pepper flakes
- 2 large (6- to 8-ounce) skinless, boneless chicken breast halves, cut into 1/4-inch strips (about 3 cups)
- 1 bunch (6–8) green onions, thinly sliced on the diagonal (about 1/2 cup)
- 4 medium garlic cloves, minced (about 2 teaspoons)
- 2 bunches broccoli, cut into florets, about 4 cups, blanched
- 1/2 cup homemade chicken stock or low-sodium chicken broth
- 2 tablespoons hoisin sauce
- 2 tablespoons rice wine vinegar
- 2 tablespoons soy sauce
- 1 tablespoon cornstarch
- Salt and freshly ground pepper
- 2 cups cooked rice
- 2 tablespoons peanuts, chopped

Heat 1 tablespoon olive oil in a wok (or large skillet) over medium-high heat. Add the ginger, red pepper flakes, and chicken to the wok and stir fry until golden, about 4–5 minutes. Remove the chicken to a platter.

Pour the remaining 1 tablespoon olive oil into the skillet. Add the green onions, garlic, and broccoli. Stir fry until golden, about 2–3 minutes.

Whisk together the chicken stock, hoisin sauce, rice wine vinegar, soy sauce, and cornstarch. Pour this mixture into the broccoli and stir. Add in the chicken and simmer until sauce thickens slightly, about 3–5 minutes. Season with salt and pepper.

To serve, ladle the chicken over white rice and sprinkle with peanuts.

On Shopping Day: Blanch the broccoli and store in an airtight container for up to 4 days.

SPAGHETTI SQUASH CARBONARA

The traditional Italian dish that this recipe is based on is prepared with linguini and a rich (cream, bacon, and egg) sauce, filled with calories and fat—so probably a no-no in a well-balanced diet; unless, of course, we substitute fresh veggies for the pasta and reduce the amount of sauce per serving. Now that's a compromise you can live with!

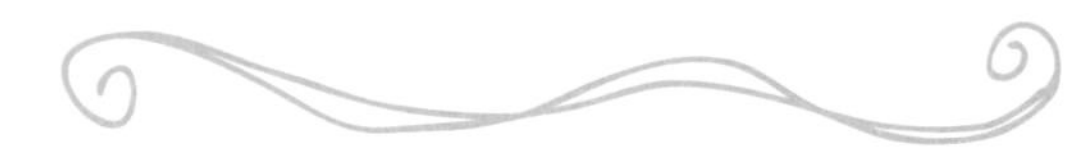

If you have SENSITIVITIES that do NOT allow you to eat RAW eggs, you might want to skip this recipe. Or you can prepare it by cooking the sauce in a double boiler over SIMMERING heat, stirring constantly, until the sauce reaches a temperature that indicates the eggs are cooked (in excess of 145 degrees).

Makes 4 main dish servings or 6 side dishes
Prep Time: 10 minutes
Cook Time: 30 minutes

For the spaghetti squash

- 1 large spaghetti squash (about 4 –5 pounds)
- 1 tablespoon olive oil

For carbonara sauce

- 4 large eggs
- 1/4 cup whipping cream
- 2 tablespoons butter
- 8 ounces pancetta, diced
- 4 ounces grated Parmesan cheese (about 1 cup)
- 1/4 cup chopped fresh parsley
- Salt and freshly ground pepper

Preheat the oven to 400 degrees. Cut the squash in half, lengthwise, and remove the seeds. Brush the cut side with olive oil and place (cut-side down) onto a baking sheet with lip. Roast until soft, about 40 minutes.

Let eggs, cream, and butter come to room temperature. Cook the pancetta in a skillet over medium heat until crisp. Use a slotted spoon to transfer to paper toweling to drain. Whisk together eggs and cream until just blended.

Use a fork to create strands of spaghetti from the hot squash. Place into a bowl and toss with the butter. Pour egg mixture over the squash and toss until well coated. Add pancetta, grated cheese, and parsley. Toss to mix. Season with salt and freshly ground pepper.

GRILLED NEW YORK STRIP STEAKS

With Garlic Herb Oil

Serve these steaks hot off the grill with a generous amount of oil for that classic steak house dish.

Makes 4 servings
Prep Time: 10 minutes
Cook Time: 12 minutes

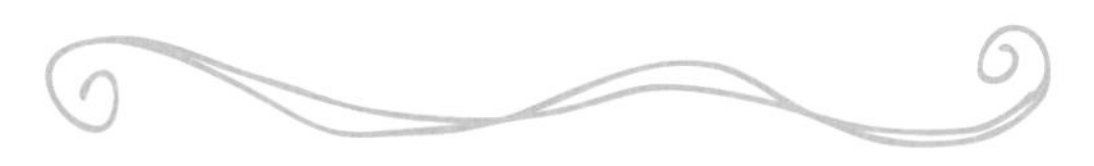

Test for DONENESS with your finger; if the meat springs back when touched, it's on its way to being well done. The less spring, the RARER the steak will be.

- 4 large shallots, peeled and separated into lobes
- 4 medium garlic cloves
- 2 tablespoons fresh chives
- 2 tablespoons fresh parsley leaves
- 2 tablespoons fresh thyme leaves
- 1/2 cup olive oil
- Salt and freshly ground pepper
- 4 8-ounce New York strip steaks, about 1 1/2 inches thick

Place the shallots, garlic, chives, parsley, and thyme into a mini food processor. Pulse to finely chop. With the blade running, pour in the olive oil. Season with salt and pepper. Set aside.

Season the steaks with salt and pepper. Heat a grill pan that has been coated with vegetable oil spray over high heat. Grill the steaks, turning once, about 6 minutes per side for medium rare.

To serve, place the steaks onto a platter. Slather each one with the seasoned oil.

On Shopping Day: Prepare the seasoned oil and store in an airtight container in the refrigerator up to 4 days.

ITALIAN-STYLE STRATA

You can prepare this dish in the morning before you leave the house and serve it for a simple, yet satisfying, supper.

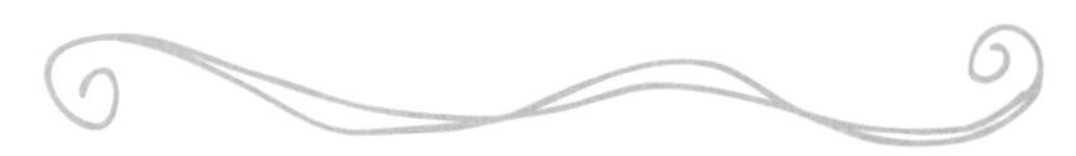

I like the combination of PANCETTA and PROSCIUTTO in this dish. Pancetta is Italian bacon cured with spices and salt, but not smoked. It is slightly salty, very tasty, and comes in a sausage-like roll. The Italian word for "ham," prosciutto is a term broadly used to describe a ham that has been SEASONED, salt-cured (but not smoked), and air-dried. The meat is pressed, which produces a firm, dense texture. You can find both at your grocer's deli counter or at the specialty market.

Makes 4 servings
Prep Time: 10 minutes
Cook Time: 30 minutes

- 2 cups reduced-fat milk
- 1 bunch (6–8) green onions, chopped (about 1/2 cup)
- 4 large eggs
- 1 tablespoon Dijon mustard
- 2 tablespoons chopped fresh oregano
- 1/2 teaspoon crushed red pepper flakes
- 1 12-ounce whole grain bread loaf, cut into 1-inch cubes
- 4 ounces prosciutto, diced
- 4 ounces smoked mozzarella cheese, grated (about 1 cup)
- 2 ounces pancetta, diced

Whisk together the milk, onions, eggs, mustard, oregano, and red pepper flakes. Add the bread cubes and submerge. Toss in the prosciutto. Pour into a baking dish. Sprinkle with cheese. Cover and chill in the refrigerator for at least one hour (or as much as overnight) to make sure that the breadcrumbs absorb the liquid.

Preheat the oven to 350 degrees. Uncover the strata. Sprinkle with pancetta and bake for 25–30 minutes or until the center is set and the cheese is bubbly.

To serve, allow the strata to rest for 5 minutes. Cut into wedges and serve with a green salad.

PORK MEDALLIONS

With Asparagus and Sweet Potatoes

Who says a one-pot meal needs to begin with a box? Using fresh veggies brightens up an everyday supper, making it very eye-appealing.

Makes 4 servings
Prep Time: 15 minutes
Cook Time: 25 minutes

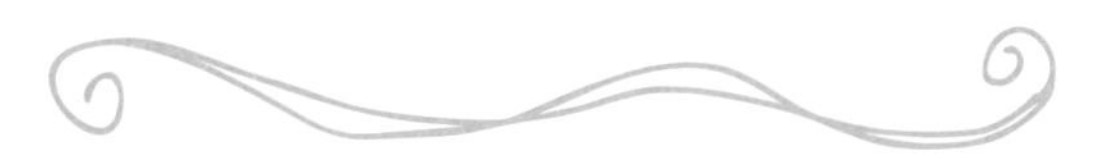

To make PORK MEDALLIONS, begin with a pork tenderloin. Lay the tenderloin onto your work surface. Cut the pork tenderloin into 4 pieces. Place each (cut-side down) onto your work surface between sheets of waxed paper. Use a meat mallet to POUND each slice into a medallion.

- 8 ounces fresh asparagus spears, ends trimmed, cut diagonally into ½-inch lengths (about 1 cup)
- 3 tablespoons olive oil, divided use
- 2 medium sweet potatoes, peeled and diced into 1-inch cubes (about 2 cups)
- Salt and freshly ground pepper
- 4 4-ounce pork medallions
- 1 teaspoon dried oregano leaves
- ⅓ cup red wine

Blanch the asparagus in boiling water until crisp-tender, about 3 minutes. Use a slotted spoon to transfer to a bowl filled with ice water. Drain and set aside.

In a skillet heat 1 tablespoon olive oil over medium-high heat. Add the potatoes, season with salt and pepper, and cook until crisp, about 10 minutes. Remove to a platter and keep warm.

Add the remaining 2 tablespoons of olive oil to the skillet. Season both sides of the pork medallions with oregano, salt, and pepper. Cook, turning once, until both sides are golden, about 7–8 minutes total.

Pour the wine into the skillet with the pork. Add the asparagus and sweet potatoes. Cook until the liquid disappears, about 3 minutes.

To serve, place the pork onto a platter. Spoon the veggies over the top.

MUSHROOM AND SPINACH–FILLED FRITTATA

Breakfast for dinner? You betcha! The concept is especially appealing when the dish is full of fresh veggies.

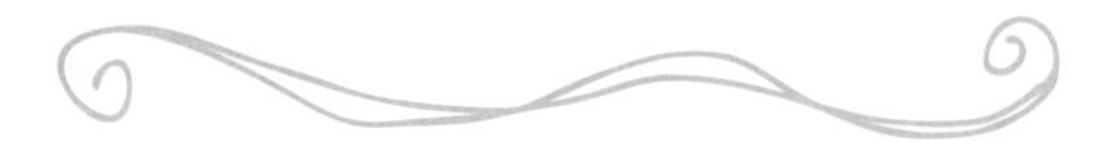

Make sure that you use a skillet with an oven-proof handle, and make doubly sure that you grab that handle with a pot holder when you are removing the frittata from the oven.

Heat 1 tablespoon olive oil in a skillet over medium-high heat. Add the onion and cook until golden, about 5 minutes. Add the mushrooms and cook until soft, about 5 minutes more. Reduce the heat to low. Stir in the spinach and chives and cook until the spinach is just wilted, about 2 minutes. Season with salt and pepper. Pour the filling into a bowl. Cool to room temperature.

In a large bowl whisk together the eggs and half and half. Season with salt and pepper. Stir in the mushroom-spinach mixture.

Preheat the oven on the broil setting. Heat 1 tablespoon olive oil in an ovenproof skillet over medium heat. Pour the egg mixture into the pan. Cook until the eggs set up, pushing the outer edges to the center, allowing the uncooked portion to run to the sides of the pan. Place the skillet on the top shelf in the oven and broil until the frittata is puffed and brown and the center set, about 5–8 minutes.

To serve, let the frittata sit in the pan for 5 minutes. Gently slide the frittata onto a serving plate. Cut into wedges.

On Shopping Day: Prepare the onion/mushroom/spinach mixture, cool, and store in an airtight container in the refrigerator for up to 4 days.

Makes 4 servings
Prep Time: 10 minutes
Cook Time: 20 minutes

For the mushroom and spinach filling

- 1 tablespoon olive oil
- 1 small red onion, peeled and diced (about 1/2 cup)
- 4 ounces shiitake mushrooms, chopped (about 1 cup)
- 4 ounces fresh spinach leaves, washed, dried, and chopped (about 2 cups)
- 2 tablespoons chopped fresh chives
- Salt and freshly ground pepper

For the frittata

- 8 large eggs
- 2 tablespoons reduced-fat half and half
- 1 tablespoon olive oil

SWEET BALSAMIC ONIONS

Serve these onions alongside a juicy steak for an incredible depth of flavor, not to mention an eyeful of delicious.

Makes 4 servings
Prep Time: 5 minutes
Cook Time: 30 minutes

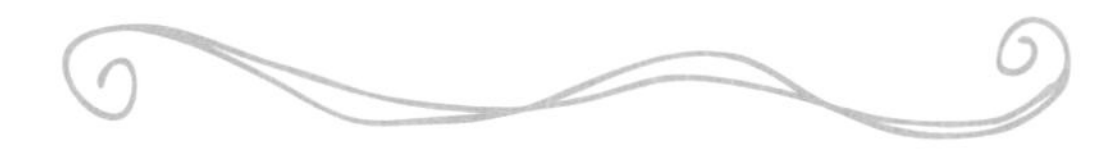

You can use any ONION for this dish.
A great variation that I offer during the holidays is made with PEARL ONIONS. Boil them in order to remove the skin, then follow the recipe.

- 1 tablespoon olive oil
- 2 large red onions, peeled and thinly sliced
- Salt and freshly ground pepper
- 1 tablespoon brown sugar
- 1 tablespoon balsamic vinegar
- 1 sprig fresh rosemary

Heat the olive oil in a skillet over medium-high heat. Add the onions. Season with salt and pepper. Stir until the onions begin to brown and soften, about 8–10 minutes. Reduce the heat to medium. Add the brown sugar and vinegar. Cook, stirring constantly, until the onions are quite brown and syrupy, about 10–15 minutes. Add the rosemary sprig and reduce the heat to low. Cook for 5 minutes more to allow the rosemary to infuse the onions.

To serve, remove the rosemary sprig and place the onions into a serving bowl.

BUTTERMILK ROLLS

With Sweet Onion Filling

These savory rolls are a delicious addition to your evening meal.

Makes 12 servings
Prep Time: 20 minutes plus dough cycle and rising
Cook Time: 30 minutes

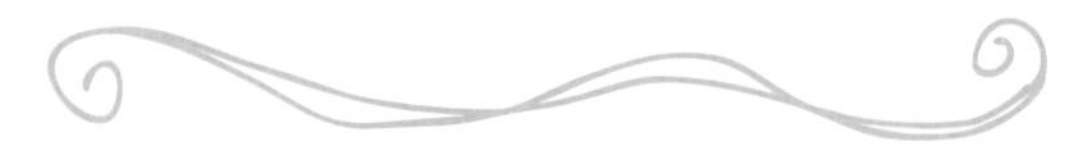

Use this recipe as a guideline to create your favorite SAVORY rolls. Use fillings such as broccoli and cheese or fresh herbs and garlic.

- 2¾ cups unbleached all-purpose flour
- ¾ cup buttermilk
- 1 tablespoon natural sugar
- 6 tablespoons unsalted butter, cut into pieces
- 1 large egg, beaten
- ½ teaspoon salt
- 2½ teaspoons active dry yeast
- 3 tablespoons olive oil, divided use
- 1 cup Sweet Balsamic Onions, chopped (see recipe on page 129)

Place the flour, buttermilk, sugar, butter, egg, and salt into the bucket of a bread machine. Place the yeast in the yeast compartment. Set the machine on the dough setting.

When the dough is prepared, turn out onto a lightly floured surface. Roll dough out to a 12 x 16-inch rectangle. Brush the dough with 2 tablespoons olive oil. Cover with chopped onions. Starting at one long side, roll up into a cylinder. Cut into 12 (1½-inch) slices. Place each slice, cut-side down, into a rimmed baking sheet that has been coated with vegetable oil spray.

Brush the rolls with the remaining 1 tablespoon olive oil. Cover with a clean towel. Let the rolls rise for 45–60 minutes. (Alternatively, cover the rolls with plastic wrap and refrigerate overnight.)

Preheat the oven to 375 degrees. Bake the rolls until golden brown about 30–35 minutes.

Serve warm rolls with a drizzle of flavorful olive oil.

ROASTED VEGGIE–STUFFED TOMATOES

I created this dish in an effort to utilize the unused veggies at the end of the week. There was a stalk of broccoli here, a loose carrot or two there, and a bunch of ripe tomatoes on the counter; the end result is a dinner side dish that's equally as good for tomorrow's lunch.

Use whatever veggies you have on hand—just make sure you chop them to about the same size. The smaller the size the faster the veggies will roast.

* * *

Since this chapter is all about the quercetin found in onions and garlic, why not use an onion for stuffing? Peel the onion and scoop out the inside. Season with salt and pepper and bake until soft. Fill the onions with the vegetable mixture. Continue to bake as directed below.

Preheat the oven to 375 degrees. Spread the veggies and mushrooms onto a baking sheet with lip. Drizzle with 2 tablespoons olive oil and season with salt and pepper. Place the rosemary sprigs into the veggies. Roast until the veggies are soft and just beginning to turn golden, about 20– 25 minutes. Remove from the oven. Discard rosemary stems.

Cut a very thin slice from the bottom of each tomato half so that it will stand without rolling in a baking dish. Remove the top and squeeze out the seeds. Season the inside of the tomatoes with salt and pepper and sprinkle with about 1 ounce of the cheese. Sprinkle the vegetables with about 2 ounces of the cheese. Use a spoon to stuff each tomato with the roasted vegetables. Place into a baking dish sprayed with vegetable oil spray. Top with the remaining cheese and drizzle with 1 tablespoon olive oil.

Bake the stuffed tomatoes until the cheese melts and begins to turn golden, about 15 minutes.

Serve one tomato as a side dish or two for a light lunch.

On Shopping Day: Prepare the dish in advance, cover with plastic wrap and refrigerate for up to 1 day.

Makes 6 servings
Prep Time: 20 minutes
Cook Time: 35 minutes

For the filling

- 1 baby eggplant, diced into 1/2-inch squares
- 2 large portobello mushrooms, diced into 1/2-inch squares
- 1 medium yellow onion, diced into 1/2-inch squares (about 1 cup)
- 1 large yellow bell pepper, seeded and cut into 2-inch dice (about 1 cup)
- 1 stalk broccoli, chopped (about 1 cup)
- 1/2 small head cauliflower, chopped (about 1 cup)
- 2 large carrots, diced into 1/4-inch squares (about 1 cup)
- 2 tablespoons olive oil
- Salt and freshly ground pepper
- 2 sprigs fresh rosemary

For the tomatoes

- 6 large beefsteak tomatoes, halved
- 4 ounces grated Parmesan cheese (about 1 cup), divided use
- 1 tablespoon olive oil

UNFRIED FRIED ONIONS

These onions crisp up once they are removed from the oil. They are perfect to serve on burgers or your favorite green bean casserole.

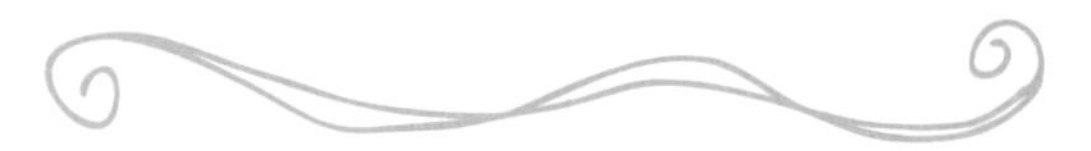

Rather than deep-fried battered onions, these are SLOWLY cooked in oil over medium heat. Watch carefully; when they begin to turn GOLDEN, they are just a few minutes away from being PERFECT.

Makes 2 servings
Prep Time: 5 minutes
Cook Time: 20 minutes

1 cup canola oil
1 large yellow onion, thinly sliced (about 2 cups)
Salt and freshly ground pepper

Pour the oil into a deep pot over medium-high heat. Bring to a boil. Carefully place the onions in the oil. Reduce the heat to medium. The onions will simmer in the oil—not fry. Cook until the onions are deep golden brown, stirring often, about 20 minutes. Use a slotted spoon to remove the onions to paper towels to drain. Season with salt and pepper.

Serve immediately.

PEAR AND STRAWBERRY CRISP

You can use your favorite fruit combinations for this dish. You can also change the topping to include whatever nuts you have on hand.

Makes 8 servings
Prep Time: 20 minutes
Cook Time: 45 minutes

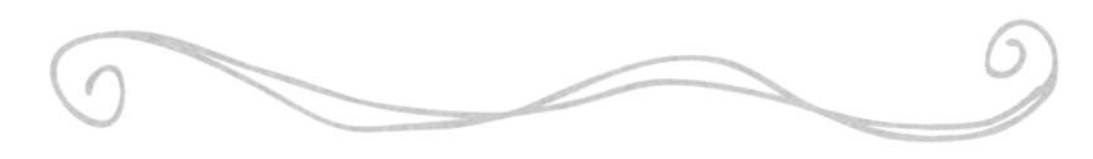

For a really, really QUICK fruit crisp, substitute prepared GRANOLA for the topping.

For the topping

- 4 tablespoons butter (1/2 stick)
- 1/2 cup old-fashioned rolled oats
- 1/3 cup walnuts, chopped
- 1/4 cup unbleached all-purpose flour
- 1/2 cup brown sugar
- 1/4 teaspoon ground allspice
- 1/4 teaspoon salt

For the filling

- 4 medium pears, peeled and sliced (about 4 cups)
- 1 quart strawberries hulled and cut in half (about 4 cups)
- 1/2 cup natural sugar
- Juice of 1 medium orange (about 1/3 cup)
- Zest of 1/2 medium orange (about 1 tablespoon)
- 2 tablespoons unbleached all-purpose flour
- 1/2 teaspoon ground cardamom

Preheat the oven to 375 degrees. Place the butter, oats, walnuts, flour, brown sugar, ground allspice, and salt into the bowl of a food processor. Pulse to form moist crumbs. Set aside.

Toss the pears and strawberries with sugar, orange juice, orange zest, flour, and cardamom. Place the filling into an 8 x 8-inch baking dish that has been coated with vegetable oil spray. Sprinkle the topping over the fruit. Bake until the top is golden brown and crispy and the fruit is bubbling, about 40–45 minutes.

To serve, cool the dish for 15 minutes. Serve warm with reduced-fat frozen yogurt.

ORANGE-GLAZED YOGURT CAKE

This rich cake uses yogurt in place of butter for a delicate texture.

Makes 12 servings
Prep Time: 20 minutes
Cook Time: 50 minutes

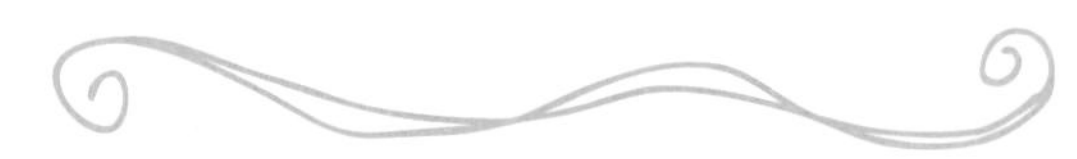

For the cake

- 1½ cups unbleached all-purpose flour
- 2 teaspoons baking powder
- ¼ teaspoon salt
- 1 cup reduced-fat vanilla-flavored yogurt
- 1 cup natural sugar
- 3 large eggs
- Zest of ½ medium orange (about 1 tablespoon)
- 1 teaspoon pure vanilla extract
- ½ cup canola oil

For the glaze

- ¼ cup orange marmalade
- Juice of ½ medium orange (about 2 tablespoons)

Preheat the oven to 350 degrees. Whisk together the flour, baking powder, and salt in a bowl. Set aside.

In a large bowl whisk together the yogurt, sugar, and eggs until fluffy. Stir in the orange zest, vanilla, and canola oil. Stir in the flour/baking powder mixture until you have a smooth, thick batter. Pour the batter into a Bundt pan that has been coated with vegetable oil spray. Bake until the cake springs back when touched and tester inserted into the center comes out clean, about 45–50 minutes. Cool the cake in the pan (on a rack) for 5 minutes. Run a knife around the edge of the pan. Carefully remove the cake from the pan by inverting onto a rack.

To make the glaze, warm the marmalade and orange juice in a pan over low heat. Brush the warm glaze over the cake. Cool.

To serve, cut the cake into slices.

CRANBERRY WEDDING COOKIES

Make these cookies on shopping day and you'll have great snacks all week long.

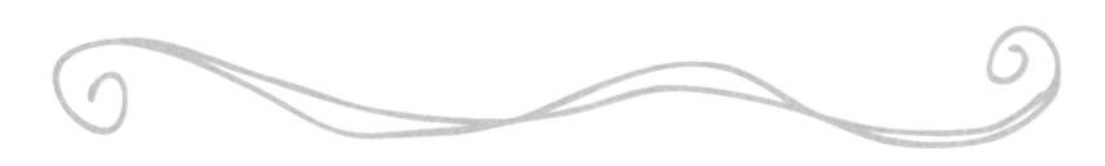

Use SWEETENED dried cranberries, available in the produce section of the grocery store for this recipe; they're SOFTER and PLUMPER than plain dried cranberries.

Makes 24 cookies
Prep Time: 10 minutes, plus chilling the dough
Cook Time: 15 minutes

- 1 cup unsalted butter, room temperature (2 sticks)
- 1/4 cup confectioners' sugar, plus extra for coating cookies
- 1/2 teaspoon lemon oil (or lemon extract)
- 2 cups unbleached all-purpose flour
- 1 cup macadamia nuts, finely chopped
- 1/2 cup sweetened dried cranberries, chopped

In a medium bowl combine the butter and sugar and beat with an electric mixer until fluffy. Stir in the lemon oil. Slowly stir in the flour. Fold in the nuts and cranberries. Remove the bowl from the mixer. Cover with plastic wrap and chill for at least 1 hour (or overnight).

Preheat the oven to 350 degrees. Roll the cookies into 1½-inch balls. Place onto cookie sheets lined with a nonstick liner or parchment paper. Bake until the cookies are golden, about 15 minutes. Roll the cookies in additional confectioners' sugar while still warm. Cool completely on a rack.

CHOCOLATE RICOTTA-FILLED CREPES

Prepare this dish for drop-by guests or a last-minute romantic rendezvous.

Makes 4 servings
Prep Time: 5 minutes

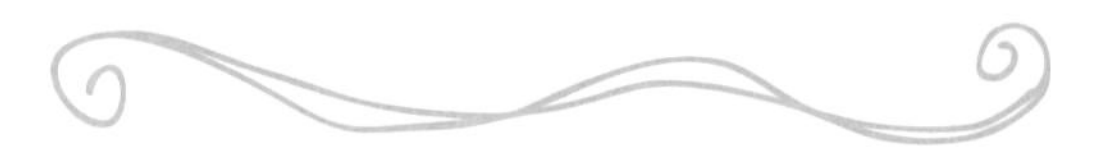

You can find PREPARED crepes in the fresh produce section of your grocery store or in the frozen food department. Better yet, find an extra few minutes on shopping day and prepare you own!

- 1 cup reduced-fat ricotta cheese
- 2 tablespoons unsweetened cocoa powder
- 2 tablespoons honey
- ½ teaspoon vanilla
- 4 prepared crepes
- Fresh raspberries (for garnish)
- Fresh mint leaves (for garnish)

Whisk together the ricotta cheese, cocoa powder, honey, and vanilla until smooth. Top each crepe with one-fourth of this mixture. Fold over the crepe.

To serve, garnish each crepe with fresh raspberries and mint.

Gorgeous Home Spa Secrets . . . for Seeing Clearly

Water retention shows up everywhere on the body, including the sensitive area around the eyes. Whether you're not sure to blame those fat bags and/or dark circles on sodium overload, too much caffeine, or PMS, we can all agree on one thing: the culprit isn't half as interesting as the cure. In addition to getting back into the lovely eyed groove of healthful, balanced eating, how do we banish signs of visible stress, fatigue, and maybe the recent hangover lingering around our eyes? Here's a few easy mix 'em up secrets lurking in the fridge at home. Soon you'll have everyone wondering: Jeepers, peepers, where'd she get those eyes?

Operation De-puff

Puffiness around the eyes is caused by a build-up of toxins or excess fluids. Press gently along the eyebrow and around the eye socket with your middle finger. This will help reduce any swelling by stimulating the lymphatic system. Soothe and de-puff eyes with the following tried-and-true home remedy: egg whites! It's a well-known fact that astringent egg whites tighten pores and reduce puffiness; their high concentration of vitamin B reduces inflammation and promotes circulation. Use your fingers to dab ½ teaspoon of raw egg white on the clean skin around your eye; let it sit and dry for 15 minutes, and then rinse the area well with warm water.

Let There Be Light

To lighten dark circles under your eyes, wrap a grated raw potato in cheesecloth and apply to eyelids for 15–20 minutes. Wipe off the residue and then apply your favorite over-the-counter eye cream; it's a compounded effort, bound to erase evidence of a hard day.

Banishing Crow's-Feet

When it comes to dreaded crow's-feet, grapes are a serious foe. Because they contain twenty known antioxidants that work together against free-radical damage, grapes contain much of the same stuff as your top-priced, touted anti-wrinkle creams. Grapes are brilliant for maintaining your good cholesterol and relaxing blood vessels, both of which can't hurt in the quest for a more youthful face. The antioxidants are concentrated in the grape's skin and seeds, and the more colorful the skin on that grape, the greater the antioxidant punch; that means red and purple grapes and purple grape juice are your best bets.

Grapes for the Face

Just cut a grape in half and gently crush it on your face and neck. Make sure that you get the crow's-feet and the lines around your mouth. Leave it on for 20 minutes or so and rinse with tepid water; then pat dry. Set aside a handful of grapes for topical application on an everyday basis, and before you know it those fine lines will start to diminish! Make sure you supplement this skin regime by drinking plenty of water, aiming for 8 hours of sleep each night, and, in the waking day, filling your grocery cart with foods from Jorj's Glam Kitchen.

Glazier Gaze

Ice really shocks the skin and increases blood circulation. To get the benefits of both, create **frozen eye pads**. Soak gauze pads in herb-and-lemon-infused water. Store in plastic bags in the freezer. In the afternoon before your big night out, lie down on the couch and cover closed eyes with a cold pad. Chill out for 15 minutes or so. Bye-bye, tired eyes.

Farsighted

Would you like to see things with a renewed perspective? Would you like to improve your ability to see the beauty that exists within the blessings all around you? Begin by volunteering with an organization that helps to improve the lives of those less fortunate. Why not check out the local volunteer opportunities for the American Foundation for the Blind (www.afb.org). You can see clearly, now.

CHAPTER 8

smile pretty

"I have witnessed the softening of the hardest of hearts by a simple smile." —Goldie Hawn

Your teeth reveal an intimate part of your personality. Your smile can be a *come-hither* asset . . . or a first-impression liability. A winning smile is more than just cosmetic. Ever heard your grandmother complain that her favorite foods "just don't taste the same" since she got dentures? Since the last thing any of us wants is to relate to those commercials featuring that symbolic string of pearls and *notorious* blueberry pie, you'll want to take care of your teeth *now*, being especially diligent about their upkeep if dental woes run in your family. The healthy but indulgent foods in this chapter go beyond the universal adage that milk is good for your teeth. All dairy contains casein—a protein precipitated from milk that protects your teeth against harmful decay. You're probably wondering how far we can take milk in terms of yummy snacks and entrees; that's why we include a variety of foods that benefit your pearly whites, like whey protein. Whey saves all of dairy's good stuff (essential amino acids) and eliminates the bad (high levels of fat and lactose), leaving you with a sugar-free, reduced-fat dairy product that tastes great in recipes. Also explored in this chapter are the vitamins we need for healthy teeth and gums. We discovered, in our quest, that Carmen Miranda may have unlocked the secret to a gorgeous smile in her edible hat. Vitamins A, E and especially C, along with bioflavonoid, selenium, and zinc are key antioxidants for gum support . . . and they just happen to run rampant in tropical fruits. So get ready to put your mouth on the mend. You'll feel like you're relaxing in the Caribbean once you set the table with these exotic dandies.

Ask Dr. Moon

The doctor is in to answer your questions.

After exploring the beautification processes for skin, hair, and eyes, at last we focus on the mouth, responsible not only for that first encounter with food but for moments of gustatory pleasure counted among the best times in a person's life. For all the positive things a mouth provides—access to gourmet flavor and interchanges ranging from standing O speeches to the merest of smiles— your sensitive mouth can be the source of *much* frustration and discomfort when things go wrong. In other words, your mouth is *much ado about everything*! To avoid teeth and mouth problems, it helps to make preemptive, daily strikes, and to do that, it helps to fully understand the function of the mouth and how to keep it sparkling clean, healthy, and above all, unafraid of your dentist.

Q: What causes tooth sensitivity, and what can be done to prevent it?

A: Tooth sensitivity is caused by the stimulation of cells found beneath the hard enamel. When enamel is worn down or gums have receded, pain can be caused by eating or drinking foods that are too hot or too cold, touching your teeth, or merely exposing them to cold air. Sensitive teeth are one of the most common complaints among dental patients. At least 45 million adults in the United States and 5 million Canadians suffer at some time from sensitive teeth. Tooth sensitivity can act up with extended usage of tartar control toothpaste, so look for American Dental Association approved "desensitizing toothpaste"—effective because its strontium chloride protects the tubules in the teeth that are connected to the nerves. But don't stop there. Other ways to decrease tooth sensitivity are reducing your intake of acid-containing foods, including and especially acidic carbonated beverages like cola, and avoiding using hard-bristled toothbrushes and/or brushing your teeth too hard, which can wear down the tooth's root surface and expose sensitive spots.

Q: Besides checking out the credentials of my dentist, are there other recommendations I should adopt?

A: Yes! The old saying *should* go: "look before you leap . . . into the dentist's chair!" Make sure your dentist has procedural literature (pros and cons) on every treatment, so you have a realistic understanding of its process, the recovery, and results. Also, be sure to "nip in the bud" all those problems (due to neglect) your hygienist admonished you for last time. The American Dental Association recommends that you brush your teeth twice a day with fluoride toothpaste, and flossing once a day as part of that regime is just as paramount. Decay-causing bacteria still linger between teeth where toothbrush bristles can't reach. Flossing removes plaque and food particles from between the teeth and under the gum line. Ideally, you should visit your dentist every six months for a professional cleaning, but once a year is acceptable *if* you brush and floss every day. Unfortunately, genetics or hard-to-floss-between back teeth wreak havoc on even the best intentions, so ask your dentist about dental sealants, a protective plastic coating that can be applied to the chewing surfaces of the back teeth where decay often starts.

Q: What are the pros and cons of cosmetic dentistry procedures?

A: Let's start with one of the most common of these: whitening. There are two main kinds of whitening available in cosmetic dentistry. **Surface whiteners** found in gums and toothpastes only act on surface staining. **Bleachers** physically change the color of your teeth. Simple in-office chemical bleaching, for example, only costs a few hundred dollars, and laser bleaching runs about one thousand dollars.

Another popular dental procedure for a "brighter smile" is **bonding**—an excellent way to repair chipped teeth or fill in large gaps between teeth. Here's how it works: a tooth doesn't grow back by itself, so it's necessary to replace any missing portions of a tooth with a composite resin. These resins are a paste to begin with, so they can be shaped and colored to look like the rest of the tooth. Once exposed to a certain wavelength of light, the resin hardens into a permanent, but thankfully natural-looking, plastic.

Here's another procedure that's thrown around dentists' offices quite a lot: **veneers**. They're another approach to enhancing the look of your teeth. They are a thin shell made of acrylic or porcelain that is cemented to the front of the tooth. A veneer can cover up stains, chips, and large gaps. Individual veneers range between $700 and $1500 per tooth, so a whole mouth restoration can run into the five-figure range.

There is also a procedure known as the **smile lift**—which builds the tips (of the sides of the teeth) out to support the lips; this results in the pink part of the lip (called the "vermillion border") rolling up, making the lip appear fuller—an interesting alternative to collagen injections in the lip itself.

Q: Are cavities preventable?

A: This question is a no-brainer. Cavities are the most common *but* preventable oral health problem in the US today. Over 50 percent of children and 95 percent of adults have one or more cavities, which are caused when the bacteria on the tooth's surface convert sugar into acid that eats away at the surface.

Q: How does sugar affect our teeth and gums?

A: First, understand that there are different kinds of sugar; some types are detrimental to your teeth, whereas others pose little threat. The carbohydrate sucrose is most harmful because oral bacteria (already in your mouth), convert sucrose into dental plaque faster than any other type of sugar. Lactose (milk sugar), by contrast, is less harmful. The form and frequency of carbohydrate-containing foods also influence plaque formation and the potential to create cavities. The longer the teeth are exposed to the sugar-containing food, the more opportunity the bacteria have to do damage. Sugar in a sticky form (dried fruit, toffee) and eaten frequently is more harmful than sugar that is rapidly cleared from the mouth, like milk.

Q: What threatens a sparkling, clean mouthful of teeth?

A: Soda can be your teeth's worse enemy. The acid in soft drinks can erode the tooth's enamel and cause cavities. If you must drink soda, try sugar-free or use a straw. A straw allows less sugary, tooth-staining liquids to reach your front teeth. Coffee and teas are no friend of teeth either; they can stain a naturally white smile. The heat from the coffee can also cause small fractures in your teeth's surfaces. Try drinking cooler coffee and use a straw or brush your teeth after drinking coffee or tea. But we have yet to reveal the worst foe of all . . . drum roll please . . . *smoking*! Smoking will cause a build up on teeth that results, eventually, in yellow to orange colored staining; these stains can take longer to lighten than color damage caused by the other culprits.

Q: How does aging affect the appearance of the mouth?

A: As we age, the perioral area surrounding the mouth develops fine lines at the corner. Your lips may appear thinner due to the underlying contraction of muscles.

Q: What is the relationship between dairy food and a great smile?

A: Milk and cheese have been proven to protect teeth against harmful decay. Their casein (a protein precipitated from milk) decreases bacteria's ability to stick to teeth. Because of milk's ability to buffer oral acids, remineralization of tooth enamel is possible. If you like your milk sweet, take heart in the fact that chocolate milk causes fewer cavities than other sucrose-containing liquids.

Q: Is there a tooth-loving beverage that has all of milk's good things but less of its bad, like fat and lactose?

A: Yes, and it's called whey protein. You can find it in any health food store or organic supermarket where it is sold as a powder. Simply mix it with water and treat it as you would an ordinary serving of milk. From a nutritional perspective, whey protein isolates are complete and high-quality; they originate from cows' milk and provide the body with all of the essential amino acids it requires. Whey protein isolates contain more than 90 percent protein on a dry weight basis with negligible amounts of fat, lactose, and minerals. The low levels of fat and lactose in whey protein isolates make them ideal ingredients for formulating sugar-free, low-fat, or fat-free dairy foods.

Q: Are there particular vitamins that we need for our gums?

A: Yes, and the biggest helping of these vitamins can be found in a bowl of tropical fruit. Your gums are the tooth's support system and must *never* be neglected. Recent studies suggest that even minor vitamin C deficiencies may increase the risk of serious gum disease. Vitamins A and E, bioflavonoids, selenium, and zinc are key antioxidants for nutritional support for the gums and run deliciously rampant in tropical fruits.

Jorj's Smile Pretty Glam Kitchen

Start building a better smile today by making sure you include plenty of dairy and fruit in your everyday diet. Oh, and drink your favorite carbonated and caffeinated beverages through a straw—your teeth's prelude to pearly!

Milk Maids

Given the benefits of dairy, one has to wonder if the residents of Wisconsin have thousand-watt smiles that can be seen from outer space. Milk proteins phosphopeptide (quite a mouthful!) and kappa casein help fight decay and prevent the formation of plaque. Cheeses like **Swiss**, **Cheddar**, **Monterey Jack**, **edam**, **gouda**, **Muenster**, **mozzarella**, and **American** processed protect against root cavities by stimulating saliva flow and strengthening your enamel.

Whey Cool

Whey protein is an excellent choice for all women who value health and beauty. As defined earlier in the chapter, it's a protein isolate—the purest form available—and unsurpassed as a source of the essential amino acids required in the daily diet. Let us never forget that essential amino acids are the building blocks for all healthy body tissue, including muscles, skin, and nails. Since whey protein delivers all of that, *plus* tooth-loving calcium and casein, without the fat and calories found in cheese and milk, it's an attractive option in the vast world of nutrition. Look for your whey protein powder in a GNC or Whole Foods Market. Use as a supplement or slip some into your tropical smoothies.

Hot Tropic

Guavas, **mangos**, **papayas**, **coconuts**, **bananas,** and **avocados** rival other fruits for top honors in the fiber and phytochemicals department, not to mention for vitamins and minerals that benefit, especially, your gums—the support system for your teeth. Ingesting the proper amount of vitamin C can get awfully boring if it appears in the diet as orange juice alone, so start cooking with a hint of tropical island flair . . . the recipes to come will show you how.

Start Your Day

Main Plates

On the Side

Snacks & Sweets

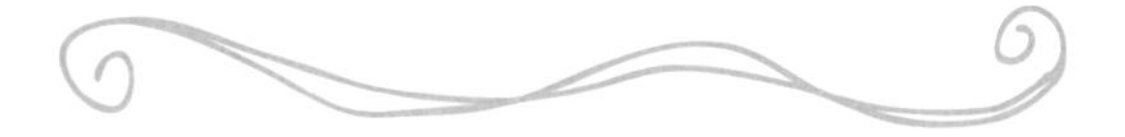

SPICY ROASTED VEGGIE AND SHRIMP SALSA

With Fried Egg and Warm Cheese Sauce

The combination of protein-rich shrimp and good-for-you veggies gets your day off to a terrific start. The sauce has just enough dairy to bring out that sly smile.

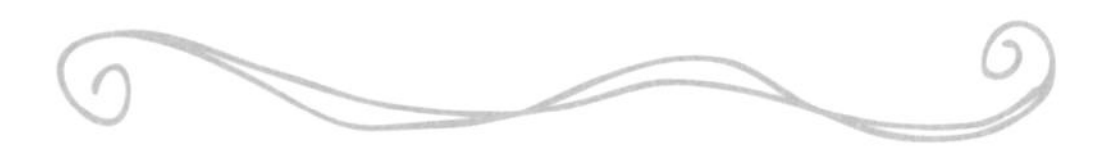

Really pour on the GOOD-FOR-YOU aspect of this dish by adding a few slices of GUAVA to each plate as a garnish.

Preheat the oven to 450 degrees. Place the tomatoes, red onion, jalapeño peppers, and garlic cloves onto a rimmed baking sheet that has been coated with vegetable oil spray. Toss with paprika, salt, and pepper and drizzle with 2 tablespoons olive oil. Roast the veggies until they begin to char, about 10 minutes. Remove from the oven and cool to room temperature. Chop the tomatoes and red onions to about ½-inch pieces. Finely dice the jalapeno peppers and thinly slice the garlic.

Place the chopped shrimp, green onions, and oregano into a bowl. Sprinkle with lime juice. Add in the chopped veggies. Mix together and season with salt and pepper.

Heat the butter and flour in a pan over medium heat. Pour in the milk and stir until thickened, about 4 to 5 minutes. Stir in the cheese and season with nutmeg, salt, and pepper.

Crack the eggs into a large skillet that has been coated with vegetable oil spray. Cook over medium heat until the whites are opaque and the yolk is still runny, about 4–5 minutes.

To serve, divide the salsa among 4 plates. Top each serving with a fried egg. Drizzle the cheese sauce over top.

On Shopping Day: Roast the veggies, cool to room temperature, and store in an airtight container in the refrigerator for up to 3 days.

Makes 4 servings
Prep Time: 20 minutes
Cook Time: 10 minutes

For the salsa

- 6 medium plum tomatoes, cut in half lengthwise (about 1 pound)
- 1 large red onion, peeled and cut into 8 wedges (about 1 cup)
- 2 medium jalapeno peppers, seeded and halved
- 4 medium garlic cloves, peeled
- 1 teaspoon paprika
- Salt and freshly ground pepper
- 2 tablespoons olive oil
- 1 pound cooked baby shrimp, chopped
- 4 green onions, thinly sliced (about ¼ cup)
- 3 tablespoons chopped fresh oregano
- Juice of 1 medium lime (about 1 tablespoon)

For the sauce

- 1 tablespoon butter
- 1 tablespoon unbleached all-purpose flour
- 1 cup reduced-fat milk
- 2 ounces grated American cheese (about ½ cup)
- ½ teaspoon nutmeg
- 4 large eggs

FRESH PAPAYA AND GRAPEFRUIT

With Yogurt and Mint

This simple assembly of fresh ingredients is an effortless way to start your day off with a smile.

Makes 2 servings
Prep Time: 5 minutes

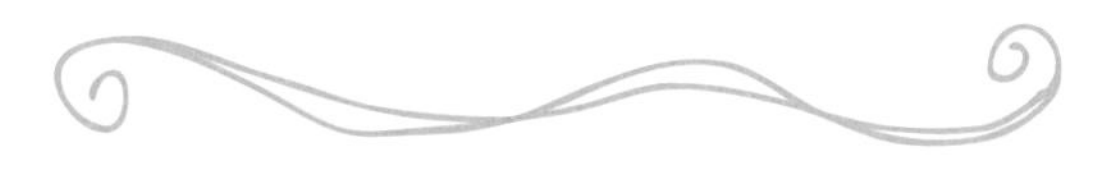

1 medium papaya, peeled, seeded, and sliced (about 1 cup)
1 red grapefruit, peeled, cut into segments
1 cup reduced-fat vanilla yogurt
1 tablespoon chopped fresh mint

To serve, divide the fruit onto 2 plates. Spoon the yogurt alongside. Sprinkle with fresh mint.

COCONUT TROPICAL SMOOTHIES

This grab-'n-go breakfast is a perfect start for your busy day.

Makes 2 servings
Prep Time: 10 minutes

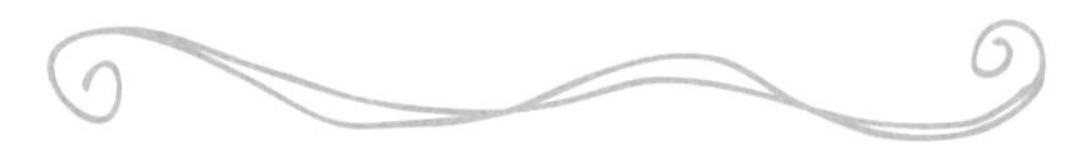

Use ANY and ALL of your FAVORITE fruits to make your perfect everyday smoothie. These are a great opportunity to add some WHEY to start your day!

- 1 large ripe mango, pitted, peeled and diced (about 1 cup)
- 1 cup fresh pineapple, cut into 1-inch cubes
- 1 cup white grape juice
- 1 cup vanilla flavored reduced-fat yogurt
- 3 tablespoons shredded fresh coconut (for garnish)

Place all of the ingredients into a blender. Add 2 cups ice cubes. Pulse until smooth.

To serve, pour the smoothie into 2 glasses. Garnish with coconut.

On Shopping Day: Prepare the fruit. Store in an airtight container for up to 4 days.

OATMEAL WITH CARAMELIZED FRUIT TOPPING

This is not your Grandma's raisin cereal. This one will keep you coming back for more and more!

Makes 2 servings
Prep Time: 10 minutes
Cook Time: 5 minutes

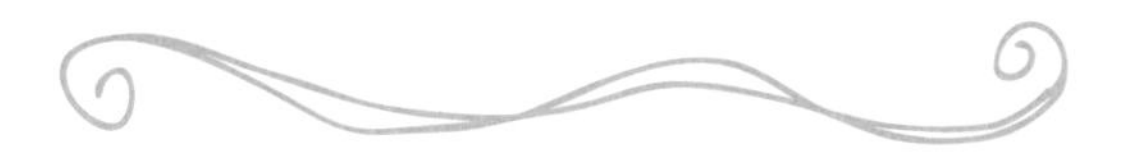

1 cup old-fashioned rolled oats
2 tablespoons unsalted butter
2 tablespoons light brown sugar
1 ripe banana, peeled and cut into 1/2-inch rounds
1 ripe peach, pitted and sliced into wedges
2 tablespoons half and half

Cook the oatmeal according to the directions on the package.

Heat the butter in a skillet over medium heat. Stir in the sugar until dissolved. Add the fruit and toss to coat. Simmer for 2 minutes.

To serve, divide the oatmeal into 2 shallow bowls. Arrange the fruit over top. Pour 1 tablespoon half and half on top of each serving.

BUFFALO CHICKEN COBB SALAD

With Buttermilk Dressing

I used flavors from my favorite snack (Buffalo wings with blue cheese dressing) to create this full-meal salad. Use your favorite snack food as an inspiration for the family's next dinner-time salad.

Makes 6 servings
Prep Time: 30 minutes
Cook Time: 10 minutes

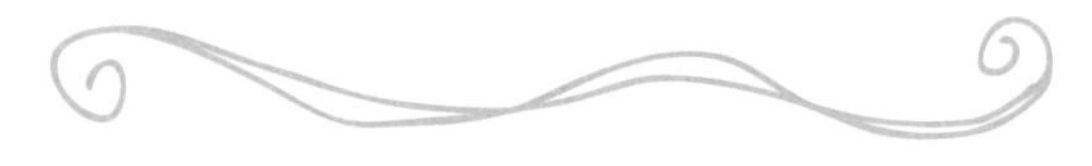

Drizzle the avocado with a little bit of LEMON (or lime) juice to prevent browning while you gather everyone around the table.

For the dressing

- 1/2 cup reduced-fat mayonnaise
- 1/2 cup buttermilk
- 1/3 cup white wine vinegar
- 4 green onions, thinly sliced (about 1/4 cup)
- Salt and freshly ground pepper

For the chicken

- 1 tablespoon olive oil
- 1 tablespoon butter
- 2 large (6- to 8-ounce) skinless, boneless chicken breast halves, cut into 1-inch pieces (about 3 cups)
- 4–6 drops hot pepper sauce

For the salad

- 1 medium head romaine lettuce, washed, dried, and torn (about 6 cups)
- 6 medium plum tomatoes, cut in half lengthwise (about 1 pound)
- 1 large avocado, peeled, pitted, and sliced (about 1 cup)
- 8 ounces bacon, cooked, drained, and crumbled
- 4 ounces Gorgonzola cheese, crumbled (about 1 cup)
- 4 medium celery ribs, sliced (about 1 cup)

Whisk together the mayonnaise, buttermilk, and vinegar until smooth. Stir in the green onions. Season with salt and pepper.

Heat the olive oil and butter in a skillet over medium-high heat. Cook the chicken in the skillet until just golden. Add hot sauce and season with salt and pepper. Use a slotted spoon to remove the chicken and drain on paper towels.

Arrange the lettuce onto a large platter. Top one section with tomatoes. Place the avocado next to the tomatoes, followed by the bacon, cheese, celery, and chicken.

To serve, drizzle the dressing over the salad and season with additional ground pepper.

On Shopping Day: Prepare the salad dressing and store in an airtight container in the refrigerator for up to 4 days.

TURKEY WITH CARAMELIZED ONION AND SMOKED GOUDA PANINI

If you were a kid who just couldn't get enough grilled cheese sandwiches, then this dish is for you!

Makes 4 servings
Prep Time: 10 minutes
Cook Time: 8 minutes per sandwich

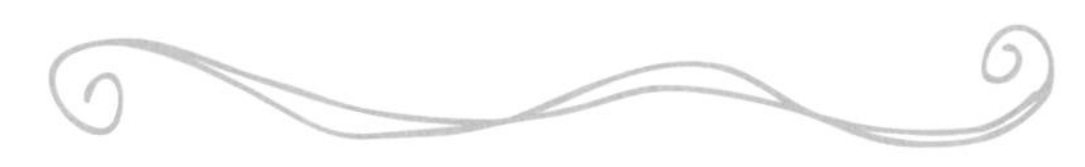

If you don't have a panini grill, use a grill pan, griddle, or skillet. PRESS down on the sandwich, WEIGHING it down with a large can of tomatoes or a skillet lid, and turn once.

For the caramelized onions

- 1 tablespoon olive oil
- 1 tablespoon butter
- 1 large red onion, peeled and thinly sliced (about 1 cup)
- 1 tablespoon balsamic vinegar
- Salt and freshly ground pepper

For the sandwiches

- 8 slices thick crusty whole grain bread
- 4 tablespoons Dijon mustard
- 3/4 pound roasted turkey, cut into 12 slices
- 1 cup frisée leaves
- 8 ounces smoked gouda cheese, cut into slices
- 2 tablespoons olive oil

Heat 1 tablespoon olive oil and butter (in a skillet) over medium-high heat. Cook the onion in the skillet until soft and brown. Stir in the balsamic vinegar and cook until the onion is syrupy. Season with salt and pepper. Remove from the heat.

Lay the bread slices onto your work surface. Brush with Dijon mustard. Layer four slices with caramelized onions, turkey, frisée, and cheese. Top with the remaining bread slices.

Heat a panini grill to medium-high heat. Brush the sandwiches with 2 tablespoons olive oil. Grill until both sides are golden and the cheese is melted, about 8 minutes.

To serve, cut each sandwich in half and serve warm.

On Shopping Day: Prepare the onions, cool to room temperature, store in an airtight container in the refrigerator for up to 4 days.

SEARED JUMBO SCALLOPS WITH HERBED BUTTER SAUCE

This is the purrfect *dish to serve for one or two; accompany it with a green salad and a crisp glass of pinot grigio!*

Makes 2 servings
Prep Time: 5 minutes
Cook Time: 10 minutes

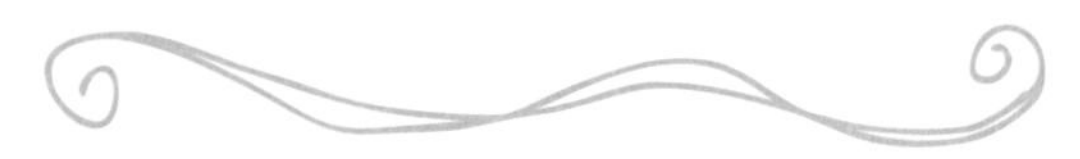

This dish is also perfect as a FIRST COURSE for your next dinner party. Allow two LARGE scallops per guest.

For the scallops

- 8 large sea scallops (about 3/4 pound)
- 1 tablespoon olive oil
- 1 tablespoon unsalted butter
- Salt and freshly ground pepper

For the sauce

- 3 tablespoons unsalted butter, divided use
- 1 large shallot, minced (about 1 tablespoon)
- 1/4 cup dry sherry
- 2 tablespoons chopped fresh dill
- 2 tablespoons chopped fresh tarragon
- Zest of 1/2 small lime (about 1/2 teaspoon)

Pat the scallops with paper towels to avoid excess moisture. Heat the olive oil and butter in a skillet over medium-high heat. Season scallops with salt and pepper. Place into the skillet. Shake the pan gently to prevent sticking. Cook until one side is golden brown and almost crisp, about 4 minutes. Use tongs to turn the scallops over and cook until the second side is golden, about 4 minutes more. Remove the scallops to a platter and keep warm. The scallops will continue cooking as they rest on the platter.

Reduce the heat to medium. Place 1 tablespoon butter into the skillet. Add the shallot and cook until soft, about 2 minutes. Pour in the sherry and stir in the dill and tarragon. Whisk in the lime zest and the remaining 2 tablespoons of butter. Reduce the heat to low. Add the scallops back into the skillet and bathe them in the warm sauce.

To serve, divide the scallops onto 2 plates. Pour the remaining sauce from the pan around the shallots. Garnish with freshly ground pepper.

DOUBLE-CHEESE AND SAUSAGE CALZONE

With Marinara Dipping Sauce

Get a head start on this dish by using refrigerated pizza dough. Another great shortcut is to stop by your local pizzeria. They will surely be happy to sell you pizza dough that you can bake at home.

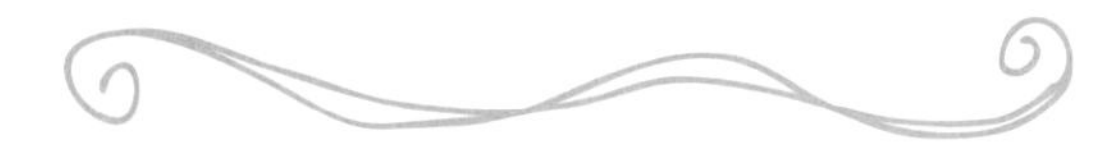

This is a great recipe to use with a PIZZA or BAKING STONE. Warm the stone in the oven and transfer the calzone by wooden paddle to bake on the stone. You will *love* the results.

* * *

Prepare MARINARA SAUCE by sautéing onion and garlic in olive oil. Add good-quality canned tomatoes, fresh BASIL, and a hint of SUGAR. Simmer and season with salt and pepper. How simple is that?!

Heat the olive oil in a skillet over medium-high heat. Cook the onion until soft. Add the sausage and cook until browned. Season with salt and pepper. Drain off any excess liquid. Cool to room temperature.

Preheat the oven to 425 degrees. Mix together the mozzarella and Fontina cheese in a bowl. Stir in the basil, red bell peppers, and sausage mixture.

Unroll the dough onto a rimmed baking sheet. Spoon the sausage mixture, crosswise, onto the lower half of the dough. Fold upper half of dough over top. Crimp the edges together. Fold in the corner to form a semicircle. Brush with olive oil. Bake until the calzone is puffed and golden, about 15–18 minutes.

To serve, cut into 4 slices. Serve with warm marinara sauce for dunking.

On Shopping Day: Prepare homemade marinara sauce, store in an airtight container in the refrigerator for up to 1 week or in the freezer for up to 1 month.

Makes 4 servings
Prep Time: 20 minutes
Cook Time: 15 to 18 minutes

1 tablespoon olive oil
1 small red onion, peeled and diced (about 1/2 cup)
8 ounces mild Italian sausage, crumbled
Salt and freshly ground pepper
4 ounces shredded fresh mozzarella cheese (about 1 cup)
4 ounces Fontina cheese, shredded (about 1 cup)
2 tablespoons chopped fresh basil
2 large roasted red bell peppers from jar, drained and diced
1 14-ounce tube refrigerated pizza dough (or make your own, if you prefer)
1 tablespoon olive oil
1 cup prepared marinara sauce

CRISPY ROASTED CHICKEN

With Penne Pasta

By using the pan drippings from the chicken, you have the beginnings of a flavorful pasta sauce. I like olives and tomatoes with penne, but you can choose your favorite veggies and pasta to create your own signature dish!

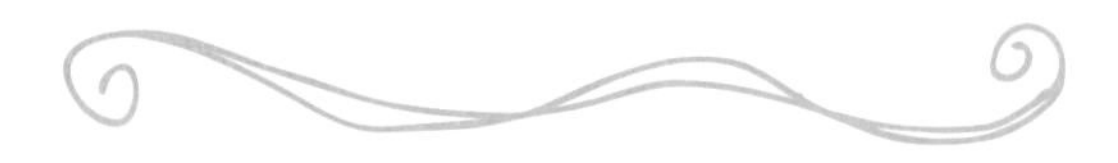

More and more FRESH PASTA and whole wheat products are available in your market. Read the package labels to find those that best fit into your gorgeous lifestyle plan.

* * *

Fewer than eight at your table?
This is a wonderful COOK-ONCE-AND-EAT-TWICE recipe. Use the second chicken for chicken salad, chicken fajitas, or chicken quesadillas. Bake the extra pasta (with the addition of a couple eggs) into a crispy pasta pie. Cut into wedges and serve with a fresh green salad for a grab-and-go lunch.

Remove the backbones from the chicken using poultry sheers or a sharp knife. Place into a shallow dish. Add the garlic, olive oil, and lemon juice. Use your hands to coat both sides of the chickens. Cover and marinate at least 1 hour or as long as overnight.

Preheat the oven to 450 degrees. Remove the chickens from the marinade. Place onto a broiler pan, skin-side up. Season with red pepper flakes, paprika, salt, and pepper. Place the rosemary sprigs alongside the chicken. Roast for 30 minutes or until the chickens are mostly cooked. Remove from the oven and change the temperature to broil.

Place the tomatoes, onions, and olives into a bowl. Drizzle with 1 tablespoon olive oil. Season with salt and pepper and toss. Place the veggies around the chicken. Return to the oven and broil until the skin is crispy and the veggies are charred, about 10–15 minutes more. Remove from the oven and check the chickens for doneness by inserting a fork into the thickest part. If the juices run clear, the chicken is done. (You can also insert a meat thermometer, which should read 165–170 degrees.)

Meanwhile, bring a large pot of water to a boil. Add salt and cook the pasta until al dente. Drain, reserving 2 cups of the pasta water.

Place the chicken onto a cutting board to rest. Place the broiler pan with the vegetables and juices onto the stovetop over medium heat. Add the pasta. Add 1 cup reserved pasta water. Toss to combine. (If the pasta is too dry, add additional pasta water.) Add the parsley, toss. Sprinkle with Parmesan cheese.

To serve, carve each chicken into pieces (2 breast halves with wings, 2 leg/thigh portions). Serve the chicken with the pasta.

Makes 8 servings
Prep Time: 10 minutes, marinate for at least 1 hour
Cook Time: 45 minutes

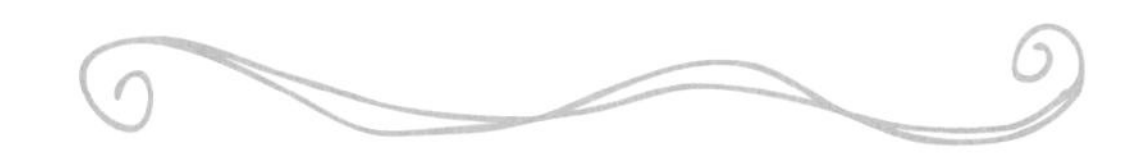

For the chicken

- 2 3 1/2-pound chickens, rinsed and patted dry
- 1 head garlic, cloves peeled and crushed
- 1/2 cup olive oil
- Juice of 2 medium lemons (about 1/4 cup)
- 1/2 teaspoon crushed red pepper
- 1 tablespoon paprika
- Salt and freshly ground pepper
- 4 sprigs rosemary

For the pasta

- 1 pint ripe cherry tomatoes or mixed baby tomatoes
- 1 bunch (6–8) green onions, thinly sliced on the diagonal (about 1/2 cup)
- 1 1/2 cups pitted black olives
- 1 tablespoon olive oil
- 1 pound penne pasta
- 3 tablespoons chopped fresh parsley
- 2 ounces finely grated Parmesan cheese (about 1/2 cup)

CHICKEN WITH BEL PAESE, PROSCIUTTO, AND CAPERS

With White Wine Pan Sauce

Creamy, melting cheese meets salty prosciutto and capers atop chicken breasts in this versatile dish—elegant enough for Saturday night's company or just plain delicious enough for Tuesday's simple supper.

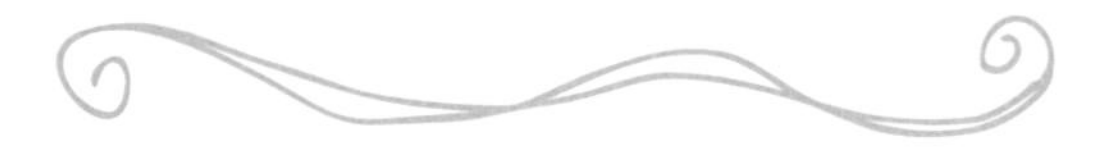

Bel Paese cheese comes from the LOMBARDY region of Italy. It is a modern, creamy, semisoft cheese and has a light, milky AROMA. The name means "beautiful land." It is available in major grocery stores and specialty Italian markets. You can SUBSTITUTE with FRESH MOZZARELLA.

Makes 4 servings
Prep Time: 20 minutes
Cook Time: 10 minutes

- 4 4- to 5-ounce skinless, boneless chicken breast cutlets
- Salt and freshly ground pepper
- 1/4 cup unbleached all-purpose flour
- 2 tablespoons olive oil
- 4 ounces Bel Paese cheese
- 4 ounces prosciutto, thinly sliced
- 1 cup dry white wine
- 2 tablespoons capers, drained and rinsed
- 2 tablespoons chopped fresh sage (plus garnish)
- 2 tablespoons unsalted butter

Use a meat mallet to pound the chicken cutlets to 1/4-inch thickness. Season with salt and pepper. Dredge in flour, shaking off excess.

Preheat the oven to 375 degrees. Heat olive oil in a skillet over medium-high heat. Add the chicken breasts and cook until golden, about 3 minutes; turn and cook the other side until golden, about 2 minutes more. Transfer to a rimmed baking sheet. Top the chicken with slices of cheese and prosciutto. Roast the chicken in the oven until cooked through, about 5 minutes.

Pour the wine into the skillet, stirring to remove brown bits. Stir in capers and fresh sage. Simmer until the sauce reduces to about ⅔ cup. Remove the skillet from the heat. Stir in the butter and season with salt and pepper.

To serve, place the chicken breasts onto a platter. Pour the pan sauce over top. Garnish with fresh sage leaves.

GRILLED SWORDFISH STEAKS

With Hot Papaya Relish and Herbed Compound Butter

Fresh grilled fish is enhanced with rich, melting butter and a zippy relish in this surprisingly enticing dish.

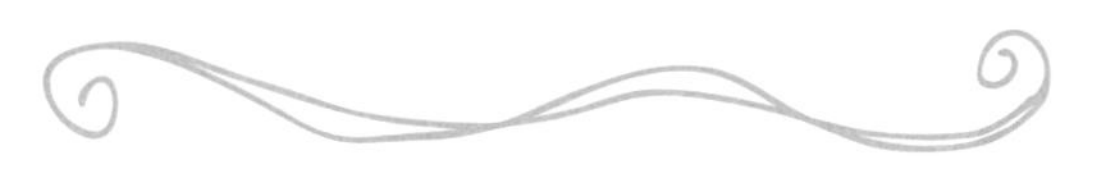

Create your own FLAVORED BUTTER with your favorite herbs, spices, and fruit.

Mash the garlic with the blade of a knife. Sprinkle with ½ teaspoon salt. Continue to mash until the garlic becomes a paste. Place into a medium bowl. Whisk in the rice wine vinegar, sugar, and hot pepper sauce. Toss the sauce with the papaya, red onion, and cilantro. Season with pepper. Chill.

Place the butter into the bowl of a food processor. Pulse until smooth. Add the parsley and Worcestershire sauce. Season with salt and pepper. Pulse until just combined. Transfer the butter to a sheet of waxed paper. Roll into a 2-inch log. Refrigerate for at least 1 hour or for several days.

Heat a grill pan over medium-high heat. Drizzle the swordfish steaks with olive oil and lime juice. Season with salt and pepper. Grill until just opaque in the center, about 4 minutes per side.

To serve, cut 4 (¼-inch) round slices of the butter from the log. Top each swordfish steak with 1 slice butter. Spoon 1 tablespoon relish on the side.

On Shopping Day: Prepare the relish and herbed butter. Store separately in airtight containers for up to 4 days. You may freeze extra butter for up to 1 month. Thaw in the refrigerator before slicing.

Makes 4 servings (reserving about half of the butter for later use)
Prep Time: 20 minutes plus chilling
Cook Time: 8 minutes

For the relish

- 2 medium cloves garlic, minced (about 1 teaspoon)
- ½ teaspoon salt
- 3 tablespoons rice wine vinegar
- 2 teaspoons natural sugar
- 6–8 drops hot pepper sauce
- 1 medium papaya, peeled, seeded, finely diced (about 1 cup)
- 1 small red onion, peeled and thinly sliced (about ½ cup)
- 3 tablespoons chopped fresh cilantro
- Freshly ground pepper

For the herbed butter

- ½ cup unsalted butter, room temperature (1 stick)
- 1 tablespoon fresh parsley, finely chopped
- 1 teaspoon Worcestershire sauce

For the swordfish

- 4 6-ounce swordfish steaks, about 1½-inch thick
- 1 tablespoon olive oil
- Juice of 1 medium lime (about 1 tablespoon)

LEMON VEAL

With Sautéed Spinach, Pine Nuts, and Goat Cheese

Lemony veal melts in your mouth. The tart spinach is combined with smooth cheese and a nutty crunch; this blend of flavors makes a satisfying yet easy mid-week meal.

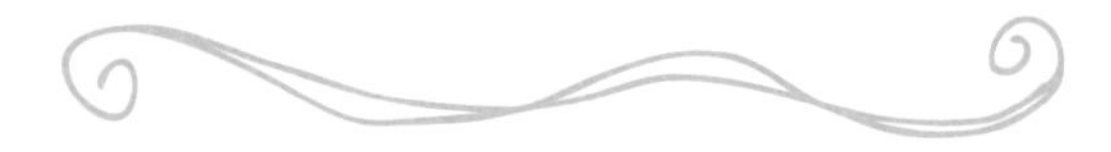

Veal scaloppini are thin CUTLETS of veal. If they are not readily available in your grocery store, ask the butcher to prepare them for you.

* * *

Toast PINE NUTS by placing them on a rimmed baking sheet. Bake at 350 degrees until they just begin to turn golden, about 5 minutes. Watch carefully so they do not burn.

Use a meat mallet to pound the veal cutlets (between sheets of waxed paper) to ¼-inch thickness. Season with salt and pepper and dredge in flour, shaking off the excess. Heat 2 tablespoons olive oil in a skillet over medium-high heat. Place the veal cutlets into the skillet. Squeeze lemon juice over top. Cook until golden, about 2 minutes. Turn, squeeze lemon juice and cook until golden, about 2 minutes more. Use additional oil if needed to cook all of the veal. Use a slotted spoon to remove the veal to a platter. Keep warm.

Heat 1 more tablespoon olive oil in the skillet. Add the onion and cook until just beginning to brown, about 5 minutes. Add the spinach and cook until wilted, about 2 minutes. Stir in the sherry vinegar. Season with salt and pepper. Remove from the heat.

To serve, toss the spinach with pine nuts and goat cheese. Mound the spinach mixture on top of the veal. Garnish with lemon wedges.

Makes 4 servings
Prep Time: 15 minutes
Cook Time: 10 minutes

For the veal

1 pound veal scaloppini
Salt and freshly ground pepper
2 tablespoons unbleached all-purpose flour
2 tablespoons olive oil
Juice of 1 medium lemon (about 2 tablespoons)

For the spinach

1 tablespoon olive oil
1 large red onion, peeled and thinly sliced (about 1 cup)
6 ounces fresh spinach leaves, washed, dried, and torn (about 4 cups)
2 tablespoons sherry vinegar
½ cup pine nuts, toasted
1 ounce goat cheese, crumbled (about ¼ cup)
Lemon wedges (for garnish)

SHRIMP SALAD

With Mango and Cucumber

Prepare this light dish on a warm summer night or for your next all-girl luncheon.

Makes 6 servings
Prep Time: 20 minutes

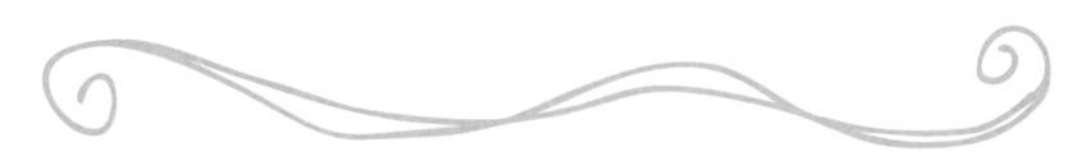

Save some DOLLARS by purchasing frozen shrimp. Thaw by placing the shrimp under running water. Plunge them into a pot of boiling water until just opaque. Rinse under cold water, drain, and chill in the refrigerator. The extra steps will save you some BIG BUCKS!

For the salad dressing

- 3 tablespoons champagne vinegar
- 2 tablespoons natural sugar
- 1/3 cup Dijon mustard
- 1/3 cup mayonnaise
- Salt and freshly ground pepper

For the salad

- 2 large cucumbers, peeled, seeded, and diced (about 2 cups)
- 1 large mango, pitted, peeled, and diced (about 1 cup)
- 1 pound cooked medium shrimp
- 2 tablespoons chopped fresh dill
- 4 cups mesclun lettuce mix

Whisk the vinegar and sugar together in a small bowl until the sugar dissolves. Whisk in the mustard and mayonnaise. Season with salt and pepper. Cover and chill in the refrigerator.

In a large bowl toss together the cucumbers, mango, shrimp, and dill. Pour all but 1 tablespoon dressing over top. Season with salt and pepper and toss again. Toss the mesclun leaves with the remaining dressing.

To serve, divide the lettuce among 4 plates. Top each with one-fourth of the salad.

On Shopping Day: Make the salad dressing and store in an airtight container in the refrigerator for up to 4 days.

SWISS CHEESE WAFERS

You can make this dough in advance, slicing off just what you need for guests; or you can bake all of the wafers, cool, and store in an airtight container for afternoon treats.

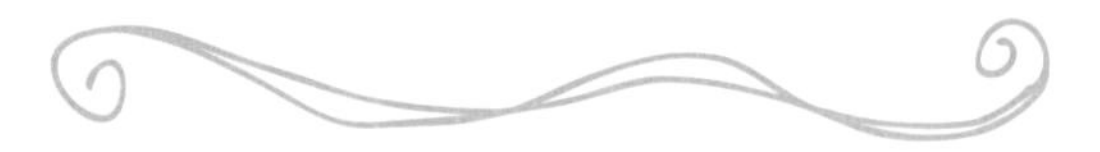

Serve these spicy wafers with a sweet jam for an irresistible SWEET and HOT taste combo. They go well with Cherry Ginger Chutney on page 389.

Makes about 3 dozen wafers
Prep Time: 10 minutes
Cook Time: 18 minutes

1 cup unbleached all-purpose flour
½ teaspoon salt
¼ teaspoon ground cayenne pepper
8 ounces grated Swiss cheese (about 2 cups)
½ cup butter, room temperature (1 stick), cut into pieces

Place the flour, salt, and cayenne pepper into the bowl of a food processor. Pulse to combine. Add the cheese and butter. Pulse to form dough. Transfer the dough to a sheet of waxed paper. Roll into a log about 2 inches in diameter. Refrigerate until chilled, at least 2 hours.

Preheat the oven to 400 degrees. Cut the log into ¼-inch slices and arrange on baking sheets lined with parchment paper (or a non-stick liner). Bake until golden, about 16–18 minutes. Transfer to a rack to cool.

BLUE CHEESE DIP

With All Kinds of Dippers

If blue cheese is not on hand, no worries! You can use any type of cheese for this quick dip. The food processor does all of the work. You need only arrange the dippers.

Makes 6 servings
Prep Time: 5 minutes

- 6 ounces blue cheese, crumbled (about 3/4 cup)
- 1/4 cup ricotta cheese
- 1 tablespoon balsamic vinegar
- 2 tablespoons olive oil
- Salt and freshly ground pepper
- Carrot slices
- Celery sticks
- Endive leaves
- Breadsticks
- Granny Smith apple wedges
- Candied spice nuts
- Swiss Cheese Wafers (see recipe on pg. 160)

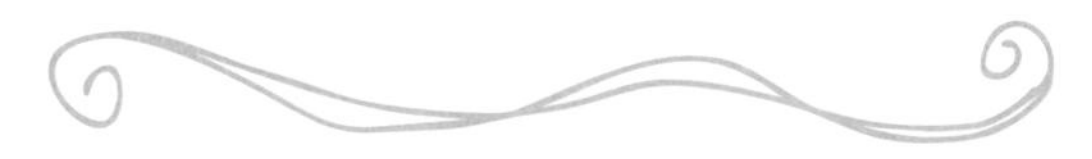

Be creative with the VEGGIES that you offer as well as the WAY you offer them. Cut radishes into FLOWERS and cauliflower florets into SLICES. Serve with grilled Portobello mushroom slices and blanched green beans. Choose whatever you find fresh in the market.

Place the blue cheese, ricotta, vinegar, and olive oil into the bowl of a food processor. Pulse to combine. Season with salt and pepper. Spoon into a serving dish.

To serve, surround the dip with your favorite veggies and breadsticks.

On Shopping Day: Prepare the veggies for the dish and store separately in airtight containers. Prepare the dip and store in an airtight container. Refrigerate both the dip and the veggies for up to 4 days.

ARTICHOKE AND ASIAGO CROSTINI

Prepare the components of this easy snack on shopping day, and it will come together in just minutes.

Makes 4 servings
Prep Time: 20 minutes
Cook Time: 10 minutes

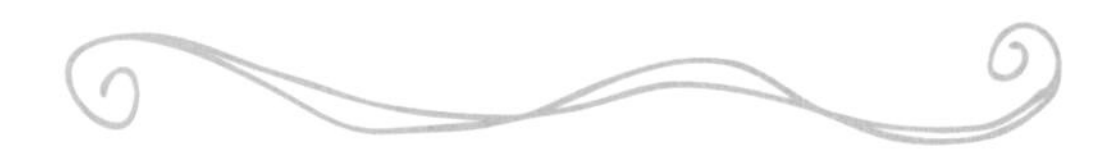

ASIAGO cheese is available in large grocery stores or specialty markets. It is strong and salty. Feel free to substitute with Parmesan if you prefer.

* * *

These are great HEATED and served WARM as well.

For the crostini

- 8 ¼-inch-thick slices French bread baguette
- 2 tablespoons olive oil
- ½ teaspoon ground garlic powder

For the topping

- 1 6.5-ounce can artichoke hearts, drained and chopped
- ¼ cup minced oil-packed sun-dried tomatoes, drained
- 2 ounces finely grated Asiago cheese (about ½ cup)
- 1 tablespoon chopped fresh basil
- 1 tablespoon olive oil
- Freshly ground pepper

Preheat the oven to 350 degrees. Diagonally slice the baguette and place the bread slices onto a baking sheet. In a small bowl mix together 2 tablespoons olive oil and garlic powder. Brush both sides of the bread with oil mixture. Bake until the tops are golden, about 4 minutes. Turn and bake the other side until golden, about another 4 minutes. Cool to room temperature.

Mix together the artichokes, sun-dried tomatoes, Asiago, and fresh basil in a small bowl.

To serve, divide the artichoke mixture onto each crostini. Drizzle with the 1 tablespoon olive oil and garnish with fresh ground pepper.

On Shopping Day: Prepare the crostini and store in an airtight container for up to 3 days. Prepare the artichoke topping; store in an airtight container in the refrigerator for up to 3 days.

Orange and Tarragon–Infused Crème Brûlées

With Sliced Bananas

This dessert is a showstopper—especially *on a Tuesday night!*

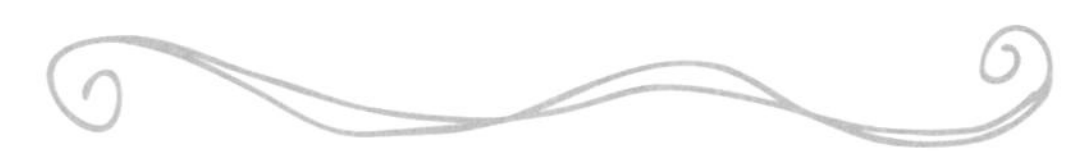

If you don't have a kitchen blow torch, preheat the oven on the BROILER setting. Carefully place the ramekins onto a baking sheet and set under the broiler until the sugar begins to BUBBLE. Use tongs or a pot holder to transfer the ramekins to a serving plate.

In a small pan whisk together the half and half, orange zest, and tarragon. Cook over medium heat until bubbles appear on the side of the liquid. Do not boil. Remove from the heat, cover, and allow the flavors to blend for 15 minutes. Strain the liquid to remove solids.

In a medium bowl whisk together sugar, egg yolks, and eggs. Stir in the vanilla and pour in the strained milk mixture. Pour this mixture back into the pan and cook over medium-low heat until thickened, about 5 minutes. The mixture should be the texture of thin pudding.

Preheat the oven to 325 degrees. Divide the custard evenly among 4 (6-ounce) ramekins. Place the ramekins into a baking dish. Pour hot water into the baking dish until it reaches halfway up the ramekins. Bake until the center is just set, about 30 minutes. Carefully remove the ramekins from the pan and cool to room temperature. Place into the refrigerator and chill for at least 1 hour or overnight.

To serve, layer the slices of banana in a circle on top of each custard. Sprinkle with brown sugar. Use a kitchen blowtorch to heat the sugar until bubbling.

Makes 4 servings
Prep Time: 20 minutes
Cook Time: 30 minutes

1½ cups half and half
Zest of 1 medium orange (about 2 tablespoons)
1 teaspoon chopped fresh tarragon
½ cup natural sugar
3 large egg yolks
2 large eggs
1 teaspoon vanilla extract
2 ripe bananas, sliced (about 1 cup)
2 tablespoons light brown sugar

NEW YORK–STYLE CHEESECAKE

There's tons of dairy in this rich dessert. You're guaranteed a BIG smile after just one bite.

Makes 12 servings
Prep Time: 20 minutes
Cook Time: 3 hours

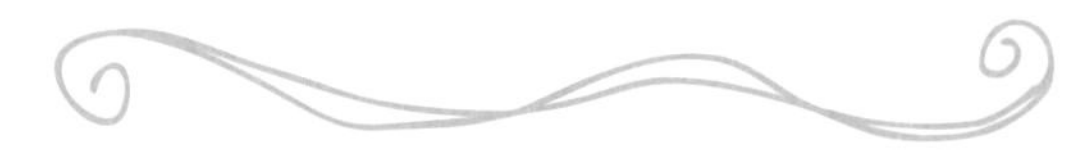

I listed REDUCED-FAT ingredients to make this dish as *smart-diet* friendly as possible. If you're ready for a walk on the wild side, go ahead and use regular ricotta, sour cream, and half and half. Just eat a SMALLER piece!

For the crust

- 1 cup graham cracker crumbs
- 3 tablespoons butter, melted

For the filling

- 3 8-ounce packages reduced-fat cream cheese
- 1 cup reduced-fat ricotta cheese
- 1/2 cup reduced-fat sour cream
- 1 cup natural sugar
- 1/3 cup reduced-fat half and half
- 3 tablespoons flour
- Juice of 1 medium lemon (about 2 tablespoons)
- Zest of 1 medium lemon (about 1 tablespoon)
- 1 tablespoon pure vanilla extract
- 3 large eggs
- Blueberries or strawberries

Preheat oven to 325 degrees. Mix together the graham cracker crumbs with the melted butter. Use a fork to press this mixture into the bottom of a 10-inch springform cake pan.

Use an electric mixer to combine the cream cheese with the ricotta cheese and sour cream until fluffy. Stir in the sugar until just combined. Mix in the half and half, flour, lemon juice, lemon zest, and vanilla. Stir in the eggs 1 at a time.

Pour the batter over the crumb crust. Use aluminum foil to cover the bottom and sides of the cake pan. Place the pan into a larger baking pan. Pour hot water into the larger pan until it comes halfway up the sides of the springform pan. Place into the oven. Bake for 1 hour. Turn off the oven and leave the cheesecake in the oven for 2 hours more. Remove the cake from the oven and remove the aluminum foil from the pan. Run a knife around the edge and chill for at least 4 hours.

To serve, cut the cake into wedges and serve with fresh blueberries or strawberries.

MANGO-WALNUT CRUMBLE

Assemble this dessert in the afternoon and bake it while you enjoy dinner. It will be warm and wonderful by the time your family is ready for dessert.

Makes 6 servings
Prep Time: 20 minutes
Cook Time: 40 minutes

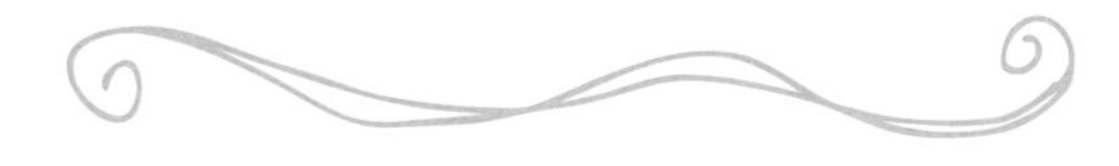

RIPE mangoes work best for this dish.

For the filling

- 3 tablespoons natural sugar
- 2 teaspoons cornstarch
- 1 teaspoon cinnamon
- 4 large mangoes, pitted, peeled, and diced (about 3 cups)
- Juice of 1 medium orange (about 1/3 cup)
- 2 tablespoons unsalted butter, melted

For the topping

- 1/3 cup unbleached all-purpose flour
- 2 tablespoons light brown sugar
- 1 teaspoon ground ginger
- 3 tablespoons unsalted butter, cut into pieces
- 1/4 cup walnuts
- Reduced-fat ice cream or whipped cream

Preheat oven to 400 degrees. Whisk together 3 tablespoons sugar, cornstarch, and cinnamon. Toss with mangoes, orange juice, and melted butter. Pour the filling into a 9-inch round baking dish that has been coated with vegetable oil spray.

Place the flour, brown sugar, ginger, butter, and walnuts into the bowl of a food processor. Pulse until the mixture resembles coarse crumbs. Sprinkle this mixture over the filling. Bake until the topping is golden and the filling is bubbling, about 35–40 minutes.

To serve, spoon the crumble into serving dishes while still warm. Top with reduced-fat ice cream or whipped cream.

EMERGENCY KEY LIME PIE

This deceptively simple recipe comes from my good pal Cindy—one of the all-star hostesses. I like it because when you need a sweet treat, this one fits the bill in no time.

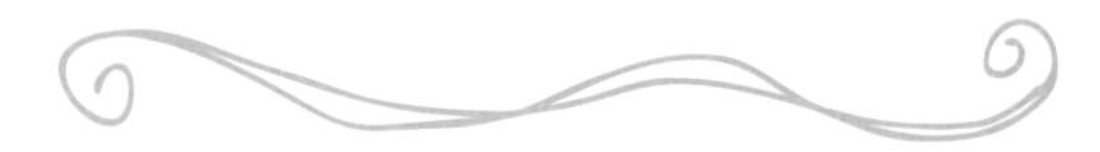

If your LOVE LIFE takes a misstep, prepare this dessert. After you've eaten a HUGE piece, things begin to look up! And you still have plenty of pie to share with someone new. Now that's something to smile about.

* * *

Prepare this simple filling and fill MINI TART SHELLS for a dessert that's sure to PLEASE at your next DINNER PARTY.

Makes 8 servings
Prep Time: 5 minutes, plus chilling

- 1 14-ounce can sweetened condensed milk
- 1 8-ounce package cream cheese
- ½–¾ cup key lime juice
- ½ teaspoon vanilla
- 1 prepared graham cracker crust
- Whipped cream
- Zest of 1 medium lime (about 1 tablespoon) (for garnish)

Use an electric mixer to combine the sweetened condensed milk, cream cheese, lime juice (begin with ½ cup and add more if you like your pie extra tart), and vanilla until smooth. Pour the filling into the crust and chill for at least 30 minutes. (If you are desperate, you can lick the bowl while you wait.)

To serve, top the pie with whipped cream and garnish with lime zest.

Gorgeous Home Spa Secrets . . . For a Come-Hither Smile

Homegrown toothpastes are no substitute for the real deal, like Crest and Aquafresh, but they are a fun, organic way to freshen up breath or brighten one's smile with novelty and good flavor to boot. Remember that scene in *Gone with the Wind* where Scarlett O'Hara received a surprise visit from Rhett? She hurriedly gargled away the bourbon on her breath with her late husband's cologne. The good news here: if you're short on mouthwash, you don't have to go *that* far. You can dash into the kitchen and get a quick, all-natural fix that you, your taste buds, and your breath will all agree upon.

Who Says You Need a Mint?

No doubt you had a great-aunt or grandmother who kept a dish of crystallized, twenty-year-old mints sitting in the foyer. You avoided finding out if they were peppermint or liquorish, knowing you stood a greater chance of cracking a tooth than freshening your breath. Rock-hard candies—whether they're Aunt Ida's or the ones on the hostess stand at your favorite steak house—aren't the best way to keep your breath fresh. What if you could whip up something to gargle with that didn't have the medicinal taste of mouthwash or the mothball quality of drugstore candy? That's where our herbal mouth fresheners come in. Go to your microwave and nuke a cup of water to boiling. While you're waiting for the *bleep*, mix 1 teaspoon each of fresh rosemary, mint, and lavender. Stir 1 teaspoon of this herbal mixture in the cup of hot water. Steep for 15 minutes, then strain. Cool and use as a mouthwash.

Catching Smiles with Vinegar

Our second simply whipped-up mouthwash possesses the additional bonus of antiseptic properties. Vinegar will dissolve deposits of tartar on your teeth, as well as wipe out bacteria in your mouth. Just combine 2 cups white wine vinegar (tastier than plain vinegar) with boiling water. Let it cool and gargle with it, as you would an over-the-counter mouthwash. Remember to gargle with plain tap water to wash away remnants of vinegar, as long-term exposure to its acidity is bad for your enamel. If you want to use regular vinegar for mouth cleansing purposes, add a touch of apple cider to improve the flavor.

Strawberry Toothpaste?

The dental cleaning regime is one that we're all familiar with—after the tartar has been scraped off and spit out, the patient gets an application of fruit-flavored grit applied to the surface of their teeth followed by the squirt-swish-and-rinse. Sounds awful, but is actually quite pleasant. Agree? It so happens fresh strawberries from home can lend the same feeling of cleanliness. Cut a fresh strawberry in half and rub your teeth and gums with it. Leave on for 15 minutes, then add some warm water and gently brush. This is not only a good cleaner but also promotes health of the gums.

Oh, to Curl Up with a Good Book

We generally like to drink something if we're curled up under a velour throw, reading in an easy chair. Having preached the teeth-staining evils of coffee and the darker caffeinated teas, we didn't get around to plugging innocuous, even *beneficial* herbal tea. It so happens that herbal tea is high in fluoride content. When you cut a wedge of lemon to go in your chamomile or rosehip tea, preserve the rind and rub your gums, massaging your upper gums downward and your lower gums upward. It's okay to go about this absently, after your tea is finished and you're into a particularly good passage of Mary Higgins Clark; this lemon rind ritual helps remove plaque and tartar.

Brush for Laughs

There's no doubt about it. The more you brush, the more you smile. Not only does your mouth feel fresh, but your smiling face invites new friendships. Smiling is good for you. You use sixteen muscles just to turn up those luscious lips. What a workout! A genuine smile increases the production of serotonin, the happy hormone. Babies as young as three weeks old respond to a smile. Smiling bonds us to each other. Remember we are designed to be social—not solitary. So start today and smile at everyone who crosses your path. Collect all of the smiles that you receive in return and watch as you become a more gorgeous you!

Smilin' and Wishin'

You can bring a smile to someone who is in desperate need of one by volunteering at your local chapter of the Make a Wish Foundation. Share your special skills to help grant someone else's wish. Start by visiting www.wish.org.

CHAPTER 9

building better bones

"Though we travel the world over to find the beautiful, we must carry it with us or we find it not."
— Ralph Waldo Emerson

Osteoporosis carries with it an image of a very old woman; ironic that it's the kind of nutritional lifestyle we lead as *young* women that determines the state of our bones in our twilight years. It's a sobering and even surprising fact, but as early as age thirty our sisters, mothers, aunts, and girlfriends all begin to lose bone density. What's key in maintaining a healthy skeletal system is stemming the tide to bone loss *before* you're in your late 50s, but take heart if you were slow to catch this boat. It's never too late to be good to your body. If you're struggling to get calcium into your daily diet and take supplements, discuss your vitamin-popping regime with your doctor—some women develop kidney stones if they're ingesting too much straight calcium and vitamin D. It's also a *great idea* to ask your doctor for a bone density scan to establish a baseline, so that you can monitor how fast or slow your bone loss is in later, more critical years. Start being good to your bones today! Really look at your daily diet. In addition to obvious sources of calcium and vitamin D (the latter not including sun exposure), are you getting enough magnesium? Your body can't absorb precious, bone-saving calcium without it. You'll see from the tasty recipes in this chapter that making your palate a friend to your bones is anything but a bitter pill to swallow.

Ask Dr. Moon

The doctor is in to answer your questions.

Osteoporosis afflicts up to 25 million Americans. To avoid becoming a member of this group, you must maintain a nutritious lifestyle in order for your bones to benefit for decades to come. In creating this book, we authors concurred: *form follows function*. We propose that how you build your bones—that is, how your skeletal structure performs based on the kind of fuel you're feeding it—determines the appearance of your structure, and structure is the *backbone* of beauty. Here, we dish with Dr. Moon about the make-or-break food and supplement choices in calcium consumption, proving almost literally that there really is "no use crying over spilt milk;" you can get your calcium in lots of other things, too!

Q: What is the role of vitamin D for strong bones, and where can I derive the healthiest doses?

A: Just like love and marriage—that is, the part about "not being able to have one without the other"—so is the relationship between vitamin D and calcium absorption: without enough of both, your skeletal system is in peril. When vitamin D is lacking, we can't form enough of the hormone calcitriol; as a result, the body must take its calcium from stores in the skeleton, weakening existing bone and preventing the formation of strong, new bone. So how do we ensure that we get enough vitamin D? Fifteen minutes in the sun is plenty of time to manufacture and store all of the vitamin D you need, but if you're working the daylight hours away or are just too fair-skinned to benefit from the great outdoors, experts recommend a daily intake of between 400 and 800 (IU), which is available in vitamin D–rich foods, like egg yolks, saltwater fish, and liver.

Q: Okay, on to the role of calcium: Why is it so important for healthy bones, and what nutritive sources are calcium cash cows?

A: Calcium is needed for our heart, muscles, and nerves to function properly and for the blood to clot. It's a well-known fact that low calcium intake throughout one's life is associated with low bone mass and high fracture rates. As we all know, milk is *fantastic* for our bones; in fact, just one glass contains about 300 milligrams of calcium. The adequate intake level for a middle-aged adult is 1,000 milligrams—so just 2 glasses of milk a day puts you well on your way to achieving the ideal. If you're not a milk person, you'll be pleased to hear that dairy is just the tip of the iceberg in terms of where one can reap the benefits of calcium. Plant foods, like spinach, potatoes, mustard greens, as well as every variation of tasty lettuce, are a good source of calcium—not to mention calcium-packed nuts, fish, beans, and tofu.

Q: What's the good news on taking calcium supplements?

A: For the more mature beauty, the news is very good. Studies have shown that supplementing with calcium increases bone density in perimenopausal women and slows bone degeneration in postmenopausal women by an average of 30–50 percent. These effects translate into a significant reduction in hip fractures. It is important for *all postmenopausal women* to note that calcium derived through food alone may not be enough for optimal bone health. You and your doctor should evaluate your unique medical history, genetics, and age; all or one of those play a part in the advocacy for supplements. These are instrumental if you expect your body to absorb the calcium coming to it from fork and plate! Your doctor may also encourage you to take a magnesium supplement along with your calcium.

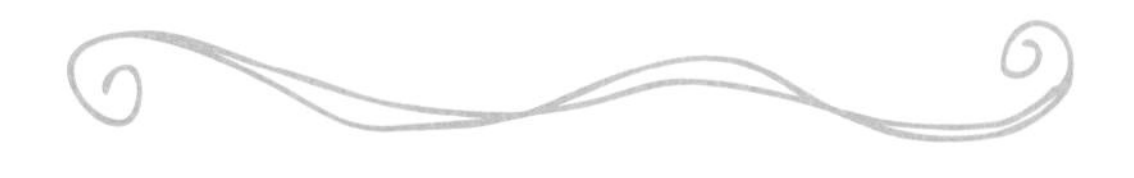

Q: Most of us can and do ensure our daily diets are calcium-enriched to combat the likelihood of bone loss, but are we leaving other nutritious stones unturned?

A: Magnesium is the fourth most abundant mineral in the body and is essential to good health. Approximately 50 percent of total body magnesium is found in bone. The other half is found predominantly inside cells of body tissues and organs. Magnesium is needed for more than 300 biochemical reactions in the body. It helps maintain normal muscle and nerve function, keeps heart rhythm steady, supports a healthy immune system, and keeps bones strong. Other nutrients are important for bone health, such as vitamin D, boron, vitamin K, vitamin C, ipriflavone, silicon, and vitamins B_6, B_{12}, and folate.

Q: What if I am not a big milk drinker—will the calcium from other food sources be enough?

A: Play your cards right, and the answer to this question is a resounding "Yes!" Enjoy a delicious salad to support your bone health. Although nondairy foods provide a large percent of your total day's calcium, when certain foods are combined, they provide *more* calcium than the amount in an 8-ounce glass of cow's milk. Let's take a salad as our example. Romaine lettuce contains 20 milligrams of calcium per cup. Using 2 cups of romaine as our salad base, we start off with 40 milligrams of calcium. A ½ cup of chard leaves would bump us up another 25 milligrams, to 65 total. Adding one-half cup of soybeans we jump up 87 milligrams—sprinkling on 2 tablespoons of sesame seeds brings us up to around 237 milligrams. To top it off, add one-third of a cup of kidney beans and we have a salad that provides a substantial 277 milligrams of calcium!

Q: How does this amount compare to a glass of 2-percent cow's milk?

A: In terms of total calcium, it's about 33 percent higher! How does it compare in calories? It's also higher here—weighing in at about 240 calories versus 120 calories for a cup of 2-percent cow's milk, but that's no real worry in this case. As we've said before "form follows function," and your body is high functioning on this big, healthy bowl of salad. Why? Because everything in this salad is something your body can use; there are no empty calories in this meal. Good function leads to good form. That being said, you are well-formed, well-*in*formed, and *gorgeous* because of it!

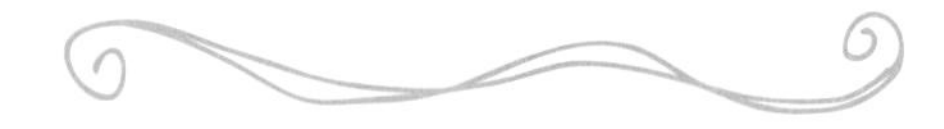

Jorj's "No Bones About It" Glam Kitchen

"Killing two birds with one stone" leaves something to be desired as an expression, but you can do just that on your next trip to the grocery store. In addition to purchasing bone-loving foods like spinach, chard, mustard and collard greens, romaine, shredded cabbage, nuts, any and all beans, gourmet seeds, and decadent dairy, there's another way to be good to your bones: it's called *exercise*, and it can be subtly (if not literally!) carried out in sacks of healthy groceries.

Skip the Gym on Shopping Day

Like muscle, bone is living tissue that constantly reforms, gaining or losing strength according to how often it is used. Without exercise, bone loses density, becomes weaker, and loses the ability to absorb enough calcium. Two types of exercises—that just happen to go hand in hand with the rigors of shopping day—are important for building and maintaining bone mass and density: (1) Weight-bearing exercise (definition: your bones and muscles work against gravity while your feet and legs bear your weight) and (2) resistance activity (definition: using muscular strength to improve muscle mass and strengthen bone). If you're parked at the far end of the parking lot, carrying and hoisting armloads of grocery bags can be *excellent* weight training! Doubly so if you have to climb stairs to reach your front door! Why not think about walking or cycling to the grocery store, dry cleaner, or drugstore. It could be your secret to a trim physique.

A Lesser-Known Fact

If you polled ten ordinary citizens about bone health, asking them to name something beyond calcium and vitamin D, I doubt many of them would know about magnesium. There's a relationship between magnesium intake and osteoporosis. Unfortunately, the best source of calcium, milk, is no "great shakes" when it comes to magnesium. Plant foods are where it's at. In other words, have some salad with dinner—serve it with cashews or almonds; always choose brown rice over white, have whole-wheat pancakes for breakfast, serve your sandwiches on rye, and discover a love for turnip greens. Loaded with magnesium, these foods will love your bones!

In English, Please . . .

In researching a diet that cuts a woman's risk for osteoporosis, one encounters intimidating medical lingo. Phrases like "decreases the serum concentration" or "increased homocysteine concentrations interfere with collagen cross-linking" don't mean much to the layperson. For our purposes, let's focus on the parts that are easily understood, such as which foods contain key nutrients for optimal bone health. They are: vitamin D, boron (fruits & veggies), vitamin K (dark leafy greens), vitamin C, soy isoflavonoids (found in **soy milk** and **edamame**), folate, and vitamins B_6 and B_{12}. An excellent source of vitamin B_6 is **bell peppers**. Strong sources of folate include **parsley**, **broccoli**, **beets**, **lentils**, and **asparagus**. **Calf's liver** and **snapper** supply a motherload of B_{12}. Nutritional notes for the more mature beauty underscore eating **apples** and using **olive oil** on her calcium-rich salads and in her daily cooking. Why? Because the phenols, which contain a unique flavonoid called phloridzin, have been shown to help protect against the inflammation-related bone loss that occurs with change of life. Okay, that's getting technical. The only things you need to remember are the **apples** and **olive oil**—along with everything else in **bold** type—and it's like being in high school again. Stay tuned for a pop quiz. . . .

Start Your Day

Main Plates

On the Side

Snacks & Sweets

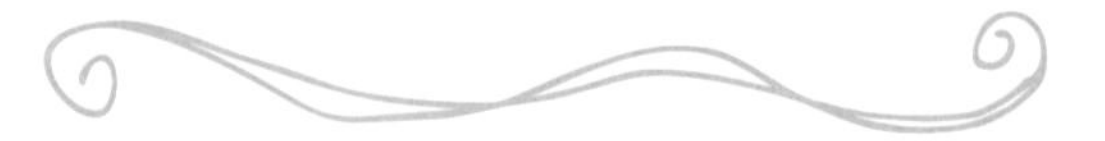

EGGS BENEDICT

With Swiss Chard and Whole Grain English Muffins

Start your day with a delicious breakfast that adds the goodness of whole grain with a dash of calcium-rich greens.

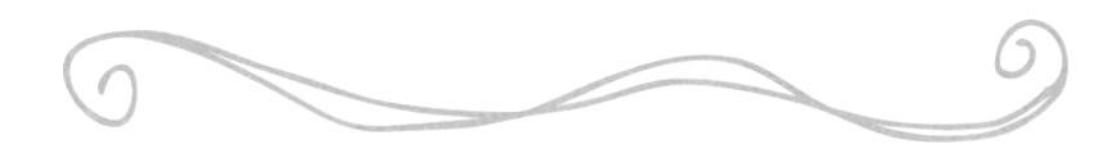

You will have more HOLLANDAISE sauce than you need for this dish. Save extra by storing in an airtight container in the refrigerator for up to 3 days. Reheat in a double boiler over slow-simmering water.

Place 3 egg yolks, lemon juice, salt, and cayenne pepper into a blender. Melt the butter in the microwave oven. (To avoid splashing, place the butter into a bowl and cover with the butter wrapper.) Microwave on high for 15 seconds at a time until it is melted and beginning to bubble.

Pulse the egg yolk mixture for 3–5 seconds. With the machine running on low speed, carefully pour in the hot butter. This should take about 30–40 seconds. By the time the butter is incorporated into the egg yolk mixture, the sauce is done. Keep the sauce warm by pouring it into a small bowl and placing that bowl over a pan of warm (not hot) water.

Heat the olive oil in a skillet over medium-high heat. Cook the Swiss chard until just beginning to wilt, about 2–3 minutes. Season with salt and pepper. Remove from the heat.

Poach the eggs in an egg poaching pan or in boiling water with a touch of vinegar. Toast the English muffin halves.

To serve, place each English muffin half onto a plate. Top with one-fourth of the Swiss chard. Gently slide one poached egg on top of the greens. Drizzle warm Hollandaise sauce over the egg. Garnish with chopped fresh parsley and a sprinkle of paprika.

Makes 4 servings
Prep Time: 30 minutes

For the Hollandaise sauce

3 large egg yolks
Juice of 1 medium lemon (about 2 tablespoons)
1/4 teaspoon salt
1/8 teaspoon cayenne pepper
1/2 cup butter, melted (1 stick)

For the Swiss chard

1 tablespoon olive oil
4 ounces Swiss chard, washed, dried, stems removed, leaves torn (about 2 cups)
Salt and freshly ground pepper

For the dish

4 large eggs, poached
2 whole grain English muffins, halved
1 tablespoon chopped fresh parsley (for garnish)
Paprika (for garnish)

SWEET POTATO AND COUNTRY HAM FRITTATA

The distinctly southern flavors of country ham and sweet potato blend with an Italian peasant dish to create a wonderful brunch or late night supper.

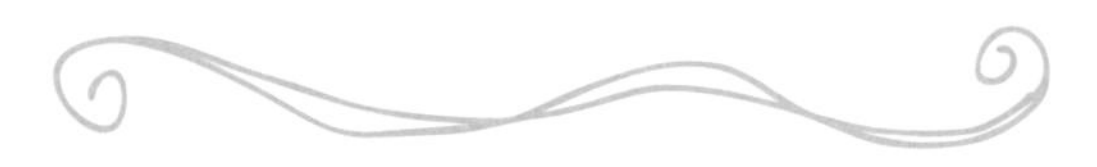

A good old-fashioned WHITE POTATO is a good substitute for the sweet potato, as is cooked bacon or sausage for the ham.

Preheat the oven to broil. Cook the potato in boiling water until fork-tender, about 8–10 minutes. Drain.

Heat olive oil in a deep ovenproof skillet (with lid) over medium-high heat. Cook the onion and bell pepper in the oil until soft, about 5–7 minutes. Reduce the heat to medium. Add the ham and sweet potato, and cook for 3 minutes more.

Add the butter to the skillet. In a small bowl whisk the eggs and Parmesan cheese until blended. Season with salt and pepper. Pour the egg mixture into the skillet. Stir. Cover the skillet with a lid, and cook until the eggs are set, about 4–5 minutes.

Remove the lid and place the skillet under the broiler. Cook until the frittata is golden, about 2 minutes. Carefully remove the skillet from the oven. Use a spatula to loosen the frittata.

To serve, transfer the frittata to a serving platter. Sprinkle with parsley and cut into wedges.

On Shopping Day: Prepare the sweet potato, cool to room temperature, and store in an airtight container in the refrigerator for up to 3 days.

Makes 4 servings
Prep Time: 20 minutes
Cook Time: 10 to 15 minutes

- 1 medium sweet potato, peeled and diced into 1/2-inch cubes (about 1 cup)
- 1 tablespoon olive oil
- 1 medium yellow onion, peeled and diced into 1/2-inch squares (about 1 cup)
- 1 large green bell pepper, seeded and diced into 1/2-inch cubes (about 1 cup)
- 1/4 pound country baked ham, cut into 1/4-inch dice
- 1 tablespoon butter
- 8 large eggs
- 1 ounce finely grated Parmesan cheese (about 1/4 cup)
- Salt and freshly ground pepper
- 2 tablespoons chopped fresh parsley (for garnish)

WHOLE GRAIN APPLE MUFFINS

With Walnut Streusel

Nothing beats a yummy muffin with your cup of morning tea (or java). These are a delicious, smart way to fuel your engine as you start the day's activities.

Makes 12 large or 15 medium muffins
Prep Time: 15 minutes
Cook Time: 20 to 25 minutes

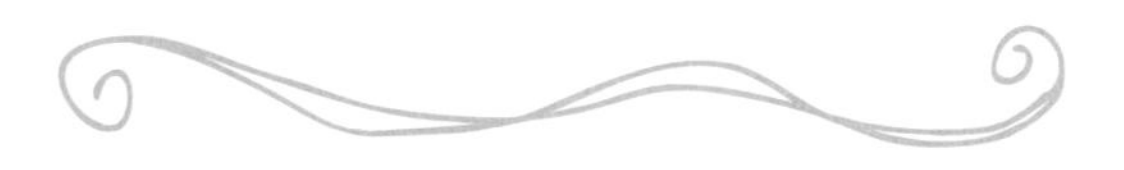

For added *appleness*, drop a spoonful of APPLESAUCE into the batter.

For the muffins

- 1 cup unbleached all-purpose flour
- 1 cup whole wheat flour
- 1 teaspoon baking powder
- 1 teaspoon baking soda
- 1/4 teaspoon salt
- 3/4 cup brown sugar
- 1/2 cup reduced-fat milk
- 1/2 cup apple juice
- 1 tablespoon butter, melted
- 1 teaspoon pure vanilla extract
- 2 large eggs, beaten
- 2 medium apples, peeled, cored, and cut into 1/4-inch cubes (about 2 cups)

For streusel

- 1/4 cup walnuts, finely chopped
- 2 tablespoons brown sugar
- 2 tablespoons butter, cut into pieces

Preheat the oven to 350 degrees. In a medium bowl whisk together the unbleached flour, whole wheat flour, baking powder, baking soda, and salt.

Place the sugar in separate large bowl. Whisk in the milk, apple juice, melted butter, vanilla, and eggs until smooth. Stir in the flour mixture until just blended. Stir in the apples. Spoon the batter into a muffin tin with paper liners.

Place the walnuts, the 2 tablespoons brown sugar, and 2 tablespoons butter into the bowl of a mini food processor. Pulse to combine. The mixture will resemble a sticky paste. Spoon the topping over the batter.

Bake until the muffins spring back when touched and a tester inserted into the center comes out clean, about 20–25 minutes. Cool on wire racks.

On Shopping Day: Prepare the muffins and store in an airtight container for up to 4 days.

BREAKFAST PANINI

With Chicken Sausage

This breakfast sandwich is way better than that one you reach for in the drive-through lane—and it's just as fast! Half a sandwich is plenty!

Makes 4 servings
Prep Time: 10 minutes
Cook Time: 3 to 5 minutes

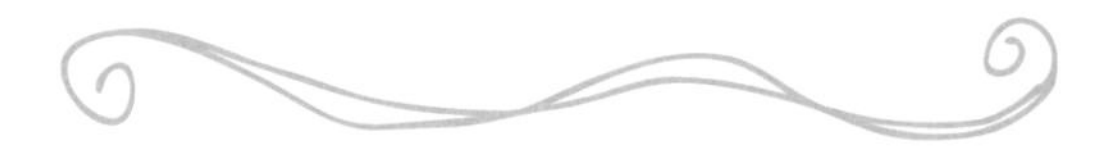

There are so many GOURMET sausages in the marketplace today. Choose your favorite flavors and check the labels to select a product that is LEAN and mean.

- 3 tablespoons olive oil, divided use
- 2 chicken and herb lean sausage links (about 6–8 ounces), cut into ½-inch slices
- 2 large eggs
- 4 slices crusty whole grain bread
- 2 ounces reduced-fat grated Monterey Jack cheese (about ½ cup)
- Salt and freshly ground pepper
- 1 cup fresh spinach leaves, washed and dried
- Sliced tomatoes

Heat 1 tablespoon olive oil in a skillet over medium-high heat. Cook the chicken sausage slices in the skillet until cooked through. Transfer to a platter and keep warm.

Fry the eggs (in batches) in the skillet, carefully turning once. (You may add a drizzle of olive oil if needed.

Heat a panini grill over medium-high heat. Place the bread slices onto your work surface. Brush 1 side of each slice with the remaining olive oil. Turn two slices of bread over. Layer both with cheese and sausage. Place one egg on top of each. Season with salt and pepper. Top with fresh spinach leaves. Lay the remaining 2 slices of bread on top with the olive oil on the outside of the sandwich.

Grill the sandwiches until the cheese melts and the bread is golden, about 3–5 minutes.

To serve, cut each sandwich in half and serve each half with sliced tomatoes.

MUSTARD-GARLIC ROASTED CHICKEN

Served with Arugula and Artichoke Salad

Roll out this dish for Sunday's supper and use the extras to create Monday's luncheon chicken salad wrap. It's a well-planned two-fer.

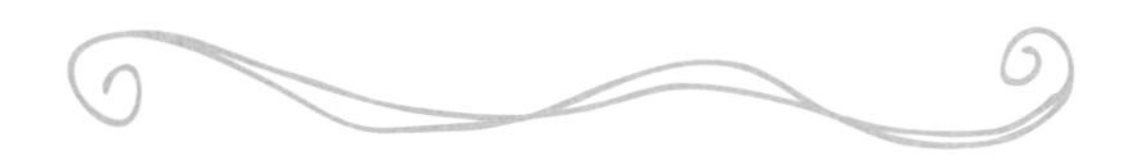

Prepare the chicken by removing it from the packaging and rinsing under cold water. Use a paper towel to pat dry before you spread on the MARINADE.

Whisk together the mustard, olive oil, minced garlic, oregano, and basil. Spread this mixture over and inside the chicken. Place into a glass baking dish. Cover with plastic wrap and marinate for at least 4 hours or overnight.

Remove the chicken from the refrigerator and bring to room temperature, about 30 minutes. Preheat the oven to 400 degrees. Season the chicken with salt and pepper. Transfer the chicken to a rack in a roasting pan. Place the rosemary sprigs on top of and inside the chicken. Roast until the juices run clear when a fork is inserted just above the thigh, about 1–1½ hours. Use a thermometer to make sure that the temperature comes up to 165–170 degrees. Let the chicken rest for 20 minutes before carving.

Combine the arugula, artichokes, and red pepper in a bowl. Toss with cheese.

In a small bowl whisk together the tarragon vinegar, lemon juice, shallot, brown sugar, and mustard until combined. Slowly whisk in the olive oil. Season with salt and pepper. Drizzle the dressing over the arugula salad and toss.

To serve, carve the chicken into 6 sections—2 breast halves, 2 thigh and legs pieces, and 2 wings. Mound the salad into the center of a platter. Place the chicken pieces around the salad.

Makes 4 servings plus extras
Prep Time: 10 minutes plus marinating
Cook Time: 90 minutes

For the chicken

- 1 cup Dijon mustard
- ¼ cup olive oil
- 1 whole head garlic, cloves peeled and minced
- 2 teaspoons dried oregano leaves
- 2 teaspoons dried basil leaves
- 1 4½- to 5-pound chicken
- Salt and freshly ground pepper
- Fresh rosemary sprigs

For the salad

- 4 ounces arugula leaves, washed and dried (about 4 cups)
- 1 14-ounce can artichoke hearts, drained and chopped
- 1 roasted red pepper (from jar), drained and diced
- 1 tablespoon grated Pecorino Romano cheese

For the vinaigrette

- ¼ cup tarragon vinegar
- Juice of 1 medium lemon (about 2 tablespoons)
- 1 large shallot, minced (about 1 tablespoon)
- 1 tablespoon brown sugar
- 1 tablespoon Dijon mustard
- 3 tablespoons olive oil

WHOLE WHEAT SPAGHETTI

With Grilled Turkey, Broccoli Rabe, Red Peppers, and Peas

A fresh-tasting pasta dish that has a twang in each bite, you'll want to include this dish in your Gorgeous Lifestyle plan—every week!

Makes 4 to 6 servings
Prep Time: 20 minutes
Cook Time: 10 minutes

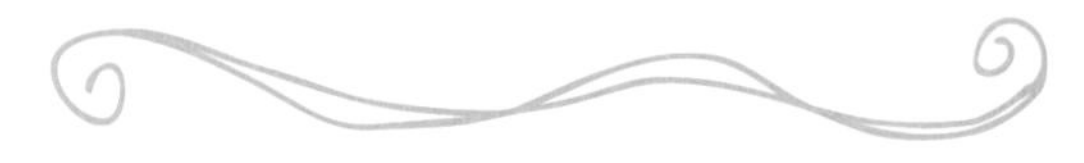

TURKEY sausage would be great in this dish, as would canned ARTICHOKES. It's a pantry pusher's dream.

- 1 large bunch broccoli rabe, chopped (about 1 pound)
- 1 1/2 pounds turkey cutlets
- Salt and freshly ground pepper
- 2 tablespoons olive oil, divided use
- 2 medium cloves garlic, minced (about 1 teaspoon)
- 1 2-ounce tin anchovies, packed in oil
- 1/2 teaspoon red pepper flakes
- 2 roasted red peppers (drained from jar), thinly sliced
- 1 15-ounce can sweet peas, drained
- 1 pound whole wheat spaghetti
- 2 ounces Asiago cheese, grated (about 1/2 cup)

Cook the broccoli rabe in salted, boiling water until just crisp-tender, about 3–4 minutes. Plunge into a bowl of ice water. Drain.

Season the turkey cutlets with salt and pepper. Heat 1 tablespoon olive oil in a grill pan over medium-high heat. Grill the turkey until golden, about 4–5 minutes per side. Remove from the grill pan to a platter.

Heat the remaining 1 tablespoon olive oil in a skillet over medium heat. Add the garlic, anchovies with oil, and red pepper flakes. Stir until the anchovies almost disappear and the garlic is golden.

Slice the turkey into strips and add to the skillet. Add the broccoli rabe, red peppers, and peas. Toss to warm through.

Bring a pot of salted water to boil in a pasta pot. Cook the whole wheat spaghetti in the pot until al dente. Pour 1–2 ladles of the pasta water into the sauce to thicken.

To serve, drain the pasta and place into a large bowl. Toss with turkey and veggies. Sprinkle cheese over all.

PARMESAN CHICKEN FINGERS

With Green Cashew and Curry Dipping Sauce

This upscale chicken finger dish is way, way better than the drive-through version, and just as quick to prepare as it is to order!

Makes 4 servings
Prep Time: 15 minutes
Cook Time: 15 minutes

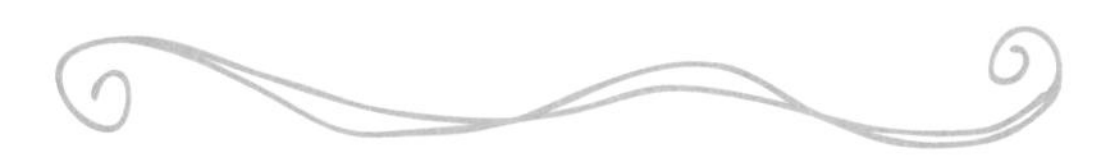

A box of CORNFLAKE crumbs can be found in the baking section of the grocery store.

For the chicken fingers

- 2 large (6- to 8-ounce) skinless, boneless chicken breast halves, cut into 1-inch strips
- Salt and freshly ground pepper
- 2 cups cornflake crumbs
- 2 ounces finely grated Parmesan cheese (about 1/2 cup)
- 2 tablespoons chopped fresh thyme leaves
- 1 teaspoon ground paprika
- 2 tablespoons olive oil
- Juice of 1 medium lemon (about 2 tablespoons)

For the sauce

- 1 1-inch piece ginger, peeled
- 1 cup cashews
- 1/2 cup reduced-fat sour cream
- 1/4 cup fresh baby spinach leaves, washed and dried
- 1 tablespoon brown sugar
- 1 teaspoon ground curry
- Lemon wedges (for garnish)

Preheat the oven to 350 degrees. Season the chicken with salt and pepper. In a shallow bowl use a fork to stir together the cornflake crumbs, Parmesan cheese, thyme, and paprika.

Heat the olive oil in a skillet over medium-high heat. Dredge the chicken pieces in the cornflake mixture. Cook in the skillet, turning once, until golden, about 4–6 minutes. Transfer to a baking dish that has been coated with vegetable oil spray. Drizzle the chicken with lemon juice. Bake in the oven until cooked through, about 15–20 minutes.

Place the ginger into the bowl of a food processor. Pulse until minced. Add the cashews and pulse until smooth. Add the sour cream, spinach leaves, brown sugar, and curry. Pulse until well combined. Season with salt and pepper. Transfer to a serving bowl.

To serve, place the chicken fingers onto a platter garnished with lemon wedges. Serve the curry sauce on the side for dipping.

On Shopping Day: Prepare the sauce and store in an airtight container in the refrigerator for up to 4 days.

GRILLED LAMB CHOPS

With White Bean Salad

Velvety white beans enhanced with snappy green onions and fragrant Italian parsley are the perfect accompaniment to tender lamb chops.

Makes 4 servings
Prep Time: 15 minutes
Cook Time: 10 to 14 minutes

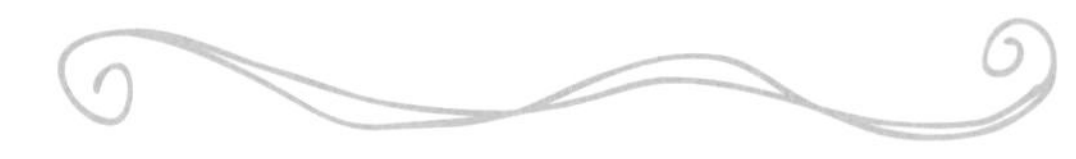

Choose LOIN lamb chops over shoulder chops for this dish.

For the lamb chops

- 4 5- to 6-ounce loin lamb chops, cut 1 1/2 to 2-inches thick
- 2 tablespoons olive oil
- Juice of 1 medium lemon (about 2 tablespoons)
- 2 teaspoons dried thyme

For the salad

- 1/2 cup fresh flat leaf Italian parsley leaves, chopped
- 2 tablespoons olive oil
- Juice of 1 medium lime (about 1 tablespoon)
- 2 green onions, thinly sliced (about 2 tablespoons)
- 1 15.5-ounce can cannellini beans, drained
- Salt and freshly ground pepper
- Fresh parsley (for garnish)

Place the lamb chops into a shallow baking dish. Sprinkle both sides with olive oil, lemon juice, and dried thyme. Loosely cover with plastic wrap and marinate at room temperature for 15 minutes.

In a bowl stir together the parsley, olive oil, lime juice, and onions. Toss in the beans. Season with salt and pepper.

Heat a grill pan over medium-high heat. Season the lamb chops with salt and pepper. Grill until rare in the center, about 4–5 minutes per side.

To serve, place the lamb chops onto a serving platter. Spoon the white bean salad alongside. Garnish with additional fresh parsley.

BAKED TILAPIA

With Fresh Herbs

A simple presentation for a mildly flavored fish . . . it's just perfect for a quick weekday supper or a casual Friday with friends.

Makes 4 servings
Prep Time: 10 minutes
Cook Time: 15 minutes

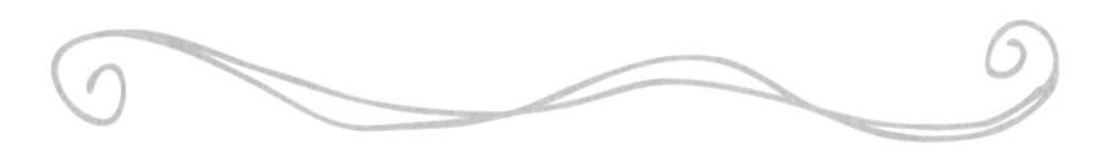

My boys are gaw-gaw over BUFFALO chicken wings. In order to get them to eat fish, I used to convince them that they were eating chicken-fish. We started with "BUFFALO CHICKEN FISH." I continue to fool them in this dish by adding hot sauce to the mayonnaise and eliminating the fresh herbs. They still love it. (Why not give it a try for your gullible crew?)

- 1½ pounds skinless tilapia fillets
- Salt and freshly ground pepper
- 3 tablespoons reduced-fat mayonnaise
- Juice of 1 medium lemon (about 2 tablespoons)
- 1 teaspoon Dijon mustard
- 1 tablespoon chopped fresh dill
- 1 tablespoon chopped fresh parsley
- 1 teaspoon chopped fresh tarragon

Preheat the oven to 375 degrees. Place the fish onto a rimmed baking sheet that has been coated with vegetable oil spray. Season with salt and freshly ground pepper.

In a small bowl whisk together the mayonnaise, lemon juice, and mustard. Whisk in the fresh herbs. Spread this mixture over the fish. Bake until the fish is opaque in the center, about 15–20 minutes depending on thickness.

To serve, place the fish onto a serving platter. Garnish with dill, tarragon, and parsley leaves.

ROSEMARY POLENTA

With Spinach, Red Beans, and Goat Cheese

This veggie dish is filled with bone building calcium and magnesium-rich ingredients—but hey, it's all about good-tasting food, and this dish is a perfect choice for your well-balanced lifestyle plan.

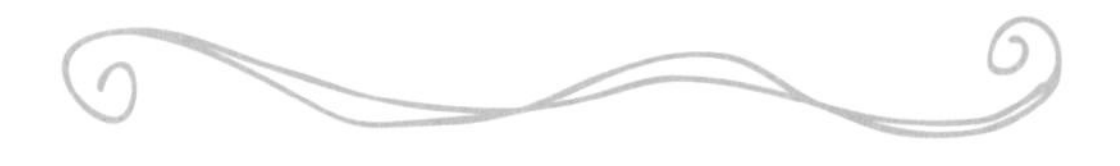

If you cannot find POLENTA in the grocery store, look for stone ground CORNMEAL.

To prepare the polenta, heat 4 tablespoons of butter and 2 tablespoons of olive oil in a deep pot over medium heat until sizzling. Add the garlic and cook until soft, about 2 minutes. Stir in the rosemary and season with salt and pepper. Pour in the chicken stock and milk and bring to a boil. Remove the pot from the heat. Reduce the heat to low. Slowly whisk in the polenta (cornmeal). Cook, stirring constantly, until the polenta is very thick and bubbling, about 6–8 minutes. Remove the pan from the heat and whisk in the cheese. Pour the polenta into an 8-inch round baking dish that has been coated with vegetable oil spray. Use a spatula to smooth the top. Cover and refrigerate until the polenta is cold and set, about 2 hours.

To prepare the topping, heat the remaining 2 tablespoons olive oil in a skillet over medium-high heat. Cook the onion until soft, about 4–5 minutes. Add the red beans and tomatoes. Stir in the cumin, and season with salt and pepper. Cook for 2–3 minutes. Stir in the spinach and cook until just wilted. Keep warm.

For the dish, cut the polenta into 6 wedges. Dust each wedge in flour. Heat 1 tablespoon butter and 1 tablespoon olive oil (in a skillet) over medium-high heat. Use a spatula to remove each wedge of polenta from the pan and place into the hot oil/butter. Cook until golden, about 2–3 minutes. Turn and cook until golden on both sides, about 2–3 minutes more. (Use additional oil and butter as needed, depending on how many wedges fit into your skillet.) Transfer to a platter and keep warm.

To serve, place each wedge of polenta into a shallow pasta bowl. Ladle the spinach mixture over the top. Top with crumbled goat cheese and fresh rosemary.

On Shopping Day: Prepare the polenta, cover, and chill for up to 4 days.

Makes 6 servings
Prep Time: 20 minutes
Cook Time: 15 minutes for the polenta, 10 minutes for the topping, and at least 2 hours for the polenta to set

For the polenta

- 5-6 tablespoons butter (¾ stick), divided use
- 5-6 tablespoons olive oil, divided use
- 2 medium cloves garlic, minced (about 1 teaspoon)
- 1 tablespoon chopped fresh rosemary leaves
- Salt and freshly ground pepper
- 1½ cups homemade chicken stock or low-sodium chicken broth
- 2 cups reduced-fat milk

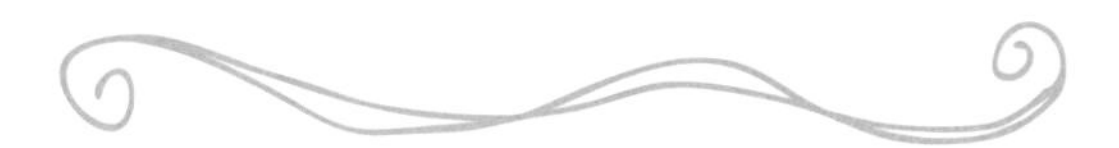

1 cup uncooked polenta
1 ounce finely grated Parmesan cheese (about 1/4 cup)
Unbleached all-purpose flour

For the topping

1 large white onion, peeled and thinly sliced (about 1 cup)
1 16-ounce can red beans, drained
1 16-ounce can diced tomatoes
1 teaspoon ground cumin
6 ounces fresh spinach leaves, washed, dried, and torn (about 4 cups)
4 ounces goat cheese, crumbled (about 1 cup)
Fresh rosemary leaves (for garnish)

PEPPERED PORK PINWHEELS

Stuffed with Swiss Chard, Sun-Dried Tomatoes, and Mozzarella

The filling is moist, full of veggie goodness, and the pinwheels are gorgeous on the plate. Serve with smashed potatoes and you have a meal your family will ask for again and again.

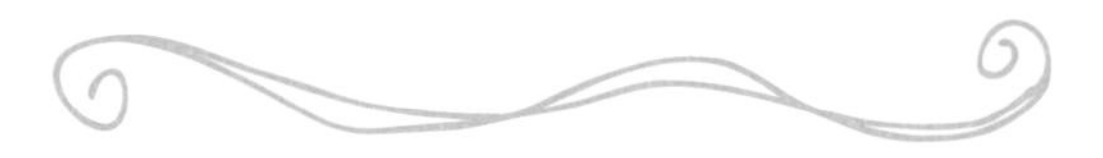

For this recipe, we're going to open the tenderloins and increase their size by three—just by slicing each one twice! Similar to BUTTERFLYING, where you cut the meat in half and then open the flaps to produce a larger, thinner piece of meat, this process we've named *tri-flying*. (You won't find this one in any culinary dictionary, but hey, it's FUN—so what the heck.)

* * *

When I demonstrated this tri-flying technique to my son, he suggested that I was cutting the pork like I was unrolling it. Essentially, he's right—kudos for good visualization!

Place one tenderloin onto a cutting board with the thick end facing away from you. Place your free hand on top to steady. Starting at the thick end and working horizontally, use a sharp knife to cut a slit about three-fourths of the way through the bottom third of the meat, from right to left. Do not cut all the way through, leave attached. Open the tenderloin. Cut a slit from the center of the meat, from right to left again, three-fourths of the way through toward the thick half. Do not cut all the way through. Open up the flap. You will have 1 large piece of meat. Repeat with the second tenderloin. Invert the second tenderloin, so that the thin end is placed next to the thick end, and overlaps slightly. Cover with plastic wrap. Use a meat mallet to pound the meat to an even thickness of about ½-inch. The two overlapping *tri-flied* tenderloins will yield a rectangular piece of meat about 10 inches by 12 inches. Place the cutting board, with the tenderloin covered with plastic, into the refrigerator to chill for at least 15 minutes.

For the chard, heat the olive oil in a large skillet over medium-high heat. Add the onion and cook until soft, about 3–4 minutes. Add half of the Swiss chard. Cook until wilted, about 4–5 minutes. Add the remaining Swiss chard and cook until wilted, about 5 minutes more. Season with salt and pepper. Cool to room temperature.

Remove the tenderloin from the refrigerator. Sprinkle the mozzarella cheese over the meat. Cover with the Swiss chard mixture. Top with sun-dried tomatoes. Carefully roll up the tenderloin around the filling. Secure with toothpicks.

Preheat the oven to 350 degrees. Brush the meat with mustard and coat generously with freshly ground pepper. Place 1 more tablespoon olive oil in the skillet over medium-high heat. Brown the pork tenderloin roll, beginning seam side down, on all sides until golden, about 5 minutes total. Place the pork roll into a baking dish. Bake until the meat is still moist and the juices are clear, about 35–45 minutes.

To serve, remove the toothpicks from the roll. Cut into 1½-inch slices.

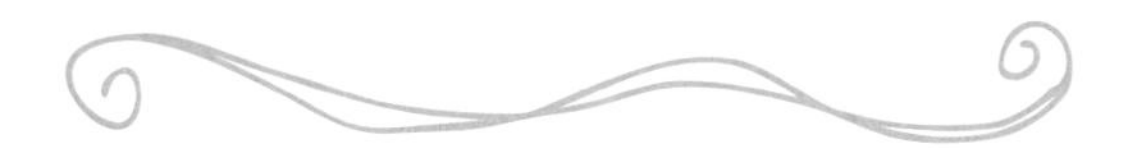

On Shopping Day: Prepare the Swiss chard filling, cool to room temperature, place into an airtight container and store in the refrigerator for up to 3 days.

Makes 6 servings
Prep Time: 30 minutes
Cook Time: 35 to 45 minutes

For the Swiss chard

- 2 tablespoons olive oil, divided use
- 1 large red onion, peeled and thinly sliced (about 1 cup)
- 1½ pounds Swiss chard, washed, dried, stems removed, leaves torn (about 8 cups)
- Salt and freshly ground pepper

For the pork

- 2 12- to 14-ounce pork tenderloins, tri-flied
- 2 ounces reduced-fat, grated mozzarella cheese (about ½ cup)
- 1 cup minced oil-packed sun-dried tomatoes, drained
- 2 tablespoons Dijon-style mustard

GREEN GAZPACHO SOUP

With Navy Bean Garnish

Bread gives this simple blender soup a velvety, thick texture.

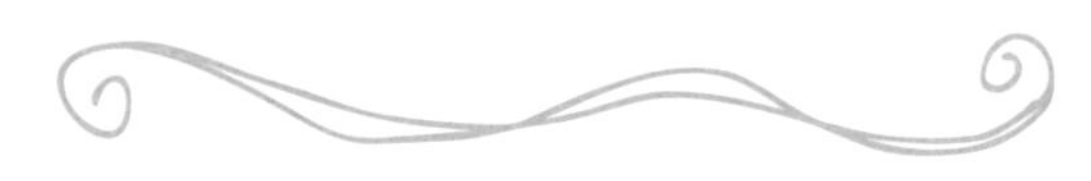

I always like a touch of SHERRY in my soup. It's a hand-me-down habit from my grandmother. Pour an ounce of sherry into the blender before the final pulse to see what I mean.

* * *

If your blender is not large enough to handle all of the ingredients, prepare the soup in BATCHES, or use a food processor.

* * *

If you can find a white variety of WHOLE GRAIN bread, it is perfect in this dish.

Soak the bread in the vinegar in a bowl for 5 minutes.

Heat 2 tablespoons of the olive oil in a skillet over medium heat. Add the garlic and zucchini and cook until soft, about 3–5 minutes. Remove from the heat and cool to room temperature.

Place the bell peppers, onions, peas, and cilantro into a blender. Pulse to combine. Add the zucchini mixture and pulse again. Add the bread cubes. Pulse again. Season with salt and pepper. Pour in the remaining 2 tablespoons of olive oil, chicken broth, and as much hot pepper sauce as you like. Pulse to create a smooth soup. Place into the refrigerator and chill for at least 1 hour.

Place the beans into a bowl. Stir in the lime zest and lime juice.

To serve, divide the soup into 4 bowls. Place one-fourth of the beans into the center of each bowl. Garnish with freshly ground pepper and an additional drizzle of olive oil.

On Shopping Day: Prepare the soup and store in an airtight container for up to 4 days.

Makes 4 servings
Prep Time: 10 minutes
Cook Time: 5 minutes

- 4 slices whole grain bread, crusts removed, cut into cubes
- 1/3 cup white wine vinegar
- 4 tablespoons olive oil, plus additional for garnish, divided use
- 2 medium cloves garlic, minced (about 1 teaspoon)
- 2 large zucchini, sliced into rounds
- 2 medium green bell peppers, seeded and cut into pieces (about 1 1/3 cups)
- 1 bunch (6 to 8) green onions, chopped (about 1/2 cup)
- 1 10-ounce package frozen sweet peas, thawed
- 2 tablespoons chopped fresh cilantro
- Salt and freshly ground pepper
- 1 cup homemade chicken stock or low-sodium chicken broth
- 4–6 drops hot pepper sauce
- 1 15-ounce can white navy beans, drained
- Juice of 1 medium lime (about 1 tablespoon)
- Zest of 1 medium lime (about 1 tablespoon)

PEPPERY WHITE BEAN SALSA

With Whole Wheat Pita Chips

Incorporate beans into your favorite appy and have a double dose of finger-lickin' FUN!

Makes 4 to 6 servings
Prep Time: 10 minutes
Cook Time: 12 to 14 minutes

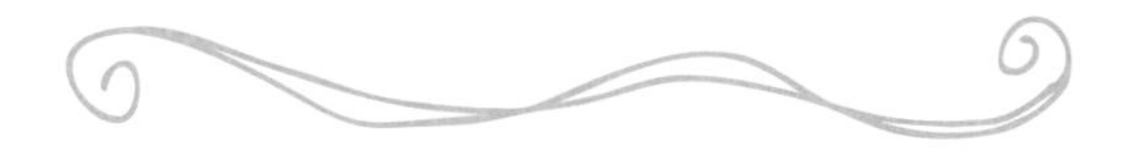

BLACK beans and white NAVY beans are also terrific in SALSA.

For the salsa

- 1 16-ounce can cannellini beans, drained
- 1 16-ounce can diced tomatoes
- 1 medium jalapeño pepper, seeded and diced (about 2 tablespoons)
- 1 small red onion, peeled and diced (about 1/2 cup)
- 2 medium cloves garlic, minced (about 1 teaspoon)
- 2 tablespoons olive oil
- 2 tablespoons red wine vinegar
- Juice of 1 medium lime (about 1 tablespoon)
- 2 tablespoons chopped fresh cilantro
- Salt and freshly ground pepper

For the pitas

- 4 whole wheat pita pockets
- 2 tablespoons olive oil
- 1 ounce finely grated Parmesan cheese

Place the cannellini beans, tomatoes, jalapeño pepper, red onion, and garlic in a bowl. Stir in the olive oil, vinegar, and lime juice. Stir in the cilantro and season with salt and pepper. Chill for at least 30 minutes.

Preheat the oven to 350 degrees. Cut pita pockets into eighths and place onto a rimmed baking sheet. Brush the tops with olive oil and sprinkle with Parmesan cheese. Bake until golden and crispy, about 12–14 minutes. Remove from oven and cool to room temperature.

To serve, place the pita chips around the salsa and dip away!

On Shopping Day: Prepare the salsa and store in an airtight container for up to 4 days.

LENTILS

With Wild Rice and Mushrooms

A perfect accompaniment to roasted chicken or beef, this earthy side dish adds a rustic flare to a meal.

Makes 6 servings
Prep Time: 10 minutes
Cook Time: 45 minutes

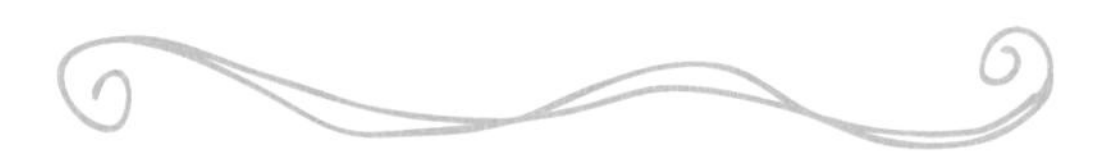

French green LENTILS would be wonderful in this recipe. They are available in most major grocery stores and many specialty markets.

- 2½ cups water, salted
- 1 cup wild rice
- 2 tablespoons olive oil
- 4 ounces baby portobello mushrooms, finely diced (about 1 cup)
- 1 small white onion, peeled and finely diced (about ½ cup)
- 1 large carrot, finely diced (about ½ cup)
- 2 medium celery ribs, finely diced (about ½ cup)
- 2 medium cloves garlic, minced (about 1 teaspoon)
- ½ teaspoon ground cloves
- Salt and freshly ground pepper
- 4 ounces pancetta, diced into ¼-inch cubes
- 1 cup dried lentils
- 2 cups homemade chicken stock or low-sodium chicken broth
- 1 bay leaf
- 2 tablespoons chopped fresh parsley (for garnish)

Heat 2½ cups salted water in a pot. Add the rice and bring to boil. Reduce heat, cover, and simmer until rice is just tender, about 45 minutes. Drain. Return rice to pan.

Meanwhile, heat the olive oil in a large skillet over medium-high heat. Add the mushrooms, onion, carrot, celery, and garlic. Cook until the veggies are just beginning to turn golden. Stir in the ground cloves and season with salt and pepper. Add pancetta and cook until crisp, about 5 minutes. Add the lentils. Cover with chicken stock. Add in the bay leaf, bring to a boil. Reduce heat, cover, and simmer until lentils are tender, about 30–35 minutes. Remove from the heat. Stir the rice into lentil mixture. Simmer until all of the liquid has been absorbed, about 5 minutes.

To serve, taste and adjust seasonings. Pour into a serving bowl and garnish with fresh parsley.

On Shopping Day: Prepare the veggies, store in an airtight container in the refrigerator for up to 4 days.

WATERCRESS SALAD

With Raspberry Vinaigrette and Blood Orange

A crisp, fresh blend of tart greens and sweet fruit makes this a salad for all occasions.

Makes 4 servings
Prep Time: 5 minutes

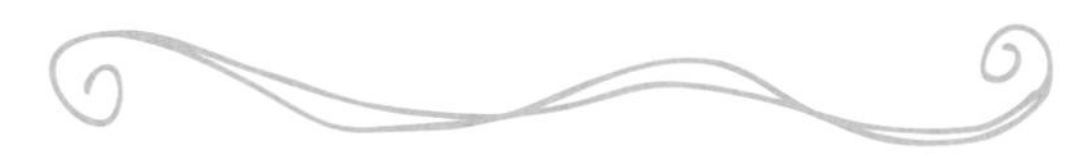

ARUGULA would be a great addition to this salad; its PEPPERY flavor is perfect with the raspberry and orange.

* * *

Blood oranges are SWEETER than navel oranges and have a DEEPER color. They are cropping up in major grocery stores and on fresh fruit stands. Substitute with your favorite orange or tangerine if you like.

For the vinaigrette

- 3 tablespoons raspberry vinegar
- 1 tablespoon honey
- Zest of 1/2 medium lime (about 1 teaspoon)
- 1/2 cup olive oil
- Salt and freshly ground pepper

For the salad

- 2 ounces mesclun lettuce mix (about 2 cups)
- 1 bunch watercress, washed, dried, stems removed (about 4 cups)
- 1 blood orange, peeled, sections separated
- 1 small red onion, peeled and thinly sliced (about 1/2 cup)
- 1/4 cup fresh raspberries (for garnish)

In a medium bowl whisk together the raspberry vinegar, honey, and lime zest. Slowly whisk in the olive oil. Season with salt and pepper.

Place the lettuce and watercress into a bowl. Toss with the orange sections and onion. Pour the dressing over top.

To serve, divide the salad among 4 chilled dishes. Garnish each with fresh raspberries.

On Shopping Day: Prepare the vinaigrette, store in an airtight container in the refrigerator for up to 3 days.

SUMMER SQUASH SALAD

With Baby Spinach, Roasted Tomatoes, and Parmesan Cheese

This blend of fresh veggies makes for a refreshing and filling salad. The dish would be gorgeous served as a layered salad in a crystal-clear trifle dish.

Makes 6 servings
Prep Time: 20 minutes
Cook Time: 1 hour

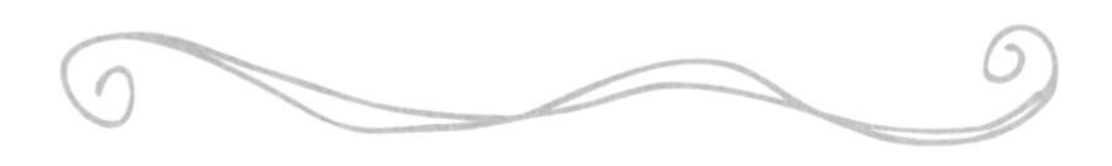

A MANDOLINE is the perfect tool to use when making paper-thin slices of veggies for arranged salads. Watch your fingers—it's sharp!

For the roasted tomatoes

- 12 medium plum tomatoes cut into quarters (about 4 cups)
- 2 tablespoons olive oil
- 2 medium cloves garlic, minced (about 1 teaspoon)
- 1 teaspoon dried oregano leaves
- Salt and freshly ground pepper

For the dressing

- Juice of 2 medium lemons (about 1/4 cup)
- 1 teaspoon Dijon mustard
- 1/2 cup olive oil

For the salad

- 2 medium zucchini, thinly sliced
- 4 medium yellow squash, thinly sliced
- 6 ounces fresh baby spinach leaves, washed and dried (about 4 cups)
- 1/2 cup fresh flat-leaf parsley
- 1/2 cup fresh basil leaves
- 2 ounces finely grated Parmesan cheese (about 1/2 cup)
- Shaved Parmesan cheese (for garnish)

Preheat the oven to 350 degrees. Toss the tomatoes with 2 tablespoons olive oil, garlic, dried oregano, salt, and pepper. Lay onto a rimmed baking sheet. Roast for 1 hour. Cool to room temperature.

In a bowl whisk together the lemon juice and Dijon mustard. Slowly whisk in ½ cup olive oil. Season with salt and pepper.

Toss the zucchini and squash with half of the dressing. Toss the baby spinach, parsley, and basil leaves with the other half of the dressing.

To serve, assemble the salad on a large serving platter. Place one-third of the spinach leaves onto the platter. Top with half of the squash and zucchini slices. Sprinkle with half of the grated Parmesan cheese. Repeat with the remaining ingredients. Top the salad with the roasted tomatoes. Garnish with shaved Parmesan cheese.

On Shopping Day: Roast the tomatoes and store in an airtight container in the refrigerator for up to 3 days.

MACADAMIA NUT BISCOTTI

Dipped in Chocolate and Coconut

My very good gal pal taught me that just a little bite of cookie can be really satisfying for dessert. Of course, it's so hard to stop at just one bite! Well . . . I like taking that "just a little bite" to new heights—so here's to you, Doreen!

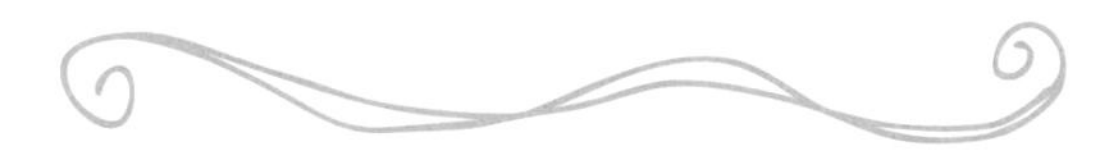

You can DIP the cookies in your favorite ingredients. Melt WHITE CHOCOLATE, CARAMEL, or BUTTERSCOTCH and dip in chopped walnuts or pecans—it's all *sooooo* good. . . .

Preheat the oven to 350 degrees. In a medium bowl whisk together the flour, baking powder, nutmeg, and salt. In a separate large bowl use an electric mixer to combine the sugar and butter until smooth and fluffy. Stir in the eggs, one at a time. Stir in the vanilla.

Stir in the flour mixture. Stir in the macadamia nuts. Divide the dough in half. Wrap each half in plastic wrap and freeze for 20 minutes. Remove the dough from the freezer. Use your hands to form each piece into a log, about 12 inches long and 3 inches wide. Place both logs on a Silpat- (or parchment-) lined baking sheet. Bake until golden brown, about 20 minutes. Remove from the oven.

Reduce the oven temperature to 300 degrees. Cool the logs for 15 minutes. Use a serrated knife to cut each log into diagonal ½-inch slices. Lay the slices onto the baking sheet cut-side up. Bake until the biscotti is golden and dry to the touch, about 30 more minutes. Cool on racks.

Melt the chocolate in a double boiler over simmering water until smooth (or melt in a microwave oven, stirring often). Place the coconut into a shallow bowl. Dip one end of each cookie into the melted chocolate and then into the coconut.

To serve, place the cookies onto a platter.

On Shopping Day: Prepare the cookies. Store in an airtight container for several days, in the fridge for several weeks, and in the freezer for several months!

Makes 30 servings
Prep Time: 20 minutes, plus chilling dough
Cook Time: 50 minutes

For the biscotti

- 2 cups unbleached all-purpose flour
- 1½ teaspoons baking powder
- ¼ teaspoon ground nutmeg
- ¼ teaspoon salt
- ¾ cup granulated sugar
- ½ cup butter, room temperature (1 stick)
- 2 large eggs
- 1 tablespoon vanilla
- 1 cup macadamia nuts, coarsely chopped

For the dipping

- 1 cup mini semisweet chocolate chips
- ⅓ cup flaked, sweetened coconut

PEANUT BUTTER SANDWICH COOKIES

Forget those prepackaged sandwich cookies! These peanut butter treats are delicious, decadent and, above all, deserving of your time.

Makes 2 dozen cookie sandwiches
Prep Time: 10 minutes
Cook Time: 15 minutes

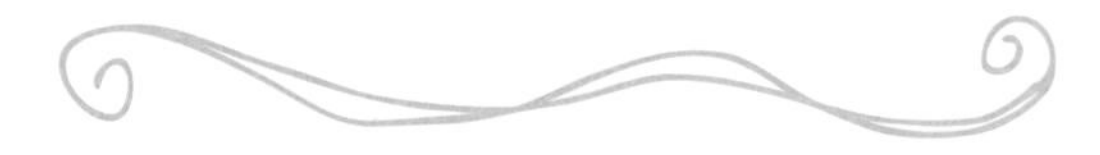

You can fill these cookies with everything from CREAM CHEESE to butter cream to GANACHE. For your next cookie buffet, fill your PEANUT BUTTER cookies with all three!

- 1 1/4 cups unbleached all-purpose flour
- 1/2 teaspoon baking soda
- 1/2 teaspoon salt
- 1/4 cup butter (1/2 stick), room temperature
- 1/4 cup vegetable shortening
- 1/2 cup brown sugar
- 1/2 cup confectioners' sugar
- 1 large egg
- 1 cup peanut butter
- 1 teaspoon pure vanilla extract
- 1 cup old-fashioned oats
- 1 13-ounce jar hazelnut/cocoa spread

Preheat the oven to 375 degrees. In a small bowl whisk together the flour, baking soda, and salt. Use an electric mixer to combine the butter, shortening, brown sugar, and confectioners' sugar until fluffy. Add the egg, peanut butter, and vanilla extract. Mix until smooth. Stir in the flour mixture on slow speed. Stir in the oats on slow speed until just blended.

Drop the dough by rounded teaspoonfuls onto a baking sheet lined with parchment paper (or Silpat liner). Flatten each round with the back side of a fork 2 times (making a cross pattern). Bake until golden, 10–12 minutes. Transfer to a rack to cool.

When the cookies have cooled, spread the bottom half of one cookie with a spoonful of the hazelnut/cocoa spread. Top with another cookie to create a sandwich. Repeat using all of the cookies and spread.

On Shopping Day: Prepare these cookies for weekday treats. Store in an airtight container for up to 1 week.

ALMOND-TOPPED RICOTTA CHEESECAKE

Being ***gorgeous*** *means you can have your cheesecake and eat it too—especially if it's topped with ultra-nutritious nuts!*

Makes 16 servings
Prep Time: 15 minutes
Cook Time: 80 minutes

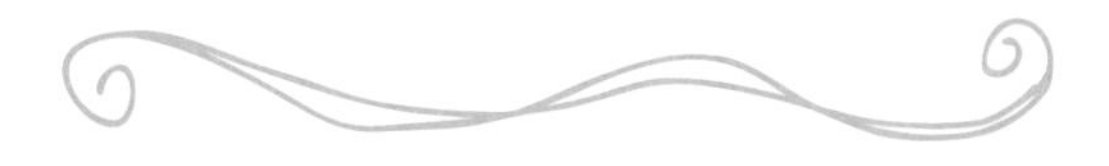

Using REDUCED-FAT ricotta cheese helps to LIGHTEN up this dish, but remember, a little goes a long way.

- 6 large eggs, separated into whites and yolks
- 2/3 cup natural sugar
- 2 teaspoons pure vanilla extract
- 2 15-ounce containers reduced-fat ricotta cheese
- Zest of 1/2 medium orange (about 1 tablespoon)
- 1 cup honey-roasted almonds, chopped
- Confectioners' sugar (for dusting)

Preheat the oven to 325 degrees. Separate the eggs, placing the whites in a large bowl and the yolks in another large bowl.

Use an electric mixer to combine the egg yolks, sugar, and vanilla until thick and fluffy. Add the ricotta and orange zest and mix until just combined. Set aside.

Clean the beaters. Use the electric mixer to beat the egg whites until soft peaks form. Fold the egg whites into the ricotta mixture. Pour into a 10-inch springform pan that has been coated with vegetable oil spray. Smooth the top with a spatula.

Bake until the cake is a deep golden brown and the sides begin to pull away from the pan, about 1 hour and 20 minutes. Transfer to a rack and sprinkle the chopped almonds over top. Let cool completely. Run a knife around the edge of the pan. Cover with plastic wrap and refrigerate for at least 4 hours or overnight.

To serve, release the sides of the springform pan, dust with confectioners' sugar, and cut into wedges.

COCKTAIL NUT COOKIE BARS

A twist on the one-nut cookie, this recipe features your favorite combination of mixed nuts in a gooey bar.

Makes 24 bars
Prep Time: 15 minutes
Cook Time: 25 to 30 minutes

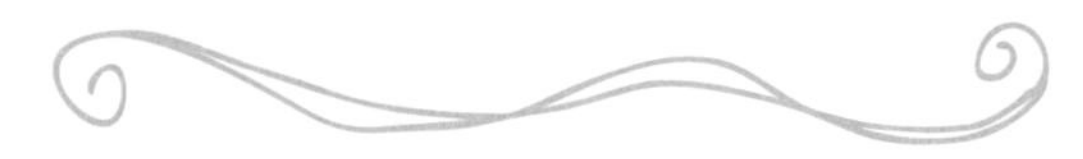

Since COCKTAIL nuts come in all shapes and sizes, coarsely chopping with a knife works better than pulsing the nuts in a food processor.

For the crust

- 1/2 cup unsalted butter (1 stick), room temperature
- 1/4 cup brown sugar
- 1 cup unbleached all-purpose flour
- 1/2 teaspoon salt

For the topping

- 3 large eggs
- 3/4 cup corn syrup
- 1/2 cup natural sugar
- 2 tablespoons butter, melted
- 1 10-ounce package semisweet chocolate chips
- 1 cup butterscotch morsels
- 2 cups mixed nuts, chopped

Preheat the oven to 350 degrees. Place the butter, brown sugar, flour, and salt into the bowl of a food processor. Pulse until coarse crumbs form. Pour the crust mixture into the bottom of an 11 x 9 x 2-inch baking dish that has been coated with vegetable oil spray. Press down with a fork to compact the crust.

In a large bowl whisk together the eggs, corn syrup, sugar, and melted butter. Add semisweet chips, chocolate chunks, and nuts. Pour this mixture over the crust. Bake until the center is set, about 25–30 minutes. Remove the pan from the heat and cool to room temperature.

To serve, cut into 24 bars.

On Shopping Day: Make the bars and store in an airtight container for up to 1 week.

Mary Ellen Weighs In

Exercise plays a significant role in the good bone equation. Like muscle, bone is living tissue that constantly reforms, gaining or losing strength according to how often it is used. Without exercise, bone loses density and becomes weaker. Good bone strength depends on balancing good exercise habits with your lifestyle.

Exercise also encourages calcium absorption into your bones. Two types of exercise are important for building and maintaining bone mass and density. The first is weight-bearing exercise in which your bones and muscles work against gravity. In weight-bearing exercise, your feet and legs are bearing your weight. These exercises include jogging or walking.

The second is resistance exercise, which uses your muscle strength to improve your muscle mass and strengthen your bones. Weightlifting using machines or free weights falls under this category. Most important to remember when beginning resistance training is *to start with a weight that you can lift with proper form and body alignment.* If you lift the weight improperly or lift a weight that is too heavy, you risk injury.

Get the help of a qualified trainer to make sure you start off on the right foot. A personal trainer will help you set achievable goals. Your personal trainer is a source of inspiration, motivation, and encouragement. She will have the latest information on health and fitness, and she'll help you make the most of your workout time.

Gorgeous Home Spa Secrets . . . For Pampering the Bone-Tired

I know we're talking about bones, but there are a few other (unmentionable) issues we have to consider when working out to build those bones. Proper feminine hygiene for health is imperative. Nearly 80 percent of women exercise on a regular basis, yet as many as one-third of these women mistakenly wear their sweat-soaked clothing for hours following a workout. Appropriate workout attire like clothes made from breathable fabrics and a quick shower immediately after your workout all play an important part in a healthy active lifestyle. Don't be afraid to ask the sticky questions when shopping for the perfect workout clothing. Let us not forget the importance of good shoes, too. Proper shoes are very important in preventing injury. Look for ones that offer ankle and arch support.

After you've had a busy workout, there's tired . . . and then there's *bone-tired*—a condition that requires no less than a good hot bath. The right kind of tub-time can improve the body's circulation, rid it of toxins, and set aching joints right as rain. So what do professional spas use that can be implemented at home? Read on.

Fleur de Sel

Whether it be plain old table salt or the Frenchman's *fleur de sel* (flower of salt), it's the secret to a great bath in any form or language. Epsom and Dead Sea Salt are among the favorite types of bath salts. While these are ideal soaks for magnesium-deprived, bone-tired bodies, the list of beneficial baths hardly stops there. The silica in horsetail is a great rebuilder of bones, aiding the body in its absorption of calcium. If you're especially achy and remembered to pick up this herbal remedy, add 5 drops of it to your next bath; its concentration of silicic acid, potassium, aluminum salts, flavonoids, equisetolic acid, and alkaloids will send those *achy, breaky* joint pains swirling down the tub's drain. If your concerns are more cosmetic than physical, milk baths work wonders for the skin, cleaning so deep you could say it's "down to the bone;" the lactic and alpha hydroxy acids in a milk bath promise to whisk away every last dead skin cell.

Buzzwords, Buzz Recipes

Some doctors believe that bathing in mineral-rich waters (also known as "hydrotherapy") is beneficial to fighting disease. Mineral buzzwords like calcium, phosphorous, magnesium, iron, iodine, and sodium belong in your bath as much as the bubbles—they can only do your body good, so mention them when you visit a professional spa. If you're making your own aromatherapy bath, know that salt, baking soda, and oatmeal are key ingredients. It's those nights you make the sweet stuff that home spa treatments are imminent!

The "Ahhh" in Spa

The French have cherished salt since a hefty tax on it helped start the French Revolution. Not too long after the war, a French physician named Dr. Stephan Bonnardiere discovered that breathing ocean air and soaking in salt water and seaweed were excellent ways to maintain good health. There must have been something to Bonnardiere's philosophy because its been putting the "ahhh" in spa ever since. Elements found in salt water and seaweed are similar to the chemical makeup of human plasma, allowing us to absorb key minerals and nutrients, like potassium, calcium, and iodine—all good for your body. Two great salt baths, both of which have enough magnesium sulfate to make your bones surrender to heavenly sighs, are as follows:

Bone-Weary Beauties Only

The bone-tired have *gotta* love Epsom. It's an unspoken rule! Epsom, unlike other salts, softens the skin while reducing the swelling from muscle strain. Gather 1 cup borax,

2 cups Epsom salts, ½ cup coarse sea salt, ¼ cup baking soda, ¼ cup white clay, and lavender oil for fragrance (add as much as you want, not exceeding 10 drops). Mix the ingredients with a wire whisk, cover the mixing bowl, and leave overnight to assure there's a scent. When you're ready to luxuriate in this bath, add ½ cup of your elixir to a tubful of warm, waiting water.

Bathe Like an Egyptian Royal

Credence that hydrotherapy works is owed largely to the practice of it by ancient Egyptians and Romans, including Cleopatra. Her lactic and alpha hydroxy beauty bath is a simple concoction of 4 cups fresh buttermilk or plain milk added to the rush of pure bath water. Soak in it for twenty minutes or the length of four of your favorite songs. Use a loofah; afterward, shower off any lingering film.

You, Me, and Yoga

Strengthen those bones and your inner self by exploring the wonder of yoga. Yoga is extremely effective in increasing your flexibility because it has positions that act upon the various joints of the body, including those joints that are never really "on the radar screen," let alone exercised. Various yoga positions exercise different tendons and ligaments, which aid in bone strengthening.

Yoga is perhaps the only form of activity that massages all the internal glands and organs of the body in a thorough manner, including those that get practically no external stimulation. Yoga acts in a wholesome manner on the various body parts. Check out www.healthandyoga.com to find a qualified instructor in your area.

CHAPTER 10

champagne from a glass slipper

"My feet, they haul me round the house, they hoist me up the stairs, I only have to steer them and they ride me everywhere." —Frank Gelett Burgess

The United States leads the world in the practice of podiatric medicine. Foot-care products in every size, shape, and texture fly off the shelves to comfort our feet and ankles. We're busy bees and our patters pay the price. Some of us get pedicures to tame rough spots (caused by tottering around in those Italian heels) with a pumice stone. Feet, compared to other parts of our anatomy, possess the highest number of bones. Imagine how many joints that amounts to! When your foot's vulnerable pressure points are aggravated, corns and calluses crop up. Since feet have the first and final say when it comes to mobility, *need* transcends *want* when it comes to healthy cuisine, cutting-edge spa solutions, and shoe secrets worthy of a cobbler. We've done our homework, so by chapter's end, your feet will feel and look so pure, so buffed, and so polished that Prince Charming himself could drink champagne from your glass slipper!

Ask Dr. Moon

The doctor is in to answer your questions.

Shoe shopping is a religion for some women, and even if it isn't for you, who doesn't love the sound of rustling tissue paper in a shoebox fresh from the department store? It's a great first-time feeling to strap on new heels, lace up sneakers, or Velcro a pair of sandals. You wonder just how you'll wear them out. Maybe you'll train for a 5K, learn to waltz, volunteer somewhere, or run your new shoes ragged simply by working hard at your job. Whatever the case, shoes and how you feel walking in them are a *huge* part of your daily life, and they're a commentary on your overall health, as well. Are you eating a nutritive diet and exercising enough? Do your favorite shoes connote a fun and active lifestyle or a sedentary snooze fest? Besides appreciating what looks good on your feet, have you ever thought about what a fabulous and intricately designed body part they are? Here's a brief but thorough anatomy lesson on what's filling that Manolo Blahnik sitting pretty in your closet.

Q: Besides wearing gorgeous shoes, what is the real function of our feet?

A: Well, besides providing a foot fetish for some, your feet combine mechanical complexity and structural strength. The ankle serves as foundation, shock absorber, and propulsion engine. The foot can sustain enormous pressure (several tons over the course of a one-mile run!) and provides flexibility and resiliency.

Q: What do podiatrists do exactly?

A: Podiatrists treat the lower extremities, which are comprised, obviously, of more than just feet.

Q: What causes bunions, corns, and calluses and what are the scientific definitions of these ailments?

A: There are five well-known foot disorders: athlete's foot, bunions, corns and calluses, flat feet, and warts.

(1) Athlete's foot is a fungal infection that usually occurs between the toes. It's a prime example of how skin, even as far south as feet, can't go untended; your feet need to be thoroughly washed and cleansed after a long day in hot, oppressive footwear. Socks should never be worn two days in a row even if your job takes place in an air-conditioned office. Treat athlete's foot with an over-the-counter anti-fungal medication.

(2) A **bunion** is much more complicated and beyond the victim's control. It's true bunions are exacerbated by ill-fitting shoes, but they are due, largely, to heredity, job conditions, or arthritis. Bunions are a deformity in the joint that links the big toe to your foot; treatment is custom-made or roomy shoes that place absolutely *no pressure* on the affected area. In some cases surgery is recommended, with a recovery time of 6 to 8 weeks.

(3) Corns and calluses are caused by pressure points on the foot, which are, for most people, the balls of the feet, bottoms of the toes, and certain points on the top of the foot. Calluses are tough areas on the feet and essentially harmless; the treatment amounts to nothing more than comfortable foot wear. Corns usually occur on parts of the feet where the pressure is elliptical—a pinching sensation in your shoes is the perfect breeding ground. Both can be a cosmetic problem.

(4) Flat feet are collapsed arches—the sole of the foot lies as flat on the ground as heel and toes. The human arch develops when we're babies and is fully formed by around age 6, unless you're part of the 20 to 30 percent of flat-footed Americans. Treatment can be had in the form of arch supports and physician-recommended exercise; surgery is usually a last resort.

(5) Warts on feet are an unpleasant thing to describe, let alone suffer from. They occur on the underside of the foot in response to a viral infection. Many doctors believe these small, white warts—hard to the touch—usually flair up as a reaction to stress. They go away on their own but will more than likely recur. They can be treated with over-the-counter solutions, laser treatments, or cryosurgery.

Q: Can you give a super quick anatomy lesson on the human foot?

A: The foot and ankle contain 26 bones. The feet work together to provide the body with support, balance, and mobility. Damage to the foot's structure or malfunction in any part of the foot can result in the development of problems elsewhere in the body. The ankle/foot also has 33 joints and more than 100 muscles and tendons, as well as a network of blood vessels, nerves, skin, and soft tissue.

Q: What causes joint disease?

A: In its simplest form, joint disease is the deterioration of cartilage and is classified as osteoarthritis. The condition occurs when synovial fluid, which carries nutrients to cartilage, declines, and friction results when joints slide over one another. The problem is more prevalent in women, and the majority of its sufferers (70 percent) in the 65-and-up age range. Diagnosis is made via x-ray. Chronic sufferers should consult their personal physicians for supplemental, pharmaceutical, or surgical treatment, but for the purposes of *gorgeous*, which is about preemptive strikes for a healthier you, osteoarthritis is less of a threat when you maintain a healthy weight and exercise regularly.

Q: Feet are so ugly. Is there any getting away from this fact?

A: That's where you're wrong. With the proper diet, hygiene, and exercise, you can have beautiful feet. Choosing the right shoe and paying attention to changes in feet is paramount in their upkeep.

(1) Let's first address **diet**. You're going to need a bone-and-joint-friendly menu to lessen the chances of not only osteoporosis but also *osteoarthritis*—that crippling joint disease we mentioned earlier which affects more than 20.7 million people in the United States! Fortunately, there are nutrients and foods that can help protect you from osteoarthritis, such as cold-water fish like salmon, tuna, herring, mackerel, and halibut; organically grown fruits and vegetables; nuts and seeds; whole grains; and ginger.

(2) Now about **shoes**: Don't buy them first thing in the morning because feet tend to spread during the day. Remember that the heel takes much of our weight, so a broad base with a slight heel—no higher than about 1½ inches—is ideal. The heel counter, which is the back of the shoe that grasps the heel of the foot, is important for support. Make sure it's firm with a good lining. The upper, or main part of the shoe, should ideally be a natural material so the foot can "breathe." Pliant man-made fibers are generally better than leather for soles, as they lessen the impact of the shoe hitting the floor.

Q: Do foot baths work?

A: I believe they can bring temporary relief. If your feet are swollen, try soaking them in warm water mixed with ¼ cup Epsom salts; follow that up with a shea butter foot massage for bothersome corns and calluses. You might also try a HoMedic foot massager. These machines feature infrared heat therapy, massage rollers, and pedicure attachments, so not only are soles looked after, but so are your toenails. It all sounds very pricey, but I did some comparison shopping and found an average price between $30 and $60.

Jorj's "Could Have Danced All Night" Glam Kitchen

When you play "this little piggy" with your toes, make sure you send that big toe to the market for the right groceries; there's a lot to nourish, after all, in a pair of feet, which account for a quarter of your overall bone count. We've listed some calcium-enriched yummies, making sure to include foods that have a foothold on what makes for happy joints and muscles. Antioxidants play a major role in keeping tendons and ligaments strong as well as in repairing muscle tears and strain. Consider the miles you'll cover within the next few months. Over time cumulative distance becomes impressive—you'll need plenty of the good carbs (a.k.a. "complex carbohydrates") to log those kilometers. Get ready to fill your plate with these energy boosters.

Wok Tall

After that kickboxing class, country line dancing lesson, or night of bowling, treat your deserving feet to your favorite veggies—the fail-safe bone pleaser. Calcium-rich **broccoli**, **bok choy**, **edamame**, and **salmon** smell *fantastic* sizzling in a wok. Likewise, **rice**, in all its complex carbohydrate glory, will make you a powerhouse! So will **baked potatoes** with conservative amounts of butter. If you're looking to elevate your energy level and satisfy a hankering for Italian at the same time, look no further than **pasta** noodles. Your dessert, at least in an ideal, bone-loving, weight-conscious world, should be filled with power -giving, antioxidant-rich **berries**.

Kick Up Your Heels at Breakfast

It so happens that breakfast presents an excellent opportunity to "mix it up" with special breakfast foods. Dress up these morning staples with nutrition-packed extras. Magnesium-rich **almonds**, **sunflower seeds**, or **Brazil nuts** taste terrific in a bowl of yogurt. A classic morning favorite is poached **eggs**. Add a helping of fresh **spinach** for dancin' feet.

When a Foot Soak Isn't Enough

At least once in your life, you've soaked your bone-tired feet or headed to a Jacuzzi with that particular ailing body part in mind. Perhaps you did so because your feet felt swollen. It so happens that foods rich in Omega-3 fatty acids may help reduce inflammation and repair torn ligaments. Where can one find omega in bulk? Get thee to a **crab** shack—or in the case of setting up your glam kitchen, a fish market—and pick up **salmon**, **trout**, and **tuna**.

A Foot Note on Fruit & Zinc

The antioxidants in vitamin C–laden foods keep collagen, ligaments and tendons strong; they also promote healthy muscle repair. Get enough vitamin C in your diet, and you can most assuredly count on proper healing when you've overdone it at the gym. Add **cabbage** to your soup as well as a little **potato** and **red bell pepper**. Eat **strawberries**, **oranges**, **kiwis,** and **tangerines**. Nip muscle strain in the bud by getting plenty of zinc before your intense workouts. Zinc promotes wound and tissue repair and is essential for bone health! It's found in **barley**, **crab**, **oysters**, **wheat**, **beef**, **lamb**, **chicken**, and **turkey**.

Start Your Day

Main Plates

On the Side

Snacks & Sweets

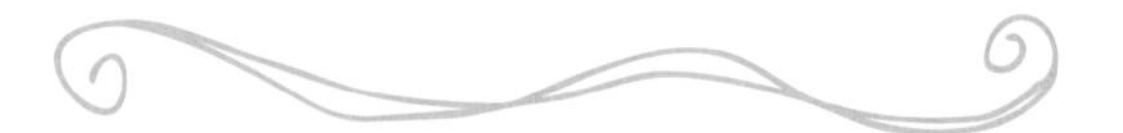

WHOLE WHEAT BRAN MUFFINS

With Golden Raisins and Walnuts

These power muffins have a little bit of everything (that's good for you!) in them. Have one to start your day and save one for later in the week as a super snack.

Makes 12 muffins
Prep Time: 10 minutes
Cook Time: 20 minutes

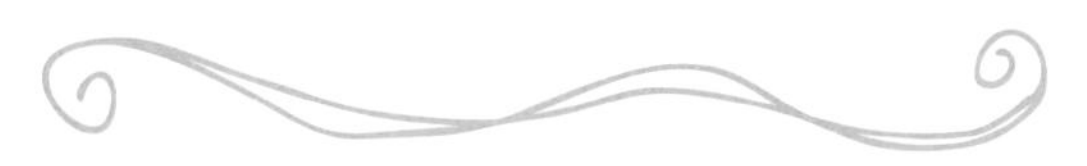

- 1 cup unbleached all-purpose flour
- 1/2 cup whole wheat flour
- 1/2 cup oat bran
- 2 teaspoons ground cinnamon
- 2 teaspoons baking powder
- 1/2 teaspoon salt
- 1 cup golden raisins
- 1/2 cup chopped walnuts
- 1/2 cup brown sugar
- 1/3 cup canola oil
- 2 large eggs
- 1 cup reduced-fat buttermilk
- 1 tablespoon pure vanilla extract
- Zest of 1/2 medium orange (about 1 tablespoon)

Preheat the oven to 400 degrees. In a medium bowl whisk together the flours, bran, cinnamon, baking powder, and salt. Stir in raisins and walnuts.

In a separate large bowl whisk together the sugar and oil. Whisk in the eggs, buttermilk, vanilla, and orange zest. Stir in the flour mixture.

Spoon the batter into a muffin tin lined with paper liners. Spray the inside of the muffin papers with vegetable oil spray to prevent sticking. Bake until the muffins spring back when touched and a tester inserted into the center comes out clean, about 18–20 minutes. Cool on wire racks.

BRUNCH FRITTATA

With Red Potatoes and Kale

A great source of calcium as well as antioxidants, kale adds a must-have dose of good stuff to this brunch.

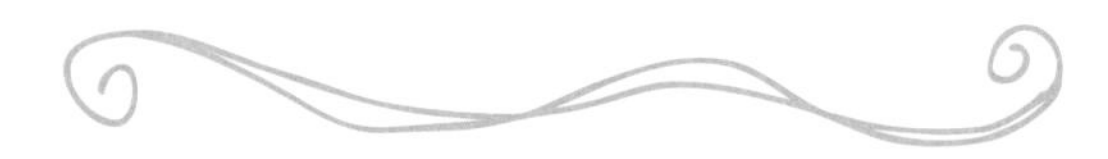

Be sure to use a skillet with an OVEN-PROOF handle and wear an oven mitt when you pull it out!

In a skillet cook the bacon over medium-high heat until crisp, about 4–5 minutes. Drain off any excess fat. Add the potatoes and onions. Cook until golden, about 5 minutes. Reduce the heat to low. Stir in the kale and cook until just wilted, about 2 minutes. Season with salt and pepper. Cool the filling to room temperature.

In a large bowl whisk together the eggs and half and half. Season with salt and pepper. Stir in the potato/kale mixture.

Preheat the oven on the broil setting. In an ovenproof skillet heat the olive oil over medium heat. Pour the egg mixture into the pan. Cook until the eggs set up, pushing the outer edges to the center and allowing the uncooked portion to run to the sides of the pan. Top the eggs with cheese. Place the skillet into the oven and cook until the frittata is puffed and brown and the center set, about 3–5 minutes.

To serve, let the frittata sit in the pan for 5 minutes. Loosen the edges with a spatula. Gently slide the frittata onto a serving plate. Cut into wedges.

On Shopping Day: Prepare the potato/kale filling, cool, and store in an airtight container in the refrigerator for up to 4 days.

Makes 4 servings
Prep Time: 10 minutes
Cook Time: 5 minutes

For the kale and potato filling

- 6 ounces bacon (about 3–4 slices), cut into 1-inch pieces
- 4–6 (2-inch) red creamer potatoes, boiled until tender, cut into quarters
- 1 bunch (6–8) green onions, chopped (about ½ cup)
- 2 ounces kale, washed, dried, stems removed, leaves torn (about 1 cup)
- Salt and freshly ground pepper

For the frittata

- 8 large eggs
- 2 tablespoons reduced-fat half and half
- 1 tablespoon olive oil
- 2 ounces finely grated Parmesan cheese (about ½ cup)

DOUBLE-BERRY WHOLE WHEAT PANCAKES

Start a special day with a special breakfast. These hearty pancakes will set you on the fast track to gorgeous.

Makes 4 servings
Prep Time: 10 minutes
Cook Time: 10 to 15 minutes

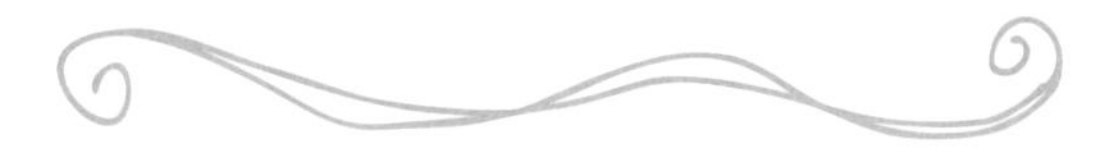

Adding ALL-PURPOSE flour lightens up the pancake batter in this recipe. Many batters incorporate both whole grain and unbleached white flours for the sake of texture.

- 1 cup whole wheat flour
- 3/4 cup unbleached all-purpose flour
- 1 tablespoon baking powder
- 1/2 teaspoon salt
- 1 1/2 cups buttermilk
- 2 large eggs
- 1 teaspoon pure vanilla extract
- 4 tablespoons butter, melted (1/2 stick)
- 1 cup fresh blueberries
- 1 cup fresh raspberries
- Canola oil
- Pure maple syrup

In a medium bowl whisk together whole wheat flour, all-purpose flour, baking powder, and salt. Stir together buttermilk, eggs, vanilla, and butter. Stir this mixture into the flour mixture. Fold the berries into the batter.

Heat a grill or skillet over medium-high heat. Coat the skillet with canola oil (about 1 tablespoon). Pour ½ cup batter into skillet (repeat with as many pancakes as will fit comfortably). Cook until bubbles form on the top (about 3–4 minutes). Use a spatula to turn each pancake. Continue cooking until both sides are golden, about 3–4 minutes more. Repeat using all of the batter and additional canola oil as needed.

To serve, place the pancakes onto a warm platter and drizzle syrup over the top.

POACHED EGGS

With Spinach and White Beans

Think a veggie-filled version of "poached eggs on potato hash," and you'll get the gist of this dish.

Makes 4 servings
Prep Time: 15 minutes
Cook Time: 12 to 14 minutes

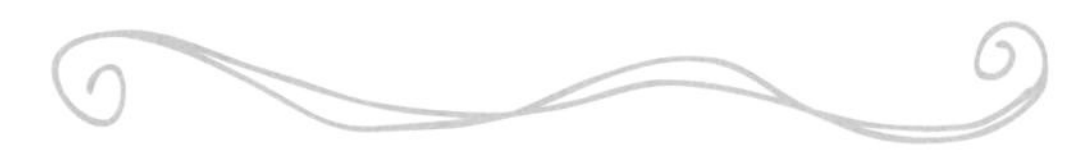

Cook the eggs for 3 1/2–4 minutes for a very SOFT center; a little longer if you want the yolks FIRM.

- 4 strips lean bacon, diced
- 1 small yellow onion, peeled and diced (about 1/2 cup)
- 4 ounces fresh spinach leaves, washed, dried, and torn (about 3 cups)
- 1 cup canned white beans, drained
- Salt and freshly ground pepper
- 4 large eggs
- 1 tablespoon chopped fresh parsley (for garnish)

In a skillet cook the bacon over medium-high heat. Add the onion and cook until soft, about 3 minutes. Add the spinach and cook until it wilts down, about 3 minutes. Stir in the white beans. Season with salt and pepper. Reduce the heat to low and keep warm.

Poach the eggs in an egg-poaching pan or in boiling water with a touch of vinegar.

To serve, place the spinach mixture onto 4 plates. Top each with a poached egg. Garnish with fresh parsley.

WILD IVORY KING SALMON FILLETS

With Macadamia Nut Crust

Also known as white king salmon, this delicate fish is making its way from the hottest restaurants to your neighborhood fishmonger. The flavor is buttery, due in part to its high oil content. Topping the fish with macadamia nuts adds another layer of richness, making this dish truly fit for a king.

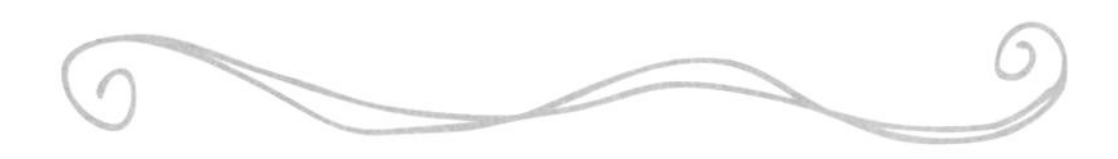

Only 1 in 100 salmon are WHITE in color, probably because their diet is rich in squid and fish rather than shrimp, krill, and crabs. Because these salmon are rare, they are more expensive than farm-raised or other wild salmon. If you are on a budget, substitute with the freshest salmon you can find.

Makes 4 servings
Prep Time: 10 minutes
Cook Time: 6 to 8 minutes

4 8- to 10-ounce center-cut fillet pieces wild ivory king salmon
Juice of 1 medium lemon (about 2 tablespoons)
1 cup macadamia nuts, chopped
Salt and freshly ground pepper
2 tablespoons olive oil

Preheat the oven to 350 degrees. Coat a baking dish with vegetable oil spray. Place the fillets into the dish. Sprinkle with lemon juice. Press the chopped nuts into the top of each fillet. Season with salt and pepper. Drizzle with olive oil.

Roast until the salmon is cooked on the outside and still rare on the inside (about 10 minutes per inch of thickness).

HOISIN BEEF AND VEGGIES

A cross between a stir fry and a stew, this fresh dish incorporates all of the veggies your family LOVES to eat!

Makes 4 to 6 servings
Prep Time: 15 minutes
Cook Time: 20 minutes

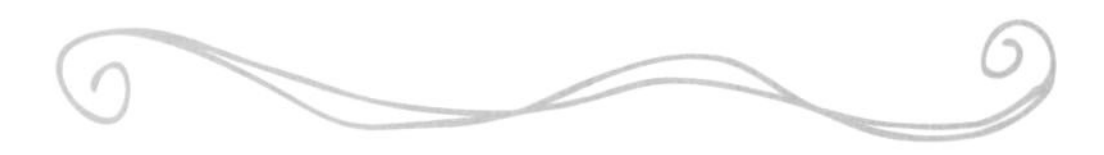

Hoisin sauce, also called PEKING sauce, is a thick, reddish-brown sauce that is SWEET and SPICY—and widely used in Chinese cooking. It's a mixture of soybeans, garlic, chili peppers, and various spices. It can be found in Asian markets and in many large supermarkets.

- 4 6-ounce New York strip steaks
- Salt and freshly ground pepper
- 1/4 unbleached all-purpose flour
- 2–3 tablespoons olive oil, divided use
- 1 bunch broccoli, stems peeled and sliced, cut into florets, about 2 cups
- 1 small head cauliflower, trimmed and cut into florets, about 2 cups
- 3 large carrots, cut into 1-inch pieces (about 2 cups)
- 1 large green bell pepper, seeded and cut into 1/2-inch pieces (about 1 cup)
- 1 large red bell pepper, seeded and cut into 1/2-inch pieces (about 1 cup)
- 1 quart homemade beef stock or low-sodium beef broth
- 1 7.25-ounce jar Hoisin sauce
- Juice of 1 medium orange (about 1/3 cup)
- Zest of 1 medium orange (about 2 tablespoons)
- 2 tablespoons soy sauce
- 2 cups cooked wild rice

Cut the steaks into 1-inch cubes. Season with salt and pepper and dredge in flour. Shake off excess. Heat 1 tablespoon olive oil in a deep pot over medium-high heat. Brown the beef (in batches) in the olive oil until golden. Use a slotted spoon to transfer to a platter. Use additional oil as needed.

Add 1 tablespoon olive oil to pot. Add the broccoli, cauliflower, carrots, and bell peppers. Stir and season with salt and pepper. Cook until the veggies begin to soften, about 4–5 minutes. Add beef stock and stir in Hoisin sauce. Add the beef back to the pot and simmer for 10 minutes. Stir in the orange juice, zest, and soy sauce. Simmer for 5 minutes more.

To serve, ladle the beef and veggies over rice.

On Shopping Day: Prepare the veggies, store in airtight containers in the refrigerator for up to 4 days.

CHARRED SIRLOIN STEAK

With Mushroom and Red Wine Sauce

A spoon full of sugar makes the well-prepared steak go down in this delicious presentation of an everyday dish.

Makes 4 servings
Prep Time: 10 minutes
Cook Time: 15 minutes

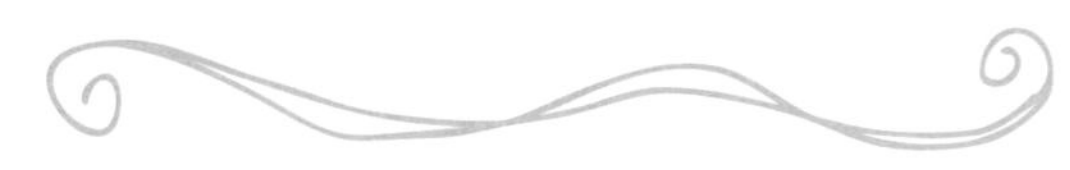

Yes, you can have your steak and eat it too! It's all about portions with red meat. A little bit of wonderful goes a long, long way.

For the steak

- 1 14- to 16-ounce $1\frac{1}{2}$-inch-thick sirloin steak
- 2 tablespoons brown sugar
- 1 teaspoon ground black pepper
- 1 teaspoon kosher salt
- 1 tablespoon olive oil

For the sauce

- 1 tablespoon olive oil
- 8 ounces baby portobello mushrooms, sliced (about 2 cups)
- $\frac{1}{2}$ cup red wine
- 2 sprigs rosemary
- 4 tablespoons chilled butter, cut into pieces ($\frac{1}{2}$ stick)
- 2 tablespoons chopped fresh parsley

Preheat oven to 400 degrees. Bring the steak to room temperature. Mix together the brown sugar, pepper, and salt. Rub this mixture over the steak. In a skillet heat the olive oil over medium-high heat. Place the steak into the pan. Cook until well browned, about 3–4 minutes per side. Place the steak into a baking dish and set in the oven to finish cooking, about 5 more minutes for rare. Remove the steak from the oven and allow to rest for 5 minutes before slicing.

For the sauce, pour 1 tablespoon olive oil into the skillet. Add the mushrooms. Season with salt and pepper. Cook until golden, about 3 minutes. Pour in the wine and add the rosemary sprigs. Cook until the mixture reduces by half. Turn off the heat. Stir in the butter.

To serve, remove the rosemary sprigs from the sauce. Remove the steak from the oven. Cut into thin slices. Pour the sauce over the steak. Top with fresh parsley. Serve family style.

OVERSTUFFED BEEFSTEAK TOMATOES

With Tortellini Salad

Fresh flavors are abundant in this recipe. Ripe tomatoes are the perfect container for spinach vinaigrette infused pasta. Wonderful for lunch or as a light summer supper, you'll make this dish again and again.

This recipe makes more pasta salad than you need for the tomatoes. Take extras to work for LUNCH the next day or serve with tomorrow night's burger.

SOPRASATTA is air-dried SALAMI found in specialty markets and major grocery stores. If you can't find it, substitute with good-quality salami.

Cook the tortellini in salted boiling water until al dente, about 10 minutes. Drain and place into a large bowl. Add the cheese, chicken breast, Soprasatta and roasted pepper.

Place the spinach leaves, onion, balsamic vinegar, lime juice, garlic, honey, and cilantro into a blender. Pulse to emulsify. Season with salt and pepper. With the machine running, slowly pour in the olive oil. Pour this mixture over the pasta salad and toss to combine. Cover and chill for at least 30 minutes or up to overnight.

Cut the tops from the tomatoes. Use a melon ball scoop to remove the seeds and pulp from each tomato. (Reserve this for another use such as marinara sauce or salsa.) Slice a thin piece from the bottom of the tomatoes so that they stand without rolling. Season the inside of the tomatoes with salt and pepper and drizzle with olive oil. Fill each tomato with pasta salad.

To serve, drizzle olive oil onto a serving platter. Grind fresh pepper over the oil. Place the tomatoes onto the platter. Garnish the tops of the tomatoes and the platter with snips of fresh dill.

On Shopping Day: Prepare the ingredients for the pasta salad and the vinaigrette and store separately in airtight containers in the refrigerator for up to 3 days.

Makes 4 to 6 servings plus extra pasta salad
Prep Time: 20 minutes
Cook Time: 10 minutes

For the pasta salad

1 pound tri-colored tortellini
10 ounces white Cheddar cheese, cut into 1/2-inch dice
1 6-ounce cooked skinless, boneless chicken breast, cut into 1/2-inch dice
8 ounces Soprasatta, cut into 1/2-inch dice
1 12-ounce jar roasted peppers, drained, cut into 1/2-inch pieces

For the vinaigrette

4 ounces fresh baby spinach leaves, about 2 cups
1/2 small onion, peeled
1/4 cup balsamic vinegar
Juice of 1 medium lime (about 1 tablespoon)
2 medium cloves garlic
1 tablespoon honey
2 tablespoons fresh cilantro leaves
Salt and freshly ground pepper
1/2 cup olive oil

For the tomatoes

4 large beefsteak tomatoes
1 tablespoon olive oil
Fresh dill (for garnish)

SEA SCALLOPS

With Blood Orange, Avocado, and Red Onion Salsa

The mild taste of simply seared sea scallops is enhanced by a spicy, exotic salsa in this dish.

Makes 4 servings
Prep Time: 15 minutes
Cook Time: 5 minutes

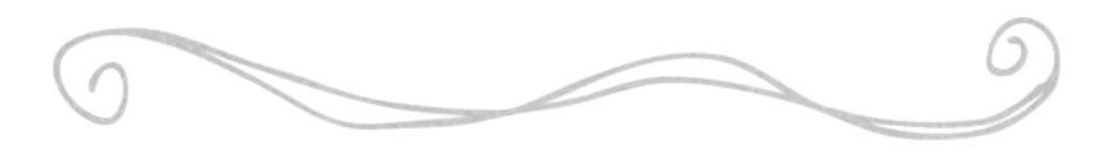

You can make this dish as a FIRST COURSE for your next dinner party. Serve 2 scallops per person.

For the salsa

- 1 blood orange
- 1 large avocado, peeled, pitted, and diced (about 1 cup)
- 1 large yellow bell pepper, seeded and cut into 1/4-inch dice (about 1 cup)
- 2 tablespoons diced red onion
- 1 medium jalapeño pepper, seeded and diced (about 2 tablespoons)
- Juice of 1 medium lime (about 1 tablespoon)
- Salt and freshly ground pepper

For the scallops

- 12 large sea scallops (about 1 pound)
- 2 tablespoons olive oil
- 2 tablespoons butter

Peel the blood orange and cut in half, horizontally. Cut away the white membranes and place the orange segments into a medium bowl. Add the avocado, bell pepper, onion, jalapeno pepper and lime juice. Season with salt and pepper. Toss and chill.

Season the scallops with salt and pepper. Heat the olive oil and butter in a skillet over medium-high heat. Place the scallops in the skillet. Cook until golden, about 2 minutes. Turn and cook until the other side is golden and the center of the scallops remain medium rare (opaque), about 2 minutes more.

To serve, place the scallops onto a platter and serve the salsa alongside.

MOJO MARINATED CHICKEN

Served over Black Beans

The combination of citrus juices and fresh garlic makes a delicious marinade for this chicken dish.

Makes 4 servings
Prep Time: 5 minutes plus marinating
Cook Time: 20 minutes

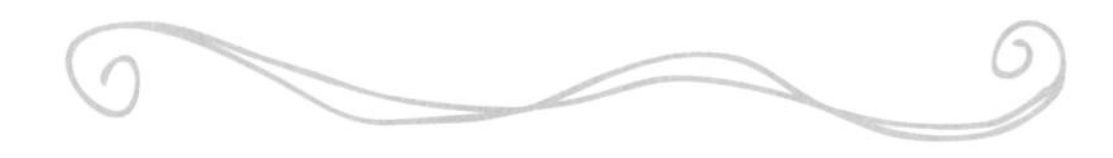

For the chicken

- 4 medium (6- to 8-ounce) skinless, boneless chicken breast halves
- Juice of 1 medium orange (about 1/3 cup)
- Juice of 3 medium limes (about 1/4 cup)
- 4 medium garlic cloves, peeled, minced (about 2 teaspoons)
- 1 teaspoon ground cumin
- 1/2 teaspoon dried oregano leaves
- 1/2 teaspoon paprika
- Salt and freshly ground pepper

For the black beans

- 1 tablespoon olive oil
- 1 small red onion, peeled and diced (about 1/2 cup)
- 1 16-ounce can black beans
- 1 teaspoon ground cumin
- 2 medium plum tomatoes, seeded and diced (about 1/2 cup)
- 2 tablespoons chopped fresh cilantro, divided use

Place the chicken into a plastic bag. In a small bowl whisk together the orange juice, lime juice, garlic, cumin, oregano, and paprika. Pour this mixture over the chicken. Seal the bag and refrigerate 30 minutes (or up to 6 hours).

Heat a grill pan that has been coated with vegetable oil spray over medium-high heat. Remove the chicken from the marinade. Season with salt and pepper. Grill the chicken, turning once, about 4–5 minutes per side. Transfer the chicken to a platter and keep warm.

Heat the olive oil in a pot over medium-high heat. Add the onion and cook until soft, about 4–5 minutes. Add the beans. Season with cumin, salt, and pepper. Cook, stirring often, until the beans begin to simmer, about 5 minutes more. Stir in the tomatoes and 1 tablespoon of the cilantro.

To serve, spoon the beans onto a platter. Cut the chicken into ½-inch thick slices and lay on top of the beans. Sprinkle the remaining cilantro over top.

BAKED POTATOES

Stuffed with Swiss Chard and Black Beans

It's soooo not about sour cream any more. Heap your baked potato with fresh veggies instead—it's the only way to enjoy that white, starchy veggie, once so forbidden.

Makes 4 servings
Prep Time: 15 minutes
Cook Time: 45 minutes

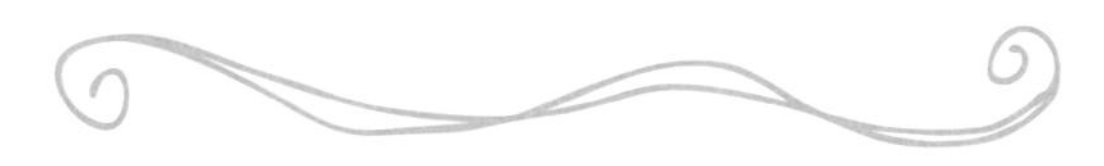

Black beans, Swiss chard, and potatoes are all excellent sources of MAGNESIUM—just what our bones need to ABSORB calcium and grow oh-so strong!

For the potatoes

2 large baking potatoes
1 tablespoon olive oil
Kosher salt

For the filling

1 tablespoon olive oil
1 large red onion, peeled and thinly sliced (about 1 cup)
1½ pounds Swiss chard, washed, dried, stems removed, leaves torn (about 8 cups)
1 16-ounce can black beans, drained
Salt and freshly ground pepper
2 tablespoons chopped fresh chives

For the garnishes

Yogurt
Jack cheese
Hot pepper sauce
Diced avocado

Preheat the oven to 350 degrees. Rub the potatoes with 1 tablespoon olive oil and season with Kosher salt. Pierce each potato with the tines of a fork. Place onto a rimmed baking sheet. Bake until soft, about 45 minutes to 1 hour. Remove from the oven and let cool slightly.

For the filling heat 1 tablespoon olive oil in a skillet over medium-high heat. Cook the onion until soft, about 5 minutes. Add the chard to the skillet and toss until it begins to wilt. Stir in the black beans and cook until heated through, about 5 minutes more. Season with salt and pepper.

Cut a slit in the top of each potato. Open slightly. Use a spoon to scoop out half of the potato keeping the shells in tact. Add the potato to the Swiss chard/black bean mixture and toss.

To serve, divide the Swiss chard filling, placing it inside and over the top of each baked potato. Top with fresh chives. Offer garnishes on the side.

BETTER VEGGIE CHILI

Crisp, fresh veggies, along with those you have stashed in your pantry, combine in just minutes for a fantastically flavored dish.

Makes 4 to 6 servings
Prep Time: 15 minutes
Cook Time: 30 minutes

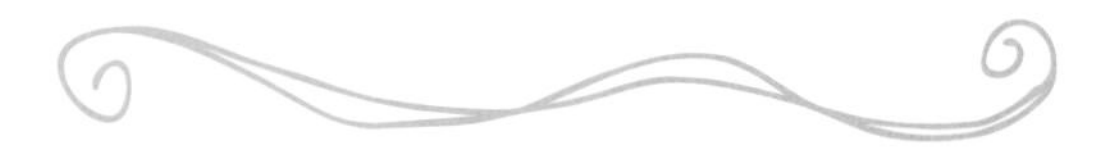

You can make this dish with any CANNED bean such as black, navy, or cannellini. Cooked lentils work well too.

- 2 tablespoons olive oil
- 1 medium yellow onion, diced into ½-inch squares (about 1 cup)
- 4 large carrots, finely diced (about 2 cups)
- 2 large red bell peppers, seeded and finely diced (about 2 cups)
- 1 large zucchini, seeded and finely diced (about 1 cup)
- 1 medium jalapeño pepper, seeded and diced (about 2 tablespoons)
- 1 28-ounce can diced tomatoes
- 1 15-ounce can corn, drained
- 1 15-ounce can red beans, drained
- 2 or more tablespoons ground chili seasoning
- 2 tablespoons tomato paste
- Salt and freshly ground pepper
- Baked tortilla chips (for garnish)
- Reduced-fat sour cream (for garnish)
- Chopped fresh cilantro (for garnish)

In a skillet heat the olive oil over medium-high heat. Cook the onion, carrots, and red bell peppers until soft, about 5 minutes. Stir in the zucchini and jalapeño pepper. Cook for 3 minutes more. Pour in the tomatoes, corn, and red beans. Stir in the chili seasoning and tomato paste. Season with salt and pepper. Reduce heat and simmer the chili for 20–30 minutes. Taste and adjust seasonings.

To serve, pour the chili into a tureen or serving bowl. Offer tortilla chips, sour cream, and cilantro to garnish.

On Shopping Day: Prepare all of the veggies. Store in an airtight container in the refrigerator for up to 4 days.

ASPARAGUS CHEESE TOASTS

Serve these rich, open-face sandwiches at your next luncheon or for a lite supper with a bowl of soup.

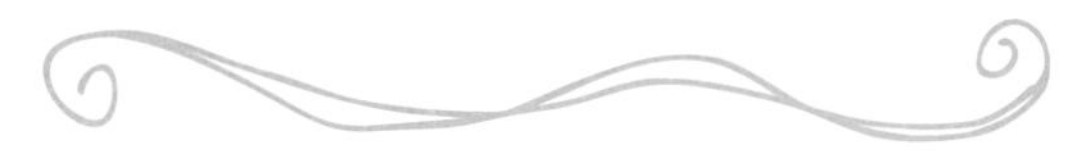

You can easily turn this recipe into an APPETIZER by substituting with small "party" bread slices and cutting the asparagus into PIECES instead of strips.

Makes 8 servings
Prep Time: 20 minutes
Cook Time: 6 minutes

- 1 pound fresh, thin asparagus spears, ends trimmed, cut to the same length as the bread
- 8 slices very thin-sliced whole grain bread
- 3 tablespoons olive oil
- 8 ounces grated, reduced-fat Swiss cheese (about 2 cups)
- 1 cup reduced-fat mayonnaise
- 2 tablespoons Dijon mustard
- 1 tablespoon prepared horseradish
- 6 ounces bacon, about 4–6 strips, cooked and crumbled
- Salt and freshly ground pepper

Blanch the asparagus in salted boiling water until tender, about 3–4 minutes. Drain and cool to room temperature under running water. Pat dry and cut in half lengthwise.

Brush both sides of the bread with olive oil. Heat a skillet over medium-high heat. Brown the bread slices until golden, about 1 minute per side. Place onto a rimmed baking sheet.

Place the Swiss cheese, mayonnaise, mustard, and horseradish into the bowl of a food processor. Pulse to mix thoroughly. Add the bacon, season with salt and pepper, and pulse again to combine.

Preheat the oven to broil. Lay the asparagus onto the toast. Spread the cheese mixture over top. Broil until the toasts are golden and bubbling, about 4–6 minutes.

To serve, cut each toast into triangles.

On Shopping Day: Blanch the asparagus, cool, and store in an airtight container in the refrigerator for up to 4 days.

ROASTED VEGGIE STACKS

With Mozzarella

Roasting veggies gives them a richer, sweeter taste and a soft texture. I like to stack the veggies because it reminds me of eating a roasted veggie sub sandwich without the bread!

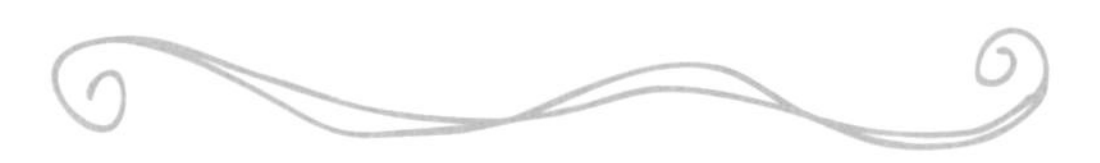

Use any VEGGIE for this recipe. A slice of tomato or a drizzle of marinara sauce adds a new component and keeps the dish FRESH.

Makes 4 servings
Prep Time: 10 minutes
Cook Time: 25 to 30 minutes

- 1 medium eggplant, sliced into (6) 1/2-inch-thick rounds
- 4 large portobello mushrooms, stem and gills removed
- 1 large red bell pepper, seeded and cut into quarters
- 1 tablespoon olive oil
- 1 teaspoon dried oregano flakes
- Salt and freshly ground pepper
- 4 1-ounce slices reduced-fat mozzarella cheese

Preheat the oven to 375 degrees. Coat a rimmed baking sheet with vegetable oil spray. Place the eggplant slices, portobello mushrooms (stem-side down), and red bell pepper pieces onto the baking sheet. Sprinkle with olive oil and season with oregano, salt, and freshly ground pepper. Roast until the veggies are soft, about 20–25 minutes. Remove from the oven.

Arrange the veggies into stacks. Flip the mushrooms so that they form shallow bowls for the remaining vegetables. Top each one with a slice of eggplant and red pepper. Place a slice of cheese on each stack. Cut the remaining 2 slices of eggplant in half and top each stack with those pieces. Place the baking sheet back into the oven and cook until the cheese has melted, about 3–5 minutes.

To serve, place the stacks of veggies on a serving platter. Garnish with a grind of fresh pepper and an additional splash of great tasting olive oil.

SWEET PEA PANZANELLA SALAD

We boost the antioxidants in this classic salad by adding extra veggies to the dressing.

Makes 8 servings
Prep Time: 20 minutes
Cook Time: 8 minutes

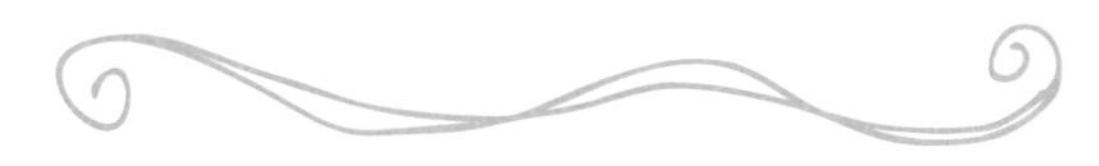

You can use FRESH peas for this salad. Simply BLANCH them in simmering water until very green, about 2 minutes.

For the Panzanella croutons

- 8 ounces whole grain crusty bread cut into 1-inch cubes
- 1/4 cup olive oil
- 4 medium garlic cloves, minced (about 2 teaspoons)
- Salt and freshly ground pepper

For the dressing

- 1 10-ounce package frozen sweet peas, thawed
- 1/2 cup reduced-fat half and half
- 1/4 cup homemade chicken stock or low-sodium chicken broth
- 1/4 cup olive oil
- Juice of 1 medium lemon (about 2 tablespoons)
- 1 tablespoon Dijon mustard

For the salad

- 1 pint ripe cherry tomatoes or mixed baby tomatoes
- 1 bunch (6 to 8) green onions, chopped (about 1/2 cup)
- Zest of 1 medium lemon (about 1 tablespoon)
- 2 ounces finely grated Parmesan cheese (about 1/2 cup)
- 2 ounces mixed lettuce leaves (about 2 cups)

Preheat the oven to 375 degrees. Place the bread cubes into a bowl. In a small pot heat the olive oil over medium heat. Add the garlic and cook until soft, about 2 minutes. Drizzle this mixture over the bread cubes. Season with salt and pepper and toss so that all of the cubes are coated. Place the bread onto a rimmed baking sheet. Bake until golden, about 5–7 minutes.

Place the dressing ingredients into the bowl of a food processor (or blender). Pulse to emulsify. Season with salt and pepper.

Place the tomatoes, green onions, and Panzanella croutons into a salad bowl. Add lemon zest and toss with the salad dressing. Sprinkle with cheese.

To serve, place the lettuce leaves onto a patter. Mound the tomato and crouton mixture over the top.

On Shopping Day: Prepare the Panzanella croutons and store in an airtight container. Prepare the dressing and store in an airtight container in the refrigerator for up to 4 days.

SLOWLY STEWED COLLARD GREENS

My pals from the South slowly cook these greens for hours and hours, so that the smoky flavor of the meat infuses into the tender leaves. You can cook the dish more quickly by reducing the liquid over a higher flame.

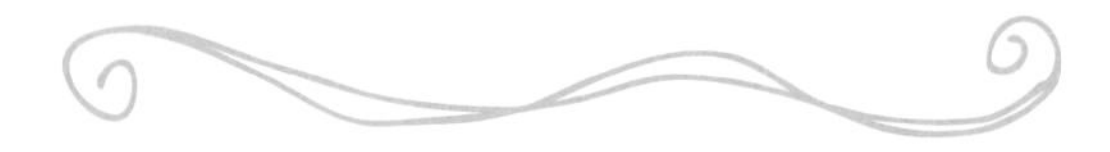

If you choose to quickly stew the collards, the meat won't be as tender, but don't worry, the flavor will still be remarkable.

Makes 4 to 6 servings
Prep Time: 15 minutes
Cook Time: 30 minutes (at least)

- 2 tablespoons olive oil
- 1 extra large white onion, thinly sliced (about 3 cups)
- 1½ pounds collard greens, washed, dried, stems removed, leaves torn (about 8 cups)
- 1 quart homemade chicken stock or low-sodium chicken broth
- 2 smoked ham hocks
- Salt and freshly ground pepper

In a saucepan heat the olive oil over medium-high heat. Add the onion and cook until soft and beginning to brown, about 5 minutes. Add the greens in handfuls and cook until wilted, about 5 minutes. Pour in the chicken broth. Submerge the ham hocks in the greens. Cover and bring to a boil. Reduce heat to low and simmer until all the liquid is absorbed and the greens are soft, anywhere from 30 minutes to several hours. The collards should be tender, but not mushy!

To serve, remove the meat from the ham hock and finely dice, discarding the fatty pieces with the bone. Add the diced meat (about 2 tablespoons) back to the greens. Season the dish with salt and pepper.

On Shopping Day: Prepare the collards, wash, dry well, and store in an airtight container for up to 5 days; or take the shortcut and purchase prewashed greens.

BLUEBERRY SHORTBREAD BARS

Grating the rich shortbread dough results in a light and crumbly cookie.

Makes 24 servings
Prep Time: 20 minutes plus chilling
Cook Time: 30 to 35 minutes

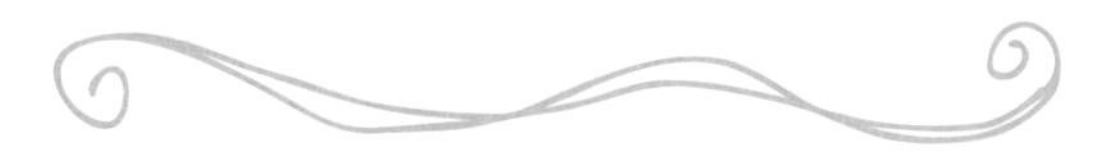

When you are looking for fruit preserves, choose one that relies on whole fruit with natural sweeteners.

- 1 cup unbleached all-purpose flour
- 1 cup whole wheat flour
- 1 teaspoon baking powder
- 1/4 teaspoon salt
- 1 cup unsalted butter, room temperature (2 sticks)
- 1 cup natural sugar
- 2 large egg yolks
- 1/2 teaspoon pure vanilla extract
- 1 cup all-natural blueberry preserves
- Confectioners' sugar

In a medium bowl whisk together the all-purpose flour, whole wheat flour, baking powder, and salt.

In another medium bowl use an electric mixer to combine the butter and sugar until fluffy. Mix in the egg yolks one at a time. Stir in the vanilla. Slowly mix in the flour mixture to form a dough. Divide the dough in half, form 2 circles, and wrap each in plastic wrap. Chill for at least 1 hour.

Preheat the oven to 350 degrees. Remove 1 circle of dough from the refrigerator. Use a box grater to grate the dough onto the bottom of a 11 x 9 x 2-inch baking dish that has been coated with vegetable oil spray. Use a spatula to gently spread the blueberry preserves evenly over the dough. Grate the remaining dough over the top of the preserves. Bake until the shortbread is golden, about 30–35 minutes.

Run a knife around the edge of the bars and cool to room temperature.

To serve, cut the shortbread into 24 bars. Use a spatula to remove from the baking dish. Sprinkle with confectioners' sugar.

On Shopping Day: Prepare the dough and refrigerate for up to 2 days.

TROPICAL STRAWBERRY TIRAMISU

Turn an Italian classic dessert into a fruit-filled favorite with just a few flavor twists.

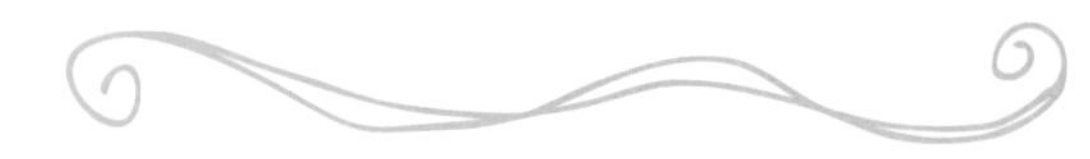

Guarantee PERFECT whipped cream by making sure that the cream is WELL CHILLED before whipping. Place the bowl and the whisk attachment (or beaters) into the freezer for 15 minutes before you begin to whip.

• • •

You can use any FLAVORINGS to create your own version of this dessert. For St. Patrick's Day, think lime juice, green grapes, and green crème de menthe liquor. For the Fourth of July, top with blueberries, and for the holidays add a layer of chopped peppermint candies.

Makes 12 servings
Prep Time: 20 minutes

- 1 8-ounce jar strawberry preserves
- 1/4 cup Cointreau (orange liquor) plus 2 tablespoons, divided use
- 1/3 cup white grape juice
- 2 8-ounce containers mascarpone cheese
- 1 cup whipping cream
- 1/3 cup natural sugar
- 1 teaspoon pure vanilla extract
- 2 pints strawberries hulled and sliced (about 4 cups)
- Zest of 1/2 medium orange (about 1 tablespoon)
- 2 packages crisp lady finger biscuits (about 48)
- 3 tablespoons flaked, sweetened coconut
- Fresh mint leaves (for garnish)

In a medium bowl whisk together the preserves, ¼ cup Cointreau, and the grape juice. Place the mascarpone cheese into a bowl. Pour in 1 tablespoon Cointreau and whisk until smooth. Pour the whipping cream into the bowl of an electric mixer. Pour in the remaining 1 tablespoon Cointreau, sugar, and the vanilla extract. Whip until soft peaks form. Fold the whipped cream mixture into the mascarpone cream. Toss the sliced strawberries with the orange zest.

To assemble, pour ½ of the strawberry preserve mixture into an 11 x 9 x 2-inch glass baking dish. Top with half of the lady finger biscuits. Top with ½ of the strawberries and ½ of the cream. Repeat with the remaining preserve mixture, ladyfingers, strawberries, and cream. Sprinkle the coconut over the top and garnish with fresh mint leaves.

Cover the dish with plastic wrap and refrigerate for at least 4 hours or overnight.

To serve, cut the tiramisu into squares and serve on chilled plates.

CHILLED BERRY SAUCE

With Lime Sherbet and Coconut Garnish

This profoundly refreshing dessert is a great way to slurp up all of those good-for-you antioxidants.

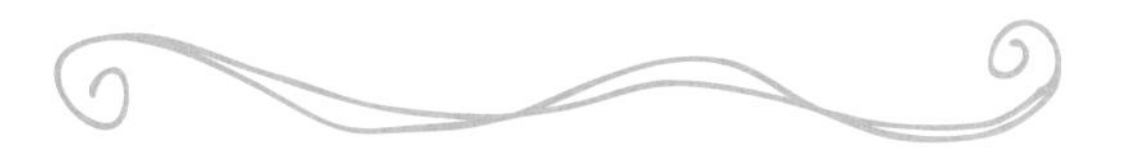

Slowly cooking the berries over BARELY simmering water works to INTENSIFY and merge the flavors.

Makes 4 servings
Prep Time: 15 minutes
Cook Time: 45 minutes, plus time for the sauce to chill

- 1 cup fresh blueberries, divided use
- 1 cup fresh raspberries, divided use
- 1 cup fresh blackberries, divided use
- 1 cup strawberries, hulled and quartered, divided use
- 1 tablespoon natural sugar
- Lime sorbet
- Flaked, sweetened coconut

Pour water into the bottom of a double boiler and heat until barely simmering. Top with another pot, making sure that the simmering water does not touch the bottom of the top pot. Place ¾ cup of each type of berry and the sugar into the pot, cover, and cook until the berries break down, about 40–45 minutes.

Use a handheld blender to emulsify the berries. (For a thinner sauce, you may strain the pureed berries through a fine sieve.) Refrigerate the sauce until chilled.

To serve, place a scoop of lime sorbet into a crystal bowl or wine glass. Surround the sorbet with the berry sauce. Garnish with reserved berries. Top with coconut.

On Shopping Day: Prepare the sauce. Store in an airtight container and chill.

PECAN GRAHAM SQUARES

This yummy bar combines good-for-you graham and nuts. It also comes together is seconds—perfect when you need just a little bit of something sweet and crunchy.

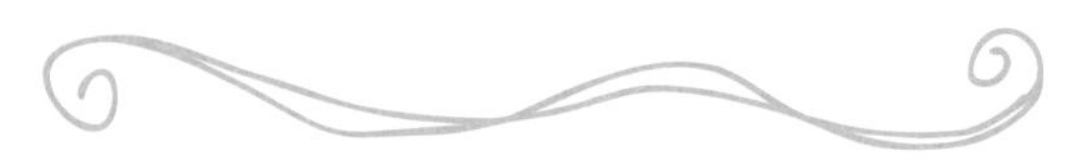

You will need about 20 graham crackers to make 1 1/2 cups of crumbs.

Makes 16 servings
Prep Time: 10 minutes
Cook Time: 35 to 40 minutes

- 1 1/2 cups graham cracker crumbs
- 1 14-ounce can sweetened condensed milk
- 1/4 teaspoon salt
- 1 1/2 cups chopped pecans
- Confectioners' sugar

Preheat the oven to 350 degrees. In a medium bowl stir together the graham cracker crumbs, condensed milk, and salt. Stir in the pecans. Spread the batter into an 8-inch square pan that has been coated with vegetable oil spray. Bake until the cookies spring back and a tester inserted into the center comes out clean, about 35–40 minutes. Cool on a rack.

To serve, dust the top with confectioners' sugar and cut into 16 squares.

Gorgeous Home Spa Secrets . . . For Cinderella-like Tootsie Toes

We engage in lots of activities that make us foot-conscious. For example, maybe you have a pilates or yoga class. In order to do Downward Facing Dog without slip-sliding across the studio floor, you can't wear socks, right? Mat-to-mat with your fellow classmates, you want your bare feet to make a good impression—especially when your instructor makes her usual rounds and decides you need help with a particular exercise. *Oh, my God, she's holding my bare feet in her hands . . .* you pray they look okay. The same goes for that annual well-woman exam. Your feet, especially if they're sockless, should look and feel as good as the rest of you. Try out these homemade "in a pinch" foot moisterizers and cleansers.

The Pampered Sole

Dry feet look worse than they feel. They inspire adjectives like "crusty," "scaly," and "tough as nails." Good thing lotion is such a popular gift. Why, there must be three bottles of moisturizer under your bathroom sink! You know . . . the ones you got for Christmas, your birthday, and that bridal shower. So why not make your own? You control the lotion quantity, preserve gas, and save a few dollars too!

Cure Dry Foot

Here's your chance to get rid of dry feet and toy with fragrances at the same time. In whisking together 1 tablespoon each almond, olive and wheat germ oil, it's the dozen or so drops of sweetness you add in the end that lends this failsafe moisturizer its unique and pleasing effect. You can choose eucalyptus, sandalwood, or other essential/fragrance oils. If you're short on natural food store supplies like these, achieve a heavenly scented moisturizer by adding a little pure vanilla extract. Add just a few squeezes of blood orange for the same beautifying quality that has enchanted Italian women for centuries. Combine the aforementioned ingredients in a bottle (an empty water bottle works!) and shake well; tip the bottle and wet a cloth so you can rub your heels and feet.

For Toes that Twinkle

You're a good steward of clean feet. You remember to wash them in the shower, reapply nail polish, and so on, but there will be days, long days, where you wore sandals and came home with less-than-fresh feet. You don't have time to take another shower. Is there a quick fix—something you could do with your feet that stops shy of hiding? The lemon juice that's always been handy in the side door of your refrigerator works wonders when you dilute a half cup of it with chilled water. Wet a washcloth and give both feet a vigorous rubdown. You'll be surprised at how refreshing it feels and impressed with the subtlety of the solution. You can steal away and wipe your feet down with a paper towel soaked in lemon juice and water.

From the Pedicure File

For a refreshing exfoliate that'll make your patters soft and smooth, mix together 8 strawberries with 2 tablespoons of olive oil and 1 teaspoon of kosher salt. Make a paste with the ingredients, using the back of a large spoon to mash. Massage it into your feet, rinse off, and dry. The strawberries in this homemade exfoliate feel just like the soothing beads in an expensive over-the-counter skin wash.

Mary Ellen Weighs In

Happy feet are more like a zone—a frame of mind. When your feet are happy, more than likely the rest of you is comfortable as well. These exercises can help every part of your foot—arches too—enter into a golden state of being. Try these movements out right after a soothing foot bath.

For happy toes, hold each of the following positions: Toe raise, toe point, toe curl, for 5 seconds. Repeat 10 times. Place toe divider sponges (the same kind used when applying nail polish) or small corks between the toes and squeeze inward for 5 seconds. Repeat 10 times. Practice picking up marbles with your toes—it keeps them flexible. Remove pain from the ball of your foot by placing a small towel on the floor; try to curl it towards you, using only your toes. If you suffer bunions try placing a thick rubberband around all your toes and spread them. Hold for 5 seconds, repeat 10 times.

Donate Your Glass Slipper Treasures

Styles change, your feet change, your needs change, and yet we continue to collect more and more shoes. Why not make someone else's Cinderella dream come true by donating those shoe treasures that are just taking up valuable space in your closet? Take an hour or so to clean out your closet and fill your trunk with treasures for others, and then take them to a thrift shop, secondhand store, or consignment store in your neighborhood.

CHAPTER 11

the white glove treatment

"You can't shake hands with a clenched fist." —Indira Gandhi

"You're soaking in it!" exclaims Madge the manicurist. Remember that? The television commercial that declared that their dish soap "softens hands while you do the dishes" is part of the collective American consciousness, demonstrating that this country's female populace cares deeply about hands—we want them soft, graceful, clean, and well-manicured. We'd do (or buy!) anything to prevent age spots, wrinkles, or knobby fingers, all of which detracts from our rings or other cherished jewelry. Worst of all, improperly cared for hands betray our age. Handshakes are an important part of first and lasting impressions. Is there a way to ensure—beyond wearing rubber gloves for housework, visiting a good manicurist, and moisturizing before slipping into bed each night—that first handshakes will be something the other person *enjoys*? Well, like everything else on a gorgeous body, diet is (or should be) your first and final answer to that question. We've dug up vitamins, minerals, and scrumptious foods that hand models must have known about all along!

Ask Dr. Moon

The doctor is in to answer your questions.

Here we sit, drumming our fingers on the tabletop, wondering what keeps nails from going brittle and looking dull. This Q&A gathers facts on the nutrients and daily practices that not only benefit our hands cosmetically but also save them from growing arthritic and weak. So what's the first thing on the table? Age spots: their cause and treatment, and how to stop them from coming in the first place. We also want to know what promotes joint function, elasticity of skin, and slows aging. If there's something wrong with your hands, it's indicative of a bigger problem concerning the whole body, right? Absolutely! Get ready to learn some surprising facts, as we talk collagen and discuss the miracle of grapes. At this segment's end, you'll want to pick Concords by the bushel—and with strong, healthy hands, why not?

Q: What are age spots, and what can I do to prevent them?

A: Age spots (a.k.a. "liver spots" or the more textbook term "solar lentigo") are collections of pigment caused by exposure to the sun. They usually occur in people age 55 and up but can appear as early as your late 30s! The spots typically show up on the hands but can appear anywhere, especially sun-exposed areas—you tennis players and swimmers know just where those vulnerable areas are! Wear protective clothing (fingerless athletic gloves are a terrific idea!) and plenty of sunscreen. Generally, an SPF 15 lotion will work, but for total protection an SPF 35 is best. Since age spots are caused by prolonged and repeated sun exposure (or sunburns) and usually don't appear until much later in adult life, early protection is the best prevention against "old-looking" hands.

Q: Can there be such a thing as spots on your hands that aren't age spots?

A: Yes—they're called *ephelides*, a ten-dollar word for freckles. Freckles are harmless and begin as superficial collections of skin pigment or melanin which accumulate within the top layer of skin (epidermis). Ephelides are flat red or light-brown spots that typically appear during the sunny months and fade in the winter; they're more prevalent in people with fair complexions and can crop up on children after brief periods of sun exposure. Age spots or lentigines (singular: lentigo) are small tan, brown, or black spots that tend to be darker than an ephelis-type freckle and which do not fade in the winter. They usually appear later in life and can occur in all skin types. Both types of pigmented spots only rarely occur in non sun exposed areas. It cannot be stressed enough: sun avoidance and the steadfast use of sun block can help lessen the appearance of both lentigines and freckles!

Q: Are there other things besides sun exposure and heredity that cause age spots?

A: Age spots can result from poor liver function and free radical damage—both aided and abetted by unhealthy lifestyle habits like smoking and eating too much red meat and/or saturated and polyunsaturated fats. Oils rich in polyunsaturated fatty acids have a greater tendency than other oils toward oxidation and rancidity (to avoid rancidity in healthy oils like olive, don't improperly store it or burn it in the pan). If we get too much bad oil in our bodies, our cells start producing lipofuscin. What is that? You could say that lipofuscin are the "wear and tear" pigments that make us look old, haggard, and peppered with age spots. Lipofuscin are found in the liver, kidneys, heart muscle, adrenals, and nerve cells. The liver spots you see on older folks are superficial dermal (meaning "skin surface") lipofuscin deposits. Some studies show lesser deposits of lipofuscin accumulate in people who eat a calorie-restricted diet. You can definitely lessen your chances of developing liver spots by eating a diet rich in carotene (e.g., carrots, yams, and leafy green vegetables). Milk thistle extract is recommended as an organic method of keeping liver function healthy. Ask your doctor about herbal teas and safe supplements.

Q: What can potassium do for hands?

A: Potassium regulates the transfer of nutrients into cells and facilitates muscle energy—very important for hand strength. Potassium also regulates water balance and aids rheumatic or arthritic conditions by causing acids to leave the joints and ease stiffness. You can get your potassium by eating lots of produce—bananas, orange juice, dried dates, and apricots. You may have heard as a kid that banana consumption helps sweaty palms; this is untrue. While potassium is great for maintaining healthy water balances in the body, sweaty palms or "palmer hyperhidrosis" is a genetic condition caused by a benign abnormality of the autonomic nervous system.

Q: Are there medical procedures that remove age spots?

A: Thankfully, yes. Since age spots involve excess melanin found in the upper layer of your skin, they are quite easy to remove by laser. Today's laser treatment approach is replacing the more invasive cryotherapy—the old "tried and true" technique for dealing with age spots. In cryotherapy, liquid nitrogen is sprayed on the spots to induce a localized frostbite. After two or three weeks, the treated age spots peel off as the underlying skin pushes to the surface, leaving a residual area of pinkness that might last weeks or months. Scarring may occur—an unpleasant possibility that led to pigment-removal lasers. Don't like either? Take heart! You may want to skip these kinds of treatments altogether and ask your dermatologist about a prescription bleaching cream.

Q: Are there ways to reduce wrinkles on your hands?

A: Perhaps the ancient Greeks and Romans knew the answer to this one: they were the first to make wines from fermented grape juice and established the age-old tradition of bringing grapes to recovering loved ones at the hospital. Why? Because grapes improve circulation, protect the skin from wrinkles and lack of elasticity, promote healing and may reduce inflammatory conditions such as arthritis. Antioxidant compounds in purple grape juice appear to have a similar effect as those in red wine, neutralizing the free radicals responsible for cellular damage. For those who wish to lose weight gently and detox at the same time, a day-long grape-fast every 10 days is recommended. Grapes are a great source of potassium and have unique cleansing properties. Since the resveratrol in grapes is both water- and fat-soluble, they're as versatile as vitamins at protecting body tissues!

Q: What part does collagen play in youthful-looking hands?

A: Collagen is the most abundant protein of connective tissue in mammals. It has much to do with elasticity in our skin. It maintains the moisture in skin cells and keeps skin smooth. We all experience loss of collagen as we grow older, which causes skin to lose moisture, wrinkle, and sag. Plenty of vitamin C can slow down collagen loss.

Q: What's the story on fingernails? Can you strengthen them with the right diet?

A: Of course you can! The primary function of our nails is to provide protection to the fingertip and a firm backing for the grip and manipulation of small objects. The nail's appearance is a barometer of health. Vertical ridges and brittleness as well as the moons, translucence, and color of the nails are all significant indicators of physical well-being. Because your nails are made of keratin (a protein), make sure you're eating enough of this nutrient in order to keep them strong.

The recommended daily amount of protein for adults is 50–63 g (the amount in about 8 ounces of cooked salmon, for example, or 1 cup of quinoa and 2 cups of cooked chickpeas).

Jorj's "Hands On" Glam Kitchen

Berries work wonders for the anatomy and function of your hands. Tending your own berry garden or going berry picking (strawberry fields dot the South, and blueberries love the Northeast) keeps you busy and blissful. You'll burn calories, take in bone-loving vitamin D under the sun (with a slather of sunscreen of course), and work the muscles in your hands for beneficial and, later on, *delicious* results. This section espouses more than just reminders about strawberries, blackberries, raspberries, and leafy greens being good for you; we dish here on their seasons, planting, and making fruit preserves. Disclaimer: a total return to wartime Victory Gardens is not what we're pluggin' here (though it'd sure be nice). We know how busy you are and that, for a lot of us, going to the grocery store every few days for fresh fruit and veggies is good enough—it has to be. We just want to remind you that the hand-friendly foods in this chapter are all about fresh fruit and veggies and, at the very least, encourage you to use your leftovers in the form of sweet breads, smoothies, and grape jam on toast . . . raisin toast if possible!

Little White Flowers in the Spring

If you're fond of little white flowers in the spring, a homegrown blueberry harvest may be right up your alley. By the time summer rolls around, your berries should be a deep blue and ripe for the pickin'. **Blueberries** are a little picky about soil chemistry, so amateur gardeners are best advised to plant blueberries in a pot, where the dirt can be monitored and manipulated easily. When you're at your local nursery, tell the staff you're looking for soil and planting tips that benefit rhododendrons and camellias; the same environment works for blueberries. Wouldn't it be great to have both blooming in your backyard?

Berry Good Notes

Plant rows of **raspberries** in late winter; that's when your local nurseries or mail order businesses start carrying them. They arrive in a bare rooted state—a freshly dug up plant in a bundle, so they will need to be planted ASAP. From June through early July, strawberries thrive. They're perfect plants for hanging baskets, and best of all, they're cheap. An excellent research tool for budding green thumbs can be found at www.bbc.co.uk/gardening. These berry experts don't neglect the veggie side of the gardening equation. Any soul looking to protect and promote their health would do well to look "across the pond" into these leafy green garden notes.

Preserve with Your Hands

Preserves don't require much in the way of resources, and for something so delicious, they are astonishingly uncomplicated. Those cute little Mason jars you're tempted to buy at Harry & David each Christmas are filled by cooking whole or large pieces of fruit in a thick sugar syrup and combining with powder or liquid pectin, sugar, and lemon juice for acidity. All you need to get these ingredients working for you are a large wooden spoon, a big open-topped sauce pan, a food scale, plastic jugs for measuring and bottling, a funnel, a handheld blender, a sieve and some of those pretty little Mason jars with lids. Consult a guide for preserving instructions. Doctors advise patients with arthritis to keep their hands busy; it helps with discomfort. Readying jars of tasty preserves may lessen the need for ibuprofen.

And if I don't want to make my own?

If you're looking to get your flavonoids (for nothing loves the human body better!) but don't want to go through the trouble of making jams and jellies, you can make small, tasty additions to everyday foods that ensure the same nutritional benefits. Sprinkle **raisins**, **flax**, **sunflower seeds**, and/or **almonds** over your yogurt and oatmeal, slice **bananas** on your **wheat bran**, patronize bakery's that use **brewer's yeast**, eat sushi made with **kelp**, enjoy sweet dried fruit like **prunes** and **cherries—emulate** that famous fruit bowl still life at the Met, the one overflowing with **plums**, **oranges**, **tangerines**, **pink grapefruit**, **apples**, **pears**, and **kiwi**. Get your free radical-fighting, age-defying nutrition in **sweet potatoes**, **cabbage**, and **red peppers**. My rule of thumb: don't postpone an invitation to dine on these foods because by eating them you might just *postpone* those age spots!

Start Your Day

Main Plates

On the Side

Snacks & Sweets

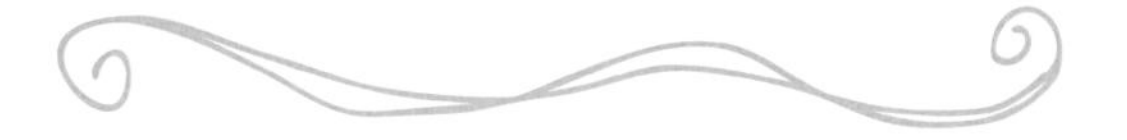

BLUEBERRY BUTTERMILK COFFEE CAKE

Topped with Granola

Serve this cake with a rich cup of java in the morning or with a cup of honeyed tea during your evening tête-à-tête.

Makes 9 servings
Prep Time: 15 minutes
Cook Time: 25 to 30 minutes

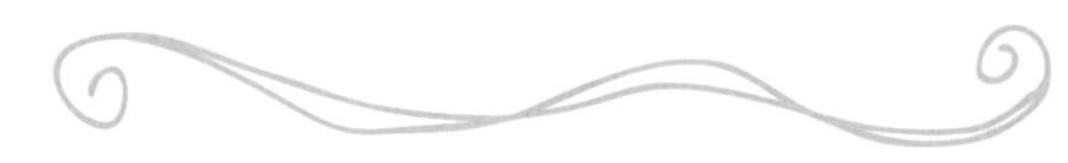

Feel free to substitute with fresh FROZEN blueberries that you keep on hand in your freezer.

* * *

Prepare the extra granola in the Fruit and Yogurt Breakfast Parfaits with Granola Crunch recipe (page 59) for use in this recipe.

For the cake

- 1 cup whole-wheat flour
- 1/2 teaspoon baking soda
- 1/2 teaspoon ground allspice
- 1/4 teaspoon ground cinnamon
- 1/4 teaspoon salt
- 1/2 cup buttermilk
- 1/2 cup brown sugar
- 2 tablespoons canola oil
- 1 teaspoon pure vanilla extract
- 1 large egg
- 4 ounces fresh blueberries (about 1 cup), divided use
- 1/2 cup prepared granola

Preheat the oven to 350 degrees. In a small bowl whisk together the flour, baking soda, all-spice, cinnamon, and salt.

In a medium bowl whisk the buttermilk, sugar, and oil together until smooth. Stir in the vanilla and egg. Stir in the flour mixture until just combined. Fold in half of the berries.

Pour the batter into an 8 x 8-inch baking dish that has been coated with vegetable oil spray. Crumble the granola over the top. Sprinkle with the remaining blueberries. Bake until the cake springs back when touched and a tester inserted into the center comes out clean, about 25–30 minutes. Cool on wire rack.

To serve, cut the coffee cake into 9 squares. Serve warm.

BANANA BREAD SNACK CAKE

Chinese five-spice lends an exotic taste to this update on banana bread. Just a hint does the trick.

Makes 12 servings
Prep Time: 10 minutes
Cook Time: 40 to 45minutes

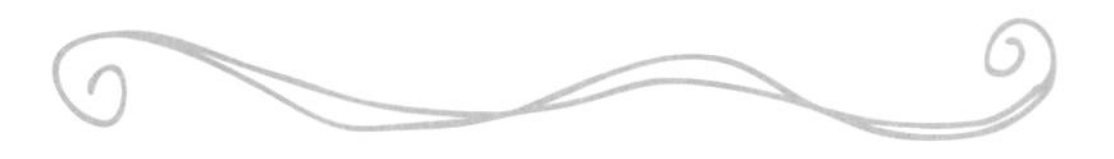

Originating in China, this spice combines equal parts of ground cinnamon, fennel, star anise, cloves, and Szechwan pepper. It's mainly used in marinades and barbecues, but I find that just a HINT of the spice added to baked goods lends an EXCEPTIONAL flavor!

- 1 1/2 cups whole wheat flour
- 3/4 cup old-fashioned rolled oats
- 2/3 cup natural sugar
- 1 1/2 teaspoons baking powder
- 1/2 teaspoon baking soda
- 1/2 teaspoon Chinese 5 Spice
- 1/4 teaspoon salt
- 2 very ripe bananas, mashed (about 1 cup)
- 1/3 cup buttermilk
- 1/4 cup vegetable oil
- 1 teaspoon pure vanilla extract
- 2 large eggs, beaten
- Honey

Preheat the oven to 350 degrees. In a medium bowl whisk together the flour, oats, sugar, baking powder, baking soda, Chinese five-spice, and salt.

In a large bowl stir together the bananas, buttermilk, and vegetable oil. Stir in the vanilla and eggs. Mix in the flour mixture. Pour the batter into an 11 x 9 x 2-inch baking dish that has been coated with vegetable oil spray. Bake until the cake springs back when touched and a tester inserted into the center comes out clean, about 30–35 minutes. Cool on wire rack.

To serve, cut into 12 squares. Serve with a drizzle of honey.

On Shopping Day: Bake the banana bread, cool to room temperature, cover with plastic wrap, and store for up to 4 days.

WALNUT-STUFFED BAKED APPLES

With Maple Syrup

The fragrant aroma when baking these apples is sure to get the whole family to the table for breakfast—even on the busiest of days.

Makes 8 servings
Prep Time: 15 minutes
Cook Time: 45 minutes

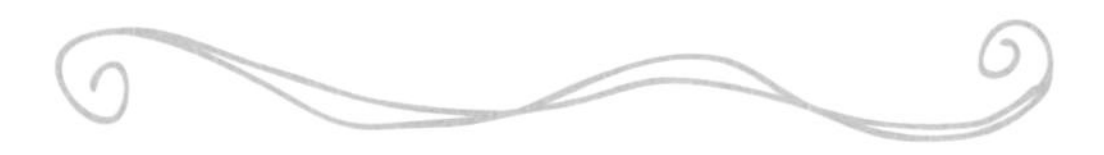

This is a great dish to prepare for guests. Instead of using apple halves, DOUBLE the amount of STUFFING (add a few oats and raisins for good measure) and fill a whole apple. It's *sooo* good.

For the filling

- 1/2 cup walnut pieces
- 1/4 cup brown sugar
- 1 tablespoon butter
- 1/2 teaspoon vanilla extract
- 1/8 teaspoon salt
- 1 large egg white

For the apples

- 4 medium Granny Smith apples
- 1 tablespoon natural sugar
- 1/2 teaspoon ground cinnamon
- 1/3 cup pure maple syrup

Preheat the oven to 350 degrees. Place the walnuts into the bowl of a food processor. Add the brown sugar, butter, vanilla, salt, and egg white. Pulse to combine.

Place the apples onto your work surface. Cut each apple in half from the stem to the bottom. Use a melon ball scoop to remove the core and seeds while creating a bowl. Cut a small slice from the rounded portion of the apple halves, so that they do not roll around. Place the apples onto a rimmed baking sheet that has been coated with vegetable oil spay. In a small bowl combine the natural sugar and cinnamon. Sprinkle this mixture into the apple centers. Fill the apples with the walnut mixture. Drizzle the maple syrup over the filling. Bake until the apples are soft and golden, about 40–45 minutes.

To serve, place the warm apples onto a platter and drizzle with any maple sauce left in the pan.

On Shopping Day: Prepare the filling for the apples and store in an airtight container in the refrigerator for up to 4 days.

GRANOLA POWER BARS

Not your everyday box of store-bought power bars, these dandies are fresh outta' the oven and prepared with the best ingredients. Wheat bran gives the bars an extra dense texture—one that your fingers *will love!*

Makes 18 servings
Prep Time: 15 minutes
Cook Time: 15 to 20 minutes

- 1 cup brown sugar
- 1 cup canola oil
- 2 large eggs
- 1 teaspoon pure vanilla extract
- 2 cups old fashioned rolled oats
- 1 cup unbleached all-purpose flour
- 1/2 cup wheat bran
- 1 teaspoon baking soda
- 1 cup raisins
- 1 cup pecans, chopped
- 1 teaspoon ground cinnamon
- 1/2 teaspoon ground nutmeg
- 1/4 teaspoon ground cloves
- 1/4 teaspoon salt

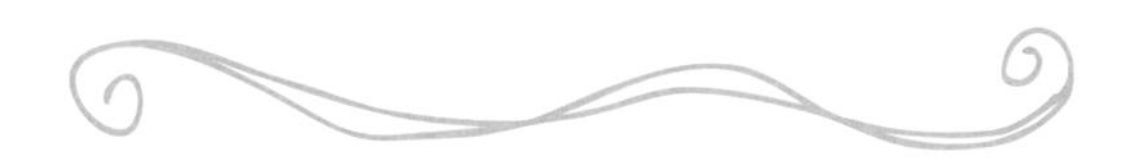

Wheat bran is an excellent source of natural food fiber and provides a healthy FULL-BODIED texture when added to baked goods.

Preheat the oven to 350 degrees. In a large bowl stir together the brown sugar, canola oil, eggs, and vanilla until smooth. Stir in the oats, flour, wheat bran, baking soda, raisins, pecans, cinnamon, nutmeg, cloves and salt.

Spread this mixture onto a rimmed baking sheet that has been coated with vegetable oil spray. Bake until golden, about 15–20 minutes. Cool to room temperature.

To serve, cut into 18 bars.

On Shopping Day: Prepare the bars, wrap in individual plastic bags, and store for up to 3 days.

POACHED SALMON IN INFUSED OLIVE OIL

With Horseradish Sauce

A double dose of good-for-you oil is found in this dish. Infusing the olive oil with fresh flavors ensures a moist and scrumptious fillet.

Makes 4 servings
Prep Time: 15 minutes
Cook Time: 10 to 12 minutes

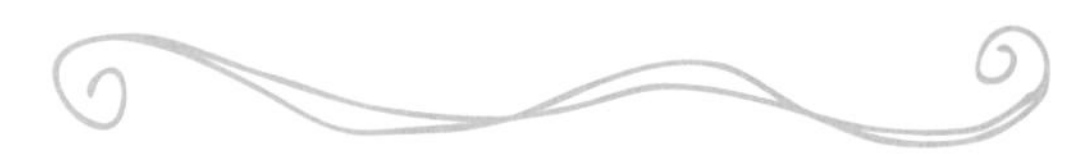

Poaching fish is an excellent way to guarantee a MOIST result. Other mediums for poaching include wine, champagne, broth—and perhaps some RED GRAPE JUICE!

For the poaching liquid

- 2 cups olive oil
- 2 large garlic cloves
- Zest of 1 medium lime (about 1 tablespoon)
- 1 tablespoon chopped fresh basil leaves
- 2 teaspoons dried thyme
- 1 teaspoon crushed red pepper flakes

For the salmon

- 4 6-ounce salmon fillets, skin removed from 1 side
- Salt and freshly ground pepper

For the sauce

- 4 tablespoons reduced-fat mayonnaise
- 2 tablespoons reduced-fat sour cream
- 2 tablespoons chopped fresh dill
- 2 teaspoons prepared horseradish

Pour the olive oil into a deep pot over medium heat. Add the garlic cloves, lime zest, basil, thyme, and red pepper flakes. Simmer the olive oil for 15 minutes to infuse the flavors.

Season the fillets with salt and pepper. Place the salmon into a deep skillet. Carefully strain the olive oil into the skillet. The salmon should be mostly covered by the oil. Simmer the salmon, over medium-low heat, turning once, until just cooked in the center, about 8–10 minutes. Do not let the oil boil.

In a small bowl whisk together the mayonnaise, sour cream, dill, and horseradish. Chill until ready to serve.

To serve, transfer the salmon to a platter. Remove the skin. Serve with a dollop of horseradish sauce.

On Shopping Day: Prepare the horseradish sauce and store in an airtight container in the refrigerator up to 2 days.

CHILLED SHRIMP SALAD

With Red Grapes

Make this refreshing salad in the evening for a simple, yet sumptuous lunch the next day.

Makes 4 servings
Prep Time: 10 minutes

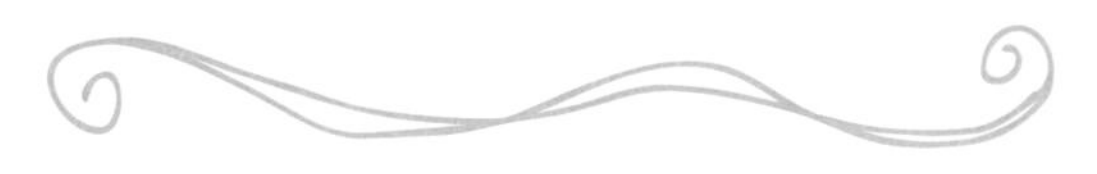

My FAVORITE way to purchase shrimp is from the FREEZER section; this way I have it on hand at all times. You can buy the shrimp cooked or uncooked. Cooking frozen shrimp requires just a few minutes—so do consider this option!

- 1 1-pound bag frozen, cooked, peeled, and deveined shrimp (about 24)
- 2 medium celery ribs, diced (about 1/2 cup)
- 4 green onions, thinly sliced (about 1/4 cup)
- 1 cup red seedless grapes, halved
- 1/2 cup reduced-fat mayonnaise
- 1 tablespoon white wine vinegar
- 1/2 teaspoon Dijon mustard
- Salt and freshly ground pepper
- 8 cups mixed greens tossed with lemon juice and freshly ground pepper
- Lemon wedges (for garnish)

Place the shrimp in a colander under cold running water until defrosted. Drain and remove the tails from the shrimp. Place into a medium bowl. Add the celery, onions, and grapes.

In a small bowl whisk together the mayonnaise, vinegar, and mustard. Pour the mayonnaise mixture into the bowl with the shrimp. Toss to coat. Season with salt and pepper. Chill in the refrigerator for at least 30 minutes or overnight.

To serve, mound the shrimp salad over mixed greens. Garnish with lemon wedges.

On Shopping Day: Prepare the shrimp salad and store in an airtight container in the refrigerator for up to 24 hours.

CHICKEN AND RICE MEATBALL HOAGIES

By using lean protein and whole grains you can update a family favorite and give it a healthful spin.

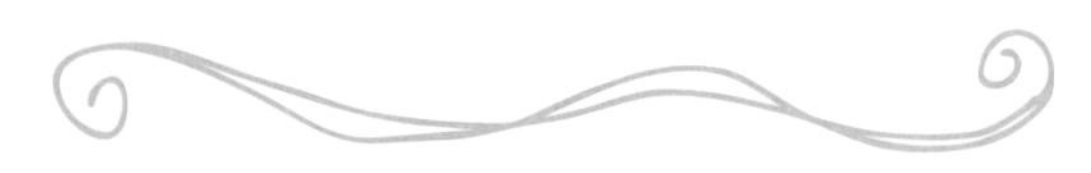

Ask your butcher to GRIND chicken for you (if you don't find it in the meat case); or prepare your own by using the meat grinder attachment on your high-powered mixer. This works best with VERY COLD poultry—a mixture of white and dark meat yields the best flavor.

* * *

Leftover rice will work well in this recipe. If you are preparing the rice, cool to room temperature before adding to the chicken mixture.

Preheat the oven to 350 degrees. In a medium bowl place the chicken, rice, milk, egg, Parmesan cheese, and oregano. Season with salt and pepper. Gently mix together. Form into 12 meatballs. Place onto a rimmed baking sheet that has been coated with vegetable oil spray. Bake until the meatballs are cooked through, about 8 minutes.

Place the diced tomatoes into a pot over medium-high heat. Stir in the tomato paste, basil, and sugar. Season with salt and pepper. Bring to a boil. Reduce heat and simmer for 5 minutes. Place the meatballs into the sauce and simmer for 5 minutes.

To serve, toast the hoagie rolls. Fill each roll with 3 meatballs and top with 2 slices of cheese. Spoon additional tomato sauce over top and garnish with fresh basil leaves.

On Shopping Day: Prepare the meatballs and the sauce. Store in an airtight container in the refrigerator for up to 4 days.

Makes 4 servings
Prep Time: 5 minutes
Cook Time: 15 minutes

For the meatballs

- 1 pound ground chicken
- 1 cup cooked brown rice
- 1/4 cup reduced-fat milk
- 1 large egg, beaten
- 1/4 cup finely grated Parmesan cheese
- 1 teaspoon dried oregano leaves
- Salt and freshly ground pepper

For the sauce

- 1 28-ounce can diced tomatoes
- 2 tablespoons tomato paste
- 2 tablespoons chopped fresh basil
- 1 teaspoon natural sugar
- 4 whole grain hoagie rolls
- 8 1-ounce slices reduced-fat mozzarella cheese
- Fresh basil leaves (for garnish)

TURKEY MEATLOAF BURGERS

With Spicy Sweet Potato Sticks

Lean protein is a must for a hand-healthy diet. Add a bit of spice to fill the fat gap for a delicious burger meal.

Watch your potato sticks as they roast. Thinner ones will cook faster than thicker slices. Think the difference between French fries and steak fries!!

* * *

You may need more breadcrumbs to hold the burgers together, depending on the freshness and coarseness of the bread you use. Feel free to use as much as you wish. The secret is to not overwork the mixture.

In a large bowl place the ground turkey, breadcrumbs, green onions, minced garlic, chili sauce, egg, 1 tablespoon olive oil, chili powder, and ground cumin. Season with salt and pepper. Use your hands to gently mix the ingredients together. Form into 4 large patties (or 6 smaller ones).

Heat a grill pan over medium-high heat. Coat with vegetable oil spray. Grill the patties until seared on one side, about 5–7 minutes. Turn and grill until cooked through, about 5 minutes more.

Preheat the oven to 450 degrees. In a medium bowl place the potato sticks. Drizzle with the remaining 1 tablespoon olive oil, garlic powder, chili powder, salt, and pepper. Toss to coat. Spread out onto a rimmed baking sheet. Bake until golden, about 5 minutes; turn and bake until crisp and golden on both sides, about 4 to 5 minutes more, depending on thickness.

To serve, place the turkey burgers on the buns. Top with lettuce, tomato, and pickles. Serve the sweet potato sticks on the side.

On Shopping Day: Prepare the burgers, wrap in plastic, and refrigerate for up to 2 days.

Makes 4 servings
Prep Time: 15 minutes
Cook Time: 15 to 25 minutes

For the burgers

1 1/2 pounds ground turkey
1/2–1 cup fresh whole grain breadcrumbs
3–4 green onions, thinly sliced (about 1/2 cup)
2 medium garlic cloves, minced (about 1 teaspoon)
2 tablespoons chili sauce
1 large egg, beaten
1 tablespoon olive oil
2 teaspoons chili powder
1 teaspoon ground cumin
Salt and freshly ground pepper
4 whole grain hamburger buns
Leaf lettuce and tomato slices
Dill pickle chips

For the roasted potatoes

2 large sweet potatoes, sliced into thin sticks
1 tablespoon olive oil
1 teaspoon garlic powder
1/2 teaspoon chili powder

SNAPPER VERONIQUE

Veronique means "with grapes;" adding grapes to delicate fish, like snapper, is an easy gourmet enhancement your dinner guests will love.

Makes 4 servings
Prep Time: 10 minutes
Cook Time: 10 minutes

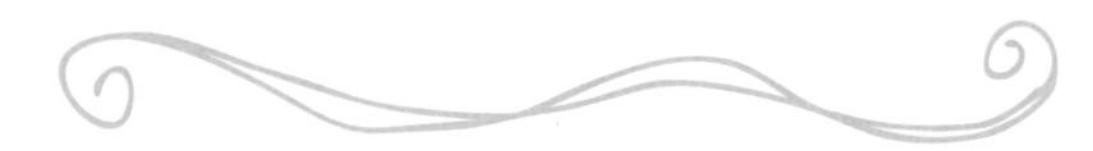

Traditionally this dish is prepared with GREEN grapes. I've taken a little liberty by substituting with RED grapes for our "hands-on" experience!

For the snapper

- 2 tablespoons olive oil
- 2 tablespoons unbleached all-purpose flour
- 4 6- to 8-ounce snapper fillets
- Salt and freshly ground pepper
- Juice of 1 medium lemon (about 2 tablespoons)

For the sauce

- 2 tablespoons olive oil
- 1 bunch (6 to 8) green onions, chopped (about 1/2 cup)
- 4 ounces button mushrooms, sliced (about 1 cup)
- 1/2 cup white wine
- 1 cup homemade chicken stock or low-sodium chicken broth
- 1 cup seedless red grapes, halved
- 2 tablespoons chopped fresh parsley (for garnish)

In a skillet heat 2 tablespoons olive oil over medium-high heat. Place the flour into a plastic bag. Add the fillets and gently shake to coat. Place the fish onto a platter. Season with salt and pepper and drizzle with lemon juice. Place the fish, skin side up, in the skillet. Cook until golden, about 3–5 minutes. Turn and cook until just opaque in the center, about 3 minutes more. Transfer to a platter.

To make the sauce, in the same skillet heat an 2 tablespoons olive oil. Add the onions and mushrooms and cook until golden, about 3–4 minutes. Add the wine and cook until most of the liquid disappears. Add the chicken broth and simmer for 2–3 minutes. Stir in the grapes. Season with salt and pepper.

To serve, spoon the sauce onto the fish. Garnish with fresh parsley.

JAMBALAYA

From the heart of New Orleans, this Creole-inspired dish is a natural comfort food!

Makes 6 to 8 servings, with extras for later in the week
Prep Time: 30 minutes
Cook Time: 1 hour (more if using a slow cooker)

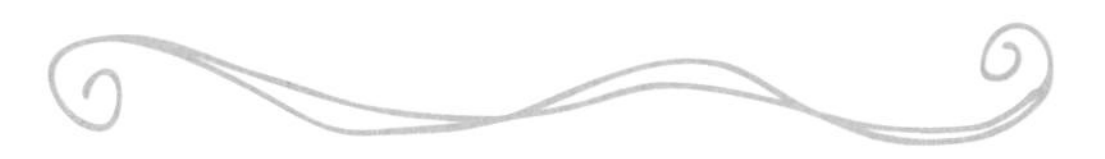

You can adapt this recipe for your SLOW COOKER. Brown the chicken in a skillet and place into the bottom of the dish. Top with the remaining ingredients and set the machine on high while you step away for the day.

- 6 chicken legs
- 6 chicken thighs
- Salt and freshly ground pepper
- 2 tablespoons olive oil
- 4 medium celery ribs, diced (about 1 cup)
- 1 large white onion, peeled and diced (about 1 cup)
- 1 large green bell pepper, diced (about 1 cup)
- 4 medium garlic cloves, minced (about 2 teaspoons)
- 1 pound smoked sausage, diced
- 8 ounces smoked ham steak, diced
- 1½ cups brown rice
- 2 cups homemade chicken stock or low-sodium chicken broth
- 1 16-ounce can tomato sauce
- 1 tablespoon tomato paste
- 1 tablespoon Worcestershire sauce
- 4–6 drops hot pepper sauce (or more if you like it hot!)
- 2 dried bay leaves
- 2 teaspoons dried thyme leaves
- Fresh parsley (for garnish)

Preheat the oven to 350 degrees. Season the chicken pieces with salt and pepper. Heat the olive oil in a Dutch oven (with lid) over medium-high heat. Brown the chicken until golden, about 6–8 minutes per side. Transfer to a platter.

Cook the celery, onion, and bell pepper in the pan until soft, about 5 minutes. Add the garlic and cook for 2 minutes more. Stir in the sausage and ham. Add the rice. Pour in the chicken stock and tomato sauce. Stir in the tomato paste, Worcestershire and hot pepper sauces, bay leaves, and thyme. Return the chicken to the pan.

Cover the pot and place in the oven. Cook until the rice is tender and the chicken is falling off the bone, about 1 hour.

To serve, ladle the jambalaya onto plates and garnish with fresh parsley.

On Shopping Day: Dice the veggies, sausage and ham. Store separately (in airtight containers) for up to 4 days.

SAUTÉED YELLOWTAIL SNAPPER FILLETS

With Braised Cabbage and Cheesy Mashed Potatoes

This is a full meal in three simple steps, served family style on one platter.

Makes 4 servings
Prep Time: 10 minutes
Cook Time: 20 minutes

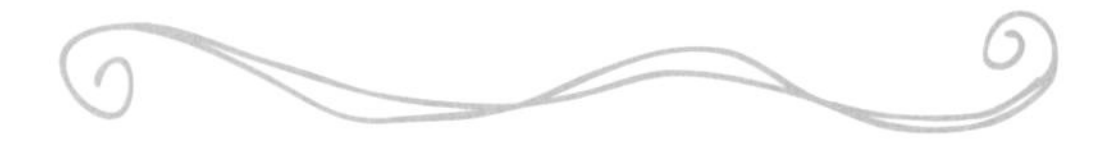

SCORE the skin sides of the fish fillets with a knife; this will prevent them from curling up on the ends.

For the cabbage

- 1 2-pound head Savoy cabbage, halved, cored, and cut into 1-inch strips
- 1 quart homemade chicken stock or low-sodium chicken broth
- 2 tablespoons olive oil
- 2 tablespoons chopped fresh dill
- Salt and freshly ground pepper

For the potatoes

- 3 medium potatoes, peeled and cut into ½-inch pieces
- 1 cup reduced-fat milk
- 2 tablespoons olive oil
- 2 ounces grated white American cheese (about ½ cup)

For the fish

- 2 tablespoons olive oil
- 6 6- to 8-ounce yellowtail snapper fillets
- Juice of 1 medium lemon (about 2 tablespoons)
- 2 tablespoons chopped fresh dill
- Lemon wedges (for garnish)
- Fresh dill (for garnish)

Place the cabbage into a deep pot. Cover with chicken broth. Bring to a boil over medium-high heat. Reduce heat to medium and simmer until the cabbage is very tender, about 15–20 minutes. Drain any excess liquid. Toss with olive oil and fresh dill. Season with salt and pepper. Keep warm.

Prepare the potatoes by boiling in salted water until fork tender, about 8 minutes. Drain and place into a bowl. Mash with milk and 2 tablespoons olive oil. Stir in the cheese. Season with salt and pepper. Keep warm.

In a skillet heat 2 tablespoons olive oil over medium-high heat. Season the fish with lemon juice, salt, and pepper. Cook the fish, skin side up, in the pan until golden, about 3–4 minutes. Use a fish spatula to turn the fillets and cook, skin side down, until just opaque in the center, about 2 minutes more. Remove to a platter.

To serve, spoon the potatoes onto a platter. Lay the cabbage alongside. Lay the fillets on top of the potatoes and cabbage. Garnish with additional fresh dill and lemon wedges.

SLICED CHICKEN BREASTS

With Red Grape Sauce

Wine is often utilized as a basis for a rich sauce. Here is an example of the virgin grape, used to recreate a sauce filled with the goodness of red wine, only lighter and fresher tasting.

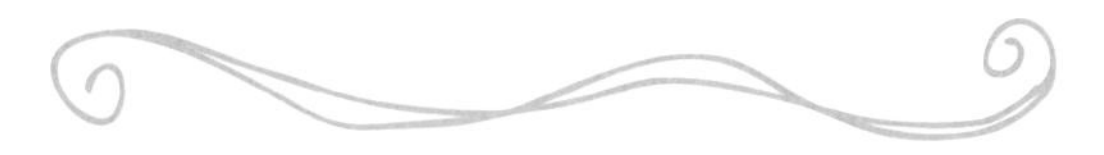

Cornstarch added to the sauce at the last moment creates a velvety SMOOTH texture. Another way to thicken the sauce is to add 1–2 tablespoons of chilled BUTTER swirled into the pan, once it is removed from the heat. Give both methods a try and see which you prefer.

Preheat the oven to 350 degrees. Season the chicken with salt and pepper. In a skillet heat 1 tablespoon olive oil over medium-high heat. Place the chicken in the skillet and cook until golden, about 4–5 minutes per side. Transfer the chicken to a baking dish and place in the oven until cooked through, about 15–20 minutes.

In the same skillet heat 1 more tablespoon olive oil over medium-high heat. Add the shallots to the pan and cook until golden, about 2 minutes. Stir in the rosemary. Pour in the grape juice and bring to a boil. Simmer until the grape juice is reduced by half, about 5–8 minutes. Pour in the chicken stock. Simmer until the sauce is reduced to about 1 cup, about 5–8 minutes more. Stir in the cornstarch and the grapes. Cook until the sauce thickens and the grapes are warmed through, about 2 minutes. Season with salt and pepper.

Transfer the chicken to a platter. Cut into slices. Pour the sauce over top and garnish with fresh rosemary sprigs.

Makes 4 servings
Prep Time: 10 minutes
Cook Time: 30 minutes

For the chicken

4 large (6- to 8-ounce) skinless, boneless chicken breast halves
Salt and freshly ground pepper
1 tablespoon olive oil

For the sauce

1 tablespoon olive oil
2 large shallots, minced (about 2 tablespoons)
1 tablespoon chopped fresh rosemary
2 cups red grape juice
2 cups homemade chicken stock or low-sodium chicken broth
2 teaspoons cornstarch mixed with 1 tablespoon cold water
1 cup red seedless grapes, cut into halves
Rosemary (for garnish)

ROASTED ASPARAGUS SALAD

With Arugula, Radishes, and Lemon Vinaigrette

This tart and sassy salad is as pleasing visually as it is to the tongue!

Makes 4 servings
Prep Time: 15 minutes
Cook Time: 8 minutes

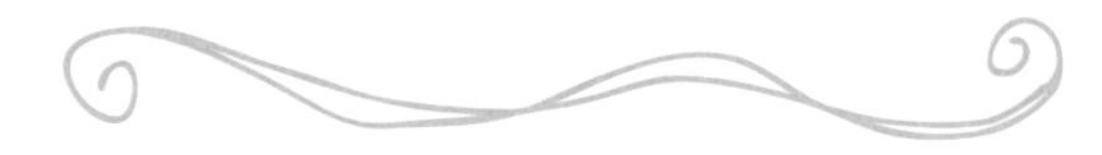

ARUGULA has a profound peppery taste. You may temper the pepper by substituting mixed greens for half of the arugula.

For the vinaigrette

- 2 large shallots, minced (about 2 tablespoons)
- Juice of 1 medium lemon (about 2 tablespoons)
- 2 tablespoons red wine vinegar
- Zest of 1 medium lemon (about 1 tablespoon)
- 1 teaspoon Dijon mustard
- 1/3 cup olive oil
- Salt and freshly ground pepper

For the asparagus

- 1 pound fresh, thin asparagus spears, ends trimmed
- 1 tablespoon olive oil

For the salad

- 2 ounces arugula leaves, washed and dried (about 2 cups)
- 6 large radishes, thinly sliced (about 1/2 cup)
- 2 tablespoons chopped fresh chives
- Parmigiano-Reggiano cheese, shaved

In a medium bowl whisk together the shallots, lemon juice, red wine vinegar, lemon zest, and Dijon mustard. Slowly whisk in the olive oil. Season with salt and pepper.

Preheat the oven to 400 degrees. Place the asparagus on a rack on a rimmed baking sheet. Drizzle with 1 tablespoon olive oil and season with salt and pepper. Roast until crisp-tender, about 8–10 minutes.

In a large bowl place the arugula, radishes, and chives. Drizzle with half of the vinaigrette. Toss.

To serve, divide the salad onto four chilled plates. Lay the asparagus spears over the top of the greens. Drizzle with the remaining vinaigrette. Shave Parmigiano-Reggiano cheese over the top.

On Shopping Day: Prepare the vinaigrette, store in an airtight container in the refrigerator for up to 2 days. Bring to room temperature before serving.

SWEET POTATO SOUFFLÉ

Light, airy, sweet, savory . . . this dish has it all—and it's so much easier to prepare than you might think!

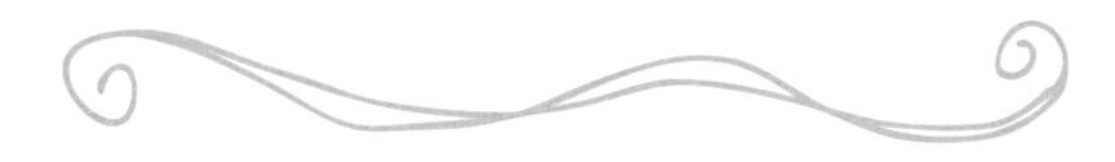

The secret to this dish is folding the egg whites into the batter. Use a large rubber spatula. Begin by stirring about a fourth of the egg whites into the sweet potato mixture. This will lighten the entire batter and make it easier for you to proceed. Pour the remaining egg whites on top of the batter. Using your rubber spatula, cut through the mixture to the bottom of the bowl and "fold" the batter on the bottom over the light ingredients at the top. Repeat this until the two are blended, but not until you've lost the fluffy texture of the light ingredients. Bottom ingredients are lifted, and then folded, gently over the top. The basic motion is lift and fold.

Preheat the oven to 375 degrees. Pierce the sweet potatoes with the tines of a fork. Place onto a rimmed baking sheet. Roast until soft, about 30–40 minutes. Cool, peel, and place into the bowl of a food processor. Add 2 tablespoons olive oil and pulse until smooth. Add the half and half, flour, brown sugar, orange juice, orange zest, cinnamon, nutmeg, thyme, salt and egg yolks. Pulse until smooth. Pour out into a large bowl.

Place the egg whites into the bowl of an electric mixer. Whip until stiff peaks form. Gently fold the egg whites into the sweet potato mixture.

Raise the temperature of the oven to 425 degrees. Pour the batter into a deep soufflé dish that has been coated with vegetable oil spray. Place onto a rimmed baking sheet. Place the soufflé into the oven and immediately reduce the heat back to 375 degrees.

Bake until the soufflé has risen, the top is golden, and the center is just set, about 1 hour.

To serve, bring the soufflé right from the oven to the table and dig in!

On Shopping Day: Bake the sweet potatoes, store in an airtight container, and store in the refrigerator for up to 3 days.

Makes 6 servings
Prep Time: 20 minutes
Cook Time: 60 minutes

- 2 large sweet potatoes (about 1 1/2 pounds)
- 2 tablespoons olive oil
- 1/2 cup reduced-fat half and half
- 1/4 cup unbleached all-purpose flour
- 1/4 cup brown sugar
- 1/4 cup fresh orange juice
- Zest of 1/2 medium orange (about 1 tablespoon)
- 1 teaspoon ground cinnamon
- 1/2 teaspoon ground nutmeg
- 1/2 teaspoon dried thyme
- 1/2 teaspoon salt
- 2 large egg yolks
- 5 large egg whites

BLACK BEAN AND ROASTED PEPPER EMPANADAS

This quick snack makes a fabulous appetizer at your next get-together or works well as an accompaniment to a great bowl of soup!

Makes 24 empanadas
Prep Time: 20 minutes
Cook Time: 8 to 10 minutes

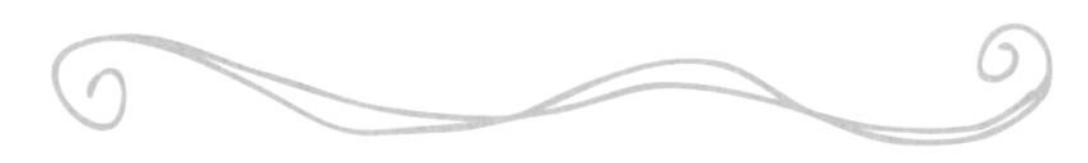

Add cooked, shredded chicken or pork to the black beans and you have an entire meal—in the palm of your hand.

For the filling

- 1 tablespoon olive oil
- 1 small white onion, diced (about 3 tablespoons)
- 2 medium cloves garlic, minced (about 1 teaspoon)
- 1 16-ounce can black beans, drained
- 2 tablespoons chopped fresh cilantro
- ½ teaspoon ground cumin
- Salt and freshly ground pepper
- 1 12-ounce jar roasted red peppers, drained and cut into strips

For the empanadas

- 1 package frozen puff pastry (2 sheets), thawed
- 4 ounces reduced-fat grated Monterey Jack cheese (about 1 cup)
- 1 egg, beaten

Heat the olive oil in a medium pot over medium heat. Add the onion and garlic and cook until just soft, about 2 minutes. Stir in the black beans and cilantro. Season with cumin, salt, and pepper. Simmer until the beans are warmed through, about 4–5 minutes. Cool to room temperature.

Preheat the oven to 425 degrees. Roll out each pastry sheet on a floured work surface to about ¼-inch thickness. Cut each into 12 squares. Sprinkle the cheese over each square. Place a tablespoon of the bean mixture onto the center of each square. Top with roasted pepper strips. Fold over to form triangles. Use the tines of a fork to seal the edges.

Place onto a rimmed baking sheet that has been coated with vegetable oil spray. Brush each triangle with beaten egg. Bake until golden, about 8–10 minutes.

To serve, place warm empanadas onto a serving platter and pass around.

On Shopping Day: Prepare the bean filling, store in an airtight container in the refrigerator for up to 4 days.

SAUTÉED RED CABBAGE

With Drunken Raisins

Perk up an everyday side dish with the addition of some fruit and wine!

Makes 4 to 6 servings
Prep Time: 10 minutes
Cook Time: 30 minutes

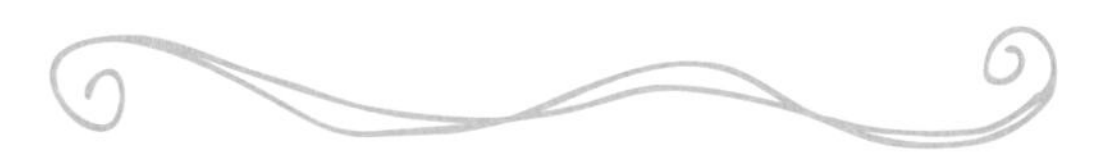

The raisins can be prepared with red grape juice if you choose.

For the raisins

- 1 cup raisins
- 1 cup red wine

For the cabbage

- 2 tablespoons olive oil
- 1 1½-pound head red cabbage, shredded (about 5–6 cups)
- 1 medium yellow onion, peeled and thinly sliced (about 1 cup)
- Juice of 1 medium lemon (about 2 tablespoons)
- 1 tablespoon balsamic vinegar
- Salt and freshly ground pepper

Place the raisins into a small bowl. Cover with red wine. Let stand for at least 15 minutes.

In a medium saucepan heat the olive oil over medium-high heat. Add the cabbage and onion and cook until beginning to wilt, about 15 minutes. Stir in the lemon juice and vinegar and cook until soft, about 10–15 minutes more. Season with salt and pepper.

Drain any excess liquid from the raisins. Add the plumped raisins to the cabbage. Stir.

To serve, pour the cabbage into a serving bowl.

STRIKE-IT-RICH CHOCOLATE PUDDING

With Chocolate Cookie Crumbles

Nothing satisfies that chocolate craving like cool, smooth pudding. You'll get a bit of a hand workout with all of the whisking involved. Keep those fingers busy!

Makes 4 servings
Prep Time: 5 minutes
Cook Time: 15 minutes, plus chilling

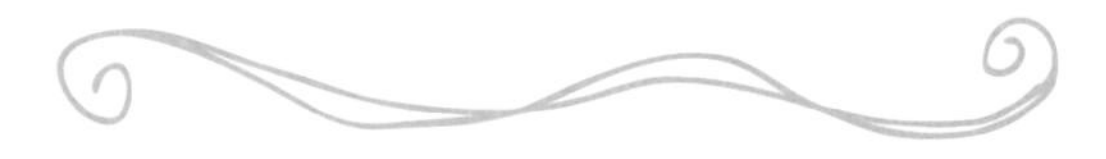

Many chocolate chip varieties are offered in your market. Choose the one with the most cocoa since it is full of good-for-you antioxidants.

- 1 cup reduced-fat milk, divided use
- 1 cup reduced-fat half and half
- ⅓ cup natural sugar
- ⅔ cup semisweet chocolate chips (the higher the cocoa content the better!)
- 3 tablespoons cornstarch
- 2 large eggs
- 2 teaspoons pure vanilla extract
- 12 chocolate wafer cookies, crumbled

Whisk together ½ cup of the milk, the half and half and the sugar in a pot over medium heat until the mixture begins to simmer and the sugar dissolves. Remove from the heat and stir in the chocolate chips until melted. Return the pot to the stove top.

In a medium bowl whisk together the remaining ½ cup milk and cornstarch until dissolved. Whisk in the eggs. Stir in 2 tablespoons of the melted chocolate mixture into the egg mixture so that you don't cook the eggs. Pour the egg mixture back into the chocolate mixture. Cook, whisking constantly until the pudding is thickened, about 4–5 minutes. Stir in the vanilla. If the mixture is lumpy, you may strain through a sieve.

Pour into 4 ramekins or custard cups. Cover each with plastic wrap to assure a smooth top. Chill for at least 1 hour or overnight.

To serve, sprinkle the crumbled cookies over the top of the pudding.

On Shopping Day: Prepare the pudding, cover with plastic wrap, and store in the refrigerator for up to 2 days.

ROASTED RED GRAPE PARFAITS

With Orange and Maple-Flavored Ricotta Cheese

*Talk about flavor-*full*, this dish has it all: the smoothness of ricotta cheese flavored with maple and orange, crumbles of gingersnaps and hazelnuts, and a big burst of roasted red grape goodness. All this—and a bunch of antioxidants, too? How good does it get?*

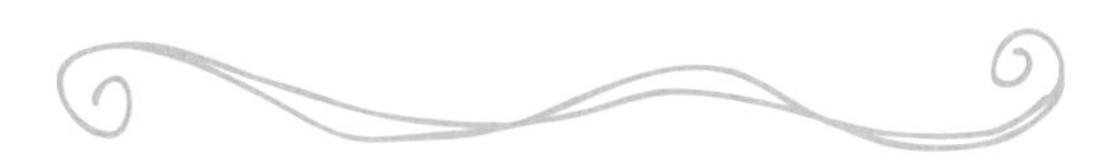

Use this recipe as an open-ended invitation to substitute whatever ingredients you have on hand. Roast plums and cherries, toast pecans and macadamia nuts, or flavor ricotta with honey or lemon zest.

Makes 4 servings
Prep Time: 10 minutes
Cook Time: 15 minutes

- 2 cups red seedless grapes
- 1 tablespoon natural sugar
- 6 gingersnaps
- 2 tablespoons hazelnuts, toasted
- 1 16-ounce container reduced-fat ricotta cheese
- 2 tablespoons maple syrup
- Zest of 1/2 medium orange (about 1 tablespoon)
- 1 teaspoon vanilla
- Fresh mint leaves (for garnish)

Preheat the oven to 450 degrees. Place the grapes onto a rimmed baking sheet. Sprinkle with sugar. Roast until the grapes begin to burst, about 15 minutes.

Place the gingersnaps and the hazelnuts into the bowl of a food processor. Pulse to form crumbs.

In a medium bowl whisk together the ricotta cheese, maple syrup, orange zest, and vanilla until smooth.

To serve, spoon half of the ricotta mix into 4 parfait glasses or oversized red wine goblets. Top with half of the gingersnap/hazelnut crumbs. Spoon half of the grapes over top. Continue layering, reserving a spoonful of ricotta mix to top each dish. Garnish with mint leaves.

SIMPLE ZUCCHINI CAKE

With Vanilla Glaze

In this easy recipe, a spoonful of sugar glaze dresses up a simple snack cake without taking you over to the dark side.

Makes 9 servings
Prep Time: 15 minutes
Cook Time: 40 to 45 minutes

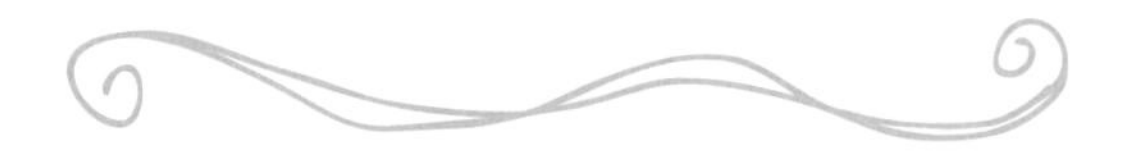

The fine shred disk attachment for your food processor is the perfect tool for readying zucchini.

For the cake

- 1 cup unbleached all-purpose flour
- 1 teaspoon baking soda
- 1 teaspoon ground cinnamon
- 1/2 teaspoon ground nutmeg
- 1/4 teaspoon salt
- 1/4 cup canola oil
- 2 large eggs
- 3/4 cup brown sugar
- 1/2 cup reduced-fat vanilla-flavored yogurt
- 1 large zucchini, finely shredded (about 1 cup)

For the glaze

- 1/2 cup confectioners' sugar
- 1 teaspoon vanilla
- 1–2 teaspoons reduced-fat milk

Preheat the oven to 350 degrees. In a medium bowl whisk together the flour, baking soda, ground cinnamon, ground nutmeg, and salt.

In another medium bowl whisk together the canola oil, eggs, and brown sugar until smooth. Stir in the yogurt. Stir in the flour mixture until just combined. Stir in the zucchini. Pour the batter into an 8-inch square cake pan that has been coated with vegetable oil spray and dusted with flour. Bake until the cake springs back when touched, and a tester inserted into the center comes out clean, about 40–45 minutes. Cool on a rack.

In a small bowl whisk together the confectioners' sugar and vanilla. Add enough milk for a thick glaze. Drizzle the glaze over the cake.

To serve, cut the cake into 9 squares.

On Shopping Day: Prepare the cake, cover, and store for easy snacking during the week.

CHOCOHOLIC'S CRUTCH

Sometimes you just gotta soothe that chocolate craving. A steamy cup of warm cocoa is just the ticket—especially when it is flavored with a fresh orange.

Makes 4 servings
Prep Time: 5 minutes
Cook Time: 10 minutes

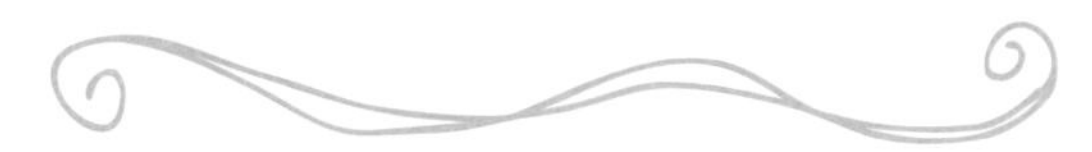

- 2 cups reduced-fat milk
- 1 cup reduced-fat half and half
- 2 tablespoons natural sugar
- 1/8 teaspoon salt
- 6 ounces bittersweet chocolate, chopped
- 3 drops orange oil
- Whipped cream
- Chocolate shavings
- Orange zest

In a saucepan warm the milk, half and half, sugar, and salt over medium heat. When the mixture begins to steam, add the chopped chocolate and stir until melted. Stir in the orange oil.

To serve, divide the hot chocolate among mugs and top with whipped cream and chocolate shavings and orange zest.

Gorgeous Home Spa Secrets . . . For White Glove Treatment

Finally, a section where the focus is on superficial beauty: where *the look* of the hands is what matters most. With dreamy manicure lingo like *soft, smooth, shiny,* and *nicely shaped,* who can resist the white-glove treatment? The easy manicure tips in this section feature nail strengthening herbal teas, vitamins, and do-it-yourself cuticle grooming, better known to your hands as that "ooh, ahh" feeling.

Moisture Retainers

You can get pure vegetable glycerin at a vitamin store or in the health food aisle at the grocery store. It costs around five dollars a bottle. **Lanolin**, similarly priced and located, is a natural oil derived from wool. A sheep's natural secretion is very close to the natural oils we secrete from our own skin, so it's the best choice for dry hands. **Glycerin** is a natural by-product of the soap-making process, and while commercial soap manufacturers remove the glycerin for use in their more profitable lotions and creams, handcrafted soap retains glycerin in each and every bar—so look for the most organic soap on the market. To prepare your own revolutionary hand cream, combine ⅓ cup glycerin with ⅔ cup water. Shake together in a bottle and then lather onto your hands.

Hangnails, defined as small, loose strips of torn skin near fingernails and toenails—don't stand a chance when your hands are properly moisturized. Because hangnails hurt so much, you'll want to avoid them by using a lanolin and glycerin-based lotion *every day*. Further protection against hangnails includes the following: don't bite your nails (something we'd *never* admit to, but may still do from time to time), and carefully remove any hang nails that *do exist* with a nail scissors. A recommended organic treatment for lessening the discomfort of hangnails is to dip fingers into a bowl of plain yogurt.

TNT—DY-NA-MITE!

For what we like to call "tough as nails tea," or TNT, drink a nail-strengthening brew comprised of two essential herbs: **nettle** (*Urtica dioica*) and **oat straw** (*Avena sativa*). This comforting beverage provides calcium, iron, and silica—the very minerals needed for healthy nails. To prepare, pour 3 cups of boiling water over 2 tablespoons each of dried nettle and dried oatstraw (available at most natural food stores). Cover, steep for 20 minutes, and strain. Drink three cups a day. You can store leftover tea for up to two days in a covered glass container.

Women Against Carpal Tunnel Syndrome (W.A.C.T.)

You could have *W.A.C.T.* me over the head with the following fact: Many people with carpal tunnel also suffer from a B_6 vitamin deficiency, which can be brought on by the uniquely female circumstances of pregnancy, menopause, or taking birth control pills. Vitamin B_6 supplementation works to strengthen the sheath surrounding the tendons in the wrist, thereby lessening the ravages of carpal tunnel. Two other B vitamins work in conjunction with B6 to make carpal tunnel treatment more effective: B_2 and B_{12}. In addition, folic acid is beneficial. Talk to your doctor about vitamin supplements or tailor (*hand*craft!) your daily diet to include these vitamins.

The "Gotta Have It!" Pre-Manicure Treatment

Before shaping and painting your nails, hydrate your hands with lotion. After that, do a warm paraffin treatment to really lock in that moisture. You'll need 3 blocks of paraffin wax, 3 oz. of vegetable oil, 20 drops of essential oil, a few drops of olive oil, and plastic sandwich bags to cover your hands later on. Start by melting the paraffin, vegetable oil, and the scented oil in a double boiler. (Be sure to use a double boiler for safety purposes!) Very carefully pour the wax into a shallow pan and wait until a skin has formed on top of the wax. When this happens, the temperature should be about right for submerging your hands. Before submersion, smooth on the olive oil and be sure to cover every inch of your hands and fingers. Dip each hand into the wax repeatedly until you have several layers of wax built up. Once your hands are covered, have a gal pal help you slip on the sandwich bags. Relax for about 30 minutes, until it's time to slip off the "white gloves" and peel the wax away; it should come off in large sections. Rinse thoroughly and have a soft terry cloth towel waiting in the wings; you'll need it for a soothing pat down. Viola! Super-soft hands!

Salon Talk in 3 Easy Steps

One cannot expect to turn her kitchen table or bathroom vanity into a nail salon without high-wattage lighting, nonacetone polish remover (the acetone ones are highly flammable and will dry out your cuticles, causing hangnails), and cotton-wrapped orange wood sticks—available in all drugstores.

1. Begin your manicure by removing the old chipped and faded polish and filing your nails to the desired shape; file them in one direction, starting at the edges and moving toward the top. After that, soak in soapy (all natural, glycerin soap!) water for a few minutes to soften cuticles.

2. Next, dot and rub in cuticle cream, using a cotton-wrapped orange wood stick to push back cuticles.

(Here's a do-it-yourself cuticle cream recipe you can make beforehand: 3 tbsp paraffin, ½ cup mineral oil, 1 tbsp coconut oil, 1 tbsp glycerin mixed together and heated in a double boiler.)

3. Wipe nails with a damp cloth; wet it with just a few drops of orange oil for a refreshing and aromatic finish. Apply a base coat of polish. Let dry for one minute. Apply two coats of your favorite color. Always apply polish by starting on the side of the nail. You should be able to cover the nail in three stokes, one on each side and one in the middle. Apply top coat.

Helping Hands

After you have groomed them to perfection, put those age-defying hands to good work. Volunteer at your local hospital, preschool, or women's shelter. Your soft touch and caring words might just change someone's life . . . as much as volunteering enhances yours. Start your search at www.volunteermatch.org.

CHAPTER 12

the truth about tummies and butts

"I've been on a constant diet for the last two decades. I've lost a total of 789 pounds. By all accounts, I should be hanging from a charm bracelet." —Erma Bombeck

What's the truth (it *hurts!*) about tummies and butts? As these body parts age, we find ourselves smack in the middle of "the middle-age spread." The truth is tummies and butts are the visible signs of how closely we watch our exercise and nutrition patterns. Wouldn't you love to stop hiding under baggy clothes, stop blaming your lumpy physique on waning youth, or stop working so much that there is no time for the gym? Well, ladies, take heart. This chapter is a way to wipe clean any erroneous beliefs that tight abs and butts are reserved for the young and unencumbered. We're offering you a fresh start—no matter how busy you are or how many kids you have—by imparting these simple how-tos: how to make tasty, high-energy recipes with low fat and calorie contents; how to get healthy doses of appetite-suppressing fiber in your everyday meal plan; how to work your way through fun tummy/butt exercises that produce nothing short of an endorphin high. We've got the lowdown on cellulite, diet myths, and what a happy digestive system can and can't live without. So show yourself some TLC by reclaiming the abs of steel God intended you to have! Whip your butt into shape today! Slip into something so very *gorgeous* that you won't believe it's you.

Ask Dr. Moon

The doctor is in to answer your questions.

Take this Q&A to heart, and you'll get the skinny (not to mention look that way yourself) on shedding excess weight—best of all, you'll learn how to keep it off FOREVER! You'll also get the hard-to-hear, but nevertheless beneficial, scoop on so-called "diet food," why you should always, *always* look at the nutrition grid on the backs of food packaging, and where to "spot train" your body's problem areas if genetics and daily diet are saddling you with saddle bags. Best of all, when we bend Dr. Moon's ear this time around, we'll be learning to sculpt our eating habits around an active lifestyle—the sole path to a perfect body. Does that kick butt or what?

Q: If I have more than 10 pounds to lose, how long (realistically!) will that take?

A: Sadly, there's no quick fix. One pound of body fat is equal to 3,500 excess calories; thus to drop as much as 14 pounds, we have to burn 49,000 extra calories. This can be done, but certainly not in one, two, or even three weeks. In order to sensibly burn excess weight, we should look to strip off between 1 and 2 pounds of body fat per *week* or the equivalent of 3500—7000 extra calories in 7 days.

Q: Does low-intensity exercise burn more fat?

A: Many people believe that low-intensity exercise (like walking) is a better fat burner than high-intensity exercise (like running). Why? Studies have shown that the body burns a large percentage of calories from fats during easy aerobic sessions. However, in order to burn excess body fat *and* lose weight, we must burn excess calories—lots of them! The harder the exercise, the more calories we burn. Period. So say someone (we'll call her Person A) exercises for 30 minutes at level 4 on a gym bike, and her friend (Person B) exercises at level 7 for the same amount of time. Who's burnt the greatest percentage of body fat? The answer is the less sweaty Person A. But before you disenable the most challenging buttons on your gym equipment, you'll want to understand how critical burning calories is to weight loss. Person B—and this is assuming that she always goes for the most exhaustive workout—is no doubt thinner than Person A.

Q: Knowing that low-cal is important to staying trim, I buy fat-free. Does "fat-free" mean no calories?

A: Some foods contain very little or no fat. But ALL foods contain calories. Just because a food suggests that its fat content is low—less than 5 percent—it hardly means that the food itself is good for you or low in calories. Low-fat snack foods are usually loaded with extra sugar—this compensates for a lack of taste left behind when the fat is either extracted or not added. Extra sugar may mean that snacks that are low in fat are actually calorie dense. Tip: Read food labels. Find out which foods are low in fat *and* in sugar!

Q: So I guess that means I should eliminate all fats from my diet?

A: Not at all. Don't fall into the trap of thinking that losing weight means eliminating all fats from your diet. When the low-fat craze seized our country's diet industry, it was understood that for every gram of fat we consume, we eat more than twice the number of calories found in protein and carbohydrates in the same weight. So at face value eliminating fats dramatically reduces the number of calories in your diet; however, some fats in our diets are very, *very* important, and to cut your body off from them is to do yourself a major disservice. Certain fats (e.g, monosaturated ones like those found in olive oil) help deliver essential vitamins to the body (vitamins A, D, E, and K) as well as delay the onset of hunger—a good tool to employ during a diet. That said, healthy fats (such as naturally occurring fats that have not been hydrogenated, processed, refined, or overheated) should make up somewhere between 15 to 25 percent of our calorie intake at each mealtime.

Q: Can I focus on losing fat from specific problem areas?

A: Each of our bodies is unique and has favorite places to store extra weight. Spot reduction is an exercise technique whereby we supposedly train a problem area (for example, the stomach) in order to lose fat solely from this area. In reality this technique cannot work. During weight loss, excess body fat is stripped from all over the body, not just areas we train. Exercising specific areas of the body can certainly help tone certain muscle groups, but performing hundreds of ab crunches may not mean that you'll lose fat from this area in double-quick time.

Q: So what if exercise and healthy diet can't get rid of my fat? What then?

A: Liposuction may be an option in these situations. It is important to note that liposuction is *not* a weight-loss method; it's elective surgery of a cosmetic nature. The average amount of fat removed is less than 10 pounds, most typically from the abdomen, thighs or buttocks—in some cases even the patient's neck. The procedure is done via a cannula, a flexible tube inserted into the body for withdrawing fluid or inserting medication, and an aspirator, a device that produces a vacuum effect. Women with muscles and skin stretched by multiple pregnancies, known colloquially as "twin skin," may find liposuction is not the best procedure to tighten those muscles and reduce loose, flabby skin. A tummy tuck may be a better alternative. For men or women who were obese at one point in their lives and still have excessive fat deposits or loose skin in the abdominal area, liposuction may be the best choice. It is important to note that liposuction is meant as a remedy for *small* bulges that are resistant to exercise; liposuction cannot remove cellulite!

Q: Will snacking sabotage my figure? Got any tips to keep it girlish?

A: Modern wisdom says snacking is the way to go. Our bodies are engines, and food is our fuel. Eating several small, healthy meals a day keeps the engine full and has us operating at optimal condition. Anyone trying to lose weight can quote one simple fact: It's the calories that count. Use these handy lists to compare the portions and calories in many of your favorite foods and perhaps find a few new favorites for snack time or mealtime. We'll break the following tasty snacks down by "calorie club."

The 50-Calorie Club

- 9 ounces of low-calorie cranberry juice cocktail
- 1 snack-size Nestlé Crunch® bar
- 1 fat-free cookie
- 20 cheddar Pepperidge Farm® Goldfish crackers
- 5 mini Quaker® apple cinnamon rice cakes
- ½ cup mashed butternut squash
- 2 small raw tomatoes
- 1 cup mixed frozen vegetables

The 100-Calorie Club

- 1 cup Kellogg's Corn Flakes®
- ⅔ Lender's Original® plain bagel
- 1¼ fresh apples
- 3 plums
- 1 medium banana
- ½ plain baked potato with skin

- 4⅓ tablespoons grated Parmesan cheese
- 2 ounces roasted round tips beef
- 3 ounces baked or broiled haddock
- ¼ cup hummus
- ½ cup vanilla soft-serve frozen yogurt

The 200-Calorie Club

- 22 thin pretzel sticks
- 1½ slices French toast
- 2¼ buttermilk pancakes
- 1 ounce Kix® cereal with 1 cup skim milk
- 2 ounces Alpine Lace® cheddar-flavored cheese
- 2 whole wheat matzo crackers
- 8 ounces flounder fillet
- 3 ounces unbreaded broiled pork center loin
- 7.5 ounces Chef Boyardee® cheese ravioli with meat sauce
- 1 cup cooked long-grain white rice
- 1 ounce dried walnuts
- 3 navel oranges

Jorj's Good-Carb, Good-Fat Glam Kitchen

The beautifying foods in this section are defined as unrestrictive, deeply satisfying, and in no way, shape, or form derived from any fad diets. These are nutrient-dense foods, chock-full of complex carbohydrates and the healthiest, most unrefined—not to mention *fast*-burning—fats. In addition to all this, the food and drink suggested here pack a powerful cocktail of amino acids as well as a rush of vitamins and antioxidants that give you the will, motivation, and most of all, desire to exercise.

It's the Digestive Tract, Stupid

It truly is your digestive system that either stands in the way of *or makes possible* a healthy lifestyle. Your stomach and colon act as a sieve when it comes to mineral and vitamin absorption, sorting out the bad and retaining only the good. Obviously we want more good than bad; to be on the other side of that equation makes for a health crisis. The 5-a-Day Challenge you see on bags of fruits and veggies wouldn't be there if daily consumption of five servings each didn't spare people from a laundry list of health problems.

With the right digestive information in hand, the whole world is your oyster—one that won't give you heartburn! Digestion, if it is to be understood in terms so brief and concise, is the chemical breakdown of solid foods into nutritive molecules that are absorbed by the bloodstream and carried to your cells. Digestion starts in the mouth. Chewed food travels to the esophagus, then to the stomach, small intestine, and colon. The digestive system tries to absorb as much fiber, carbohydrates, healthy fats, and protein as it can before nature calls; so here is your digestive wisdom in a nutshell: *You want foods as natural and unrefined as possible* for good and comfortable digestion. **Repeat your tummy's mantra:** *You Want Foods as Natural and Unrefined as Possible!!!*

B-Wise

Avoiding heartburn or colon problems is all about consuming lean meats with no trans or saturated fats. Bad fat, chiefly *animal fat,* and simple carbohydrates (found in refined, white-colored foods—the opposite of whole grain) are enemies of your digestive tract. It's a fiber-rich (the big 4 are: **wheat**, **oats**, **corn**, and **rice**) diet that includes healthy proteins, like **eggs** and **cheese**, your stomach and colon love best. If starches and sugars aren't natural, like those found in fruits and vegetables, your metabolism burns like a wet log. A diet that is fiber-rich, combined with exercise, produces a tummy and butt that complement your gorgeous body.

The Thing about Tobacco and Alcohol . . .

So *what* if the Rat Pack looked sexy smoking, giving birth to an enduring advertising campaign that has us convinced smoking is the end-all-be-all of bein' Kool? Smoking wreaks havoc on *every* body part this book talks about. It *literally* ages you from the inside out—including your digestion. Smoking contributes greatly to peptic ulcers and heartburn. Nicotine increases production of stomach acid while decreasing your body's ability to neutralize it. Women are urged to keep their alcohol consumption to no more than one drink a day. Alcohol can inflame your stomach lining and relax the valve that prevents stomach acid from backing up into your esophagus—that'll make you think twice about the meaning of Happy Hour!

Browse Through Your Area Health Food Store

People who aren't overweight and stay active have fewer occurrences of gastroesophageal reflux disease (GERD) and acid reflux. Any dietary aide as safe, relaxing, and inexpensive as a cup of tea is worth a shot, which brings us to the frontrunner on our whole foods shopping list: **green tea**. While the jury is still out on its success in promoting weight loss, it's been praised enough that some respect is due—after all, would green tea be celebrating its 3,000th year of popularity throughout Asia if it weren't a viable supplement for fit and active lifestyles? Some scientists report that green tea inhibits fat absorption and helps glucose regulation. If you choose a caffeinated brand, it's supposed to be a metabolic booster—green tea is said to burn an extra 78 calories a day for those who consume it!

While you're shopping organically, try aloe vera and citrus pectin supplements; they support digestive health. Cat's claw, another helpful tummy herb, has been used by the indigenous people of Peru for years; it cleanses the intestinal tract. You can also look for vitamins that specialize in an amino-acids formula, offering all 10 of the essentials. Amino acids are needed for enzyme production, which assists in healthy digestion. The human body cannot replenish amino acids on its own and so looks to daily food consumption. The omega fatty acids in **fish**, **soybeans**, **lamb**, and **granola**—as well as the proteins in **chicken** and **turkey**— are ideal for daily replacement of amino acids. While these nutritive gems are best sought in long, enjoyable meals with your family, their supplemental vitamin form, provided your doctor agrees, can't hurt!

Start Your Day

Main Plates

On the Side

Snacks & Sweets

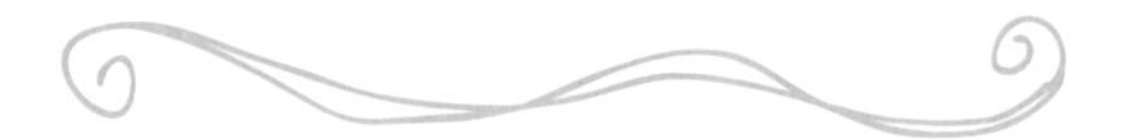

APPLE PIE FOR BREAKFAST

Just kidding. You cannot *eat apple pie for breakfast if you want a tight butt and a flat tummy. However, you* can *have all of those wonderful flavors in this delicious warm, oatmeal dish.*

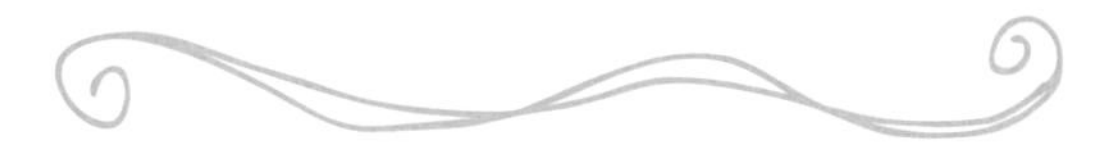

For an extra dose of protein, add a tablespoon of chopped walnuts to each bowl.

Makes 2 servings
Prep Time: 15 minutes
Cook Time: 5 minutes

For the oatmeal

- 1¾ cups reduced-fat milk
- 1 cup old-fashioned rolled oats
- ½ teaspoon ground cinnamon
- ¼ teaspoon nutmeg
- ¼ teaspoon salt

For the apples

- 1 tablespoon canola oil
- 2 medium apples, cored and thinly sliced (about 1 cup)
- 1 tablespoon honey
- ½ teaspoon ground cinnamon

Bring the milk to a boil over medium-high heat. Stir in the oats, cinnamon, nutmeg, and ¼ teaspoon salt. Reduce heat to medium and simmer until the oats are tender and most of the milk is absorbed, about 6–8 minutes. (Alternatively, you can combine these ingredients in a microwave-safe bowl, cover loosely with plastic, and cook on high for about 2–3 minutes.)

Heat 1 tablespoon canola oil in a skillet over medium-high heat. Add the apple slices and cook until tender and golden, about 2 minutes. Stir in the honey and cinnamon.

To serve, divide the oatmeal into 2 bowls. Top with apples.

BREAKFAST TACOS

Pleasing those Mexican food lovers in your household has never been so simple or *healthy. Here's a grab-and-go breakfast meal packed with protein and antioxidants. (The most deliciously deceptive part is that your tummy won't know that it's good for you!)*

Makes 2 servings
Prep Time: 5 minutes
Cook Time: 5 minutes

- 2 green onions, thinly sliced (about 2 tablespoons)
- 1/2 large red bell pepper, seeded and diced (about 1/2 cup)
- 1 large egg
- 3 large egg whites
- Salt and freshly ground pepper
- 2 6-inch corn tortillas
- 1 tablespoon reduced-fat sour cream (for garnish)
- 1 tablespoon chopped fresh cilantro (for garnish)

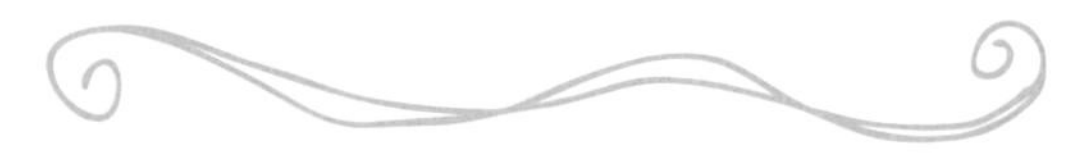

You can spice this up a bit more with the addition of hot pepper sauce or a spoonful of prepared salsa.

Coat a skillet with vegetable oil spray and heat over medium heat. Add the green onions and red bell pepper and cook until soft, about 2 minutes. In a small bowl whisk together the egg and egg whites. Pour this mixture into the skillet and cook until set, about 1–2 minutes more. Season with salt and pepper,

To serve, heat the tortillas in a microwave oven until soft. Divide the egg mixture among the tortillas. Fold in half, taco style. Garnish with sour cream and cilantro.

SAY "RICOTTA CHEESE" PANCAKES

With Very Berry Sauce

Light and fluffy pancakes are garnished with dessert toppings for this breakfast starter that is sure to get the troops up and moving!

Makes 6 servings
Prep Time: 10 minutes
Cook Time: 10 minutes

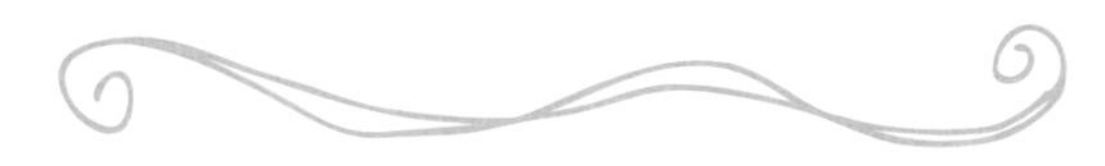

Using reduced-fat cheese is a great way to make sure that those abs and butts stay firmly in place while splurging on a sweet treat.

For the sauce

- 1 pint fresh raspberries (about 2 cups)
- 1 pint fresh blueberries (about 2 cups)
- 2 tablespoons natural sugar
- 1 teaspoon cornstarch mixed with 2 tablespoons water
- Zest of 1 medium lemon (about 1 tablespoon)

For the pancakes

- 1 cup unbleached all-purpose flour
- 1 teaspoon baking powder
- 1/4 teaspoon salt
- 1/2 cup fat-reduced milk
- 1/4 cup natural sugar
- 1 large egg
- 2 tablespoons canola oil
- 1 teaspoon vanilla extract
- 1/2 cup reduced-fat cottage cheese
- Zest of 1 medium lemon (about 1 tablespoon)
- 1/4 cup chopped walnuts (for garnish)
- 1/4 cup reduced-fat vanilla yogurt (for garnish)

Place the raspberries and blueberries in a saucepan over medium heat. Stir in the sugar, cornstarch mixture, and lemon zest. Simmer until the berries soften but do not lose their shape, about 6–8 minutes. Keep warm.

Heat a griddle over medium-high heat. Coat with vegetable oil spray. In a small bowl whisk together the flour, baking powder, and salt. In a large bow whisk together the milk, sugar, egg, canola oil, and vanilla extract. Stir the flour mixture into the milk mixture. Stir in the cottage cheese and second tablespoon of lemon zest until just blended.

Ladle the batter onto the griddle. Cook until golden and bubbly on the top, about 3 minutes. Flip and cook until golden on the second side, about 2 minutes more. Repeat using all of the batter.

To serve, place the pancakes onto a serving platter. Pour the sauce over the top. Garnish with chopped walnuts and vanilla yogurt.

On Shopping Day: Prepare the berry sauce, cool to room temperature, store in an airtight container in the refrigerator for up to 4 days.

EGG IN A FRAME

With Basil Tomatoes

Start your day with a good-for-you breakfast that balances whole grains, protein, and the antioxidants found in herbs and fruit.

Makes 2 servings
Prep Time: 5 minutes
Cook Time: 5 minutes

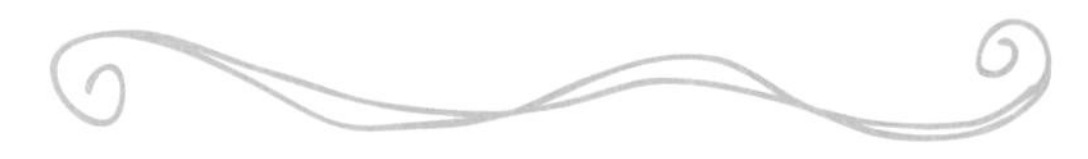

You can choose an egg substitute in this recipe to reduce the fat found in the egg yolk.

For the framed egg

2 slices thin-sliced whole grain bread
2 large eggs
Salt and freshly ground pepper

For the seasoned tomatoes

12 ripe cherry tomatoes or mixed baby tomatoes
1 tablespoon chopped fresh basil
1 tablespoon olive oil

Coat a nonstick skillet with vegetable oil spray. Cut the center from each slice of bread (this can be a circle or square depending on your artistic whim). Place the bread frames in the pan. Cook over medium heat until golden, about 1–2 minutes. Turn the bread. Crack 1 egg into the center of each bread frame. Cook until the egg is set, about 3–4 minutes. (If you like, you can carefully turn the framed egg to set the egg more firmly.) Season with salt and pepper.

In a medium bowl toss the tomatoes with basil and olive oil. Season with salt and pepper.

To serve, use a spatula to transfer each framed egg onto a plate. Spoon the seasoned tomatoes alongside.

EGGPLANT BOATS

Stuffed with Spiced Beef and Peas

Ground beef and peas were the "poor man's" version of chili in my house growing up. As with most family favorites, a little veggie update makes it a wise choice for a good-fat, good-carb meal.

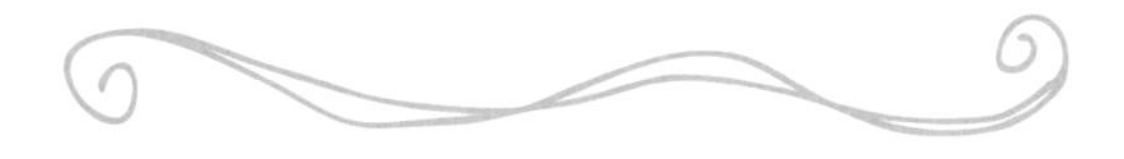

Choose lean beef for this dish. If there is any excess fat in the skillet, you can skim it off before seasoning the meat. You can also substitute ground sausage or ground turkey.

* * *

Form the eggplant boats by scooping out some of the eggplant. Be sure to leave enough so that the boat is sturdy enough to hold the filling.

Preheat the oven to 350 degrees. Remove some of the pulp from the eggplant halves to form a bowl. Cut the removed eggplant into ¼-inch dice and reserve for the filling. Place the eggplant boats onto a rimmed baking sheet. Sprinkle with 1 tablespoon olive oil and season with salt and pepper. Bake until the eggplant begins to soften, about 20 minutes.

In a skillet heat another tablespoon olive oil over medium-high heat. Add the onion and reserved eggplant. Cook until soft, about 4–5 minutes. Add the beef and cook until browned and crumbly, about 5 minutes. Stir in the Worcestershire, tomato paste, and ½ cup of the chili sauce. Reduce the heat to medium and simmer for 3–4 minutes until thickened. Stir in the peas. Season with oregano, salt and pepper.

Fill the softened eggplant halves with the meat mixture. Drizzle the remaining ½ cup chili sauce over the beef and pea filling. Sprinkle with Parmesan cheese. Bake until the eggplant is quite soft, about 10–13 minutes.

To serve, transfer the eggplant boats to a platter. Garnish with fresh herbs.

On Shopping Day: Prepare the ground beef and pea filling. Cool to room temperature, store in an airtight container in the refrigerator for up to 3 days.

Makes 4 servings
Prep Time: 20 minutes
Cook Time: 30 to 35 minutes

For the eggplant

- 2 baby eggplants, cut lengthwise, seeds removed
- 1 tablespoon olive oil
- Salt and freshly ground pepper

For the meat and peas

- 1 tablespoon olive oil
- 1 small onion, peeled and diced (about ½ cup)
- 1 pound lean ground beef
- 1 tablespoon Worcestershire sauce
- 1 tablespoon tomato paste
- 1 cup prepared chili sauce, divided use
- 1 15-ounce can sweet peas, drained
- ½ teaspoon dried oregano
- 2 tablespoons reduced-fat grated Parmesan cheese

SNAPPER FILLETS

Smothered with Caramelized Onions

Sweet onions blend with "melt in your mouth" fish to create a burst of flavor—and the best news of all? You're eating nutritious food with very little fat that's ready in just minutes! It doesn't get much better than this.

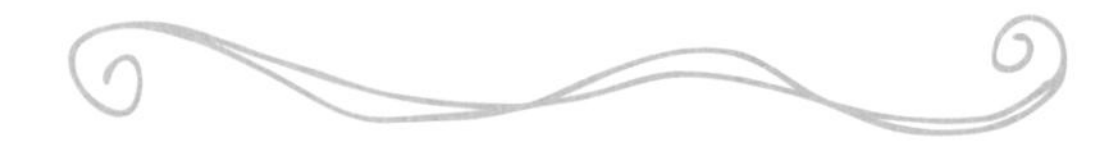

If fresh fish is not available, try this dish using boneless, skinless chicken breast or pork tenderloin medallions.

Makes 4 servings
Prep Time: 20 minutes
Cook Time: 15 minutes

1 tablespoon olive oil
2 large red onions, peeled and diced (about 2 cups)
Salt and freshly ground pepper
1 tablespoon brown sugar
1 tablespoon balsamic vinegar
4 6- to 8-ounce snapper fillets
Juice of 1 medium lemon (about 2 tablespoons)

In a skillet heat 1 tablespoon olive oil over medium-high heat. Add the onions and cook until soft, about 5 minutes. Season with salt and pepper. Stir in the brown sugar and balsamic vinegar. Reduce the heat to medium and continue cooking until the onions are quite brown and syrupy, about 5–10 minutes more.

Preheat the oven to 350 degrees. Place the fish onto a rimmed baking sheet coated with vegetable oil spray. Sprinkle with lemon juice and season with salt and pepper. Mound the onions on top of the fish. Bake until the fish is cooked through, about 15–20 minutes depending on the thickness of the fish.

To serve, use a spatula to transfer each fillet to a dinner plate.

On Shopping Day: Prepare the caramelized onions, cool to room temperature, and store in an airtight container in the refrigerator for up to 4 days.

SPICY TUNA DINNER SALAD

With Balsamic Dressing

Turn your weekday dinner salad into an entire meal with the addition of lean tuna—a good fat—and white beans—a good carb!

Makes 4 servings
Prep Time: 25 minutes
Cook Time: 10 minutes

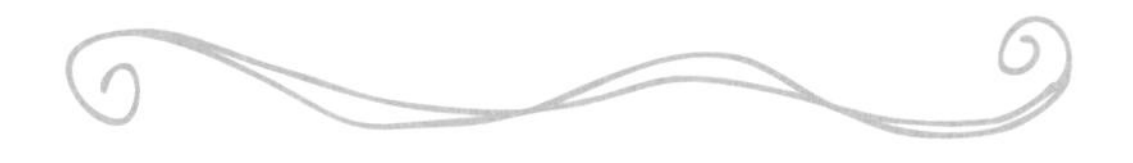

You can use this recipe plan to create a wonderful salad with the items you have in your refrigerator. Substitute flank steak or chicken for the tuna and squash, eggplant, and bell peppers for tomatoes and onions.

For the dressing

- 4 medium cloves garlic, peeled
- Juice of 1 medium lemon (about 2 tablespoons)
- 1 tablespoon Worcestershire sauce
- 1 teaspoon Dijon mustard
- 1/3 cup balsamic vinegar
- 2 tablespoons fresh cilantro leaves
- 3/4 cup olive oil
- Salt and freshly ground pepper

For the tuna

- Juice of 2 medium lemons (about 1/4 cup)
- 2 tablespoons orange marmalade
- 1 tablespoon chili powder
- 1/2 teaspoon crushed red pepper flakes
- 1 1-pound tuna steak
- 1 tablespoon olive oil
- 1 pint ripe cherry tomatoes or mixed baby tomatoes
- 1 small red onion, peeled and thinly sliced (about 1/2 cup)

For the salad

- 1 large head romaine lettuce, washed, dried, and torn (about 8 cups)
- 1 15.5-ounce can small white navy beans, drained

Place the garlic, lemon juice, Worcestershire sauce, mustard, balsamic vinegar, and cilantro into a blender. Pulse to emulsify. With the machine running, slowly add ¾ cup olive oil. Season with salt and pepper.

In a small bowl mix together the lemon juice and marmalade. Brush this mixture over the tuna. Sprinkle with chili powder and red pepper flakes. Marinate the tuna for 15 minutes. Cut the tuna into 2-inch chunks. Heat the olive oil in a skillet over medium-high heat. Sear the tuna until golden, about 2–3 minutes. Turn and add the tomatoes and onion. Cook until the tuna is seared on both sides but still rare in the center, the tomatoes have begun to turn brown, and the onion has soften. Remove from the heat.

To serve, arrange the lettuce onto 4 dinner plates. Sprinkle the beans over top. Place the tuna, tomatoes, and onions onto the salad. Drizzle the dressing over all.

On Shopping Day: Prepare the dressing, store in an airtight container in the refrigerator for up to 4 days.

GRILLED VEGGIE PANINI

With Basil Pesto Sauce

Here's another way to load your weekly menu plan with ab-friendly veggies: Add a cup of the minestrone soup, and you'll have a very figure friendly meal.

If you don't have a panini grill, you can grill the sandwiches using your grill pan. Place the sandwiches onto the hot grill pan. Top with a heavy skillet weighted down with cans of tomatoes. Cook until the sandwich is golden on the grilled side. Carefully turn, and weight down the top again with the skillet and tomato cans. Grill until the second side is golden. Voila—panini on a shoestring.

Place the basil leaves, garlic, pine nuts, and cheese into the bowl of a food processor (or blender). Pulse to combine. With the machine running, slowly pour in the olive oil. Season with salt and pepper.

Heat a grill pan over medium-high heat. Brush the vegetables with olive oil and season with salt and pepper. Grill until the veggies are golden and soft (but not mushy), turning frequently, about 5 minutes total.

Lay the bottom half of the loaf onto your work surface. Spread the cut side with pesto sauce. Place the eggplant onto the bread. Top with peppers and onion. Cut the mushrooms into strips and place on top of the vegetables. Spread the cut side of the top portion of the loaf with more pesto sauce.

Heat a panini grill. Brush the top and bottom of the sandwich with olive oil. Cut the sandwich into 4 sections. Place the sandwiches into the panini grill and heat until both sides are golden and the veggies are warmed through.

To serve, place the sandwiches onto a serving platter and serve additional basil pesto on the side.

On Shopping Day: Prepare the basil pesto, store in an airtight container in the refrigerator for up to 4 days. Grill the veggies, cool to room temperature. Store in an airtight container in the refrigerator for up to 2 days.

Makes 4 servings
Prep Time: 15 minutes
Cook Time: 6 to 8 minutes

For the pesto

- 2 cups fresh basil leaves
- 2 large cloves garlic
- 1/2 cup pine nuts
- 3 ounces grated Parmesan cheese (about 3/4 cup)
- 2/3 cup olive oil
- Salt and freshly ground pepper

For the veggies

- 2 tablespoons olive oil
- 1 medium eggplant, cut into 1/4-inch thick slices
- 4 large portobello mushrooms, stem and gills removed
- 1 large red onion, peeled and cut into 1/4-inch thick slices

For the panini

- 1 16-ounce whole grain (French bread–style) loaf, cut in half horizontally
- 4 whole roasted red peppers (drained from jar), sliced into quarters
- 2 tablespoons olive oil

BAKED CHICKEN BREASTS

With Artichoke and Sun-Dried Tomato Sauce

Mediterranean flavors combine to spice up the everyday chicken breasts in this dish.

Makes 4 servings
Prep Time: 10 minutes
Cook Time: 25 to 30 minutes

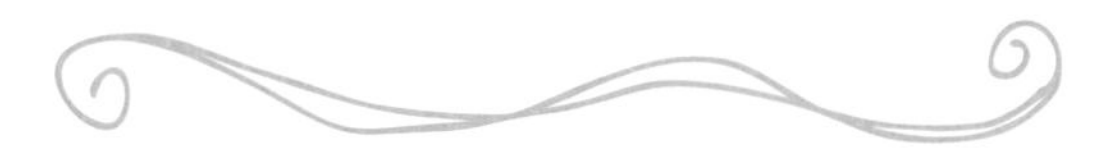

You can make this dish even more tummy-friendly by draining the oil from the sun-dried tomatoes. Add just enough of the reserved oil to easily blend the artichokes, tomatoes, and olives. Save the unused oil for your next home-prepared vinaigrette.

- 4 large (6- to 8-ounce) skinless, boneless chicken breast halves
- 1 14-ounce can artichoke hearts
- 1 7.5-ounce jar oil-packed sun-dried tomatoes, drained
- 1 7-ounce jar Kalamata olives, drained and pitted
- 2 medium cloves garlic
- 1 tablespoon balsamic vinegar
- 2 tablespoons fresh parsley leaves
- 1 tablespoon fresh tarragon leaves
- Salt and freshly ground pepper

Preheat the oven to 350 degrees. Place the chicken into a baking dish. Place the artichoke hearts, sun-dried tomatoes, olives, and garlic into the bowl of a food processor. Pulse to chop. Add the vinegar, parsley, and tarragon. Season with salt and pepper.

Spoon the sauce over the chicken. Place the dish into the oven and bake until the chicken is cooked through but not dry, about 25–30 minutes.

To serve, place the chicken breasts onto a serving platter. Spoon extra sauce from the baking dish over top.

On Shopping Day: Prepare the artichoke-and-sun-dried tomato sauce. Store in an airtight container in the refrigerator for up to 3 days.

CHICKEN PORTOBELLO

With Linguini in Butter Sauce

I know, I know, you're asking yourself, "What is she doing putting butter sauce in a tummy-flattening, butt-reducing chapter?" Well, I do so to demonstrate that just a touch of butter will give richness of flavor to an otherwise good-for-you dish. Check it out and you'll see what I mean.

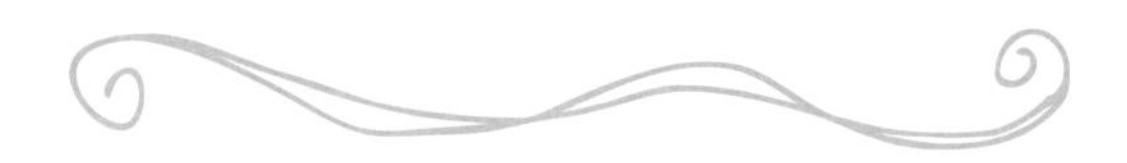

By reducing wine and chicken broth for several minutes, you increase the flavor impact. Don't worry—the alcohol cooks itself out of the sauce so it's quite good for every member of your family.

* * *

By adding meaty mushrooms to the dish, you gain a satisfying, tummy-filling component without accumulating a ton of calories.

In a large Dutch oven cook the linguini in boiling, salted water.

Preheat the oven to 350 degrees. Place each chicken breast between 2 sheets of waxed paper. Use a meat mallet to pound to ½-inch thickness. In a skillet heat 1 tablespoon olive oil over medium-high heat. Dredge the chicken in flour. Shake off the excess. Season with salt and pepper. Place the chicken into the skillet (in batches if necessary). Cook until golden, about 3–4 minutes. Turn and cook until golden on the second side, about 2 minutes more. Remove to a rimmed baking sheet, drizzle the lemon juice over top, and keep warm.

Place the remaining tablespoon of olive oil into the skillet. Cut the mushrooms into ½-inch thick strips. Season with salt and pepper. Cook the mushrooms in the skillet until golden, about 5 minutes. Transfer to the rimmed baking sheet with the chicken. Sprinkle the cheese over the chicken and mushrooms. Bake for 4–5 minutes or until the chicken is cooked through and the cheese is melted.

Remove the skillet from the heat. Pour the wine into the skillet. Return to the heat and reduce to about ½ cup, about 5 minutes. Pour in the chicken broth and reduce to 1 cup total sauce, about 10 minutes more. Reduce the heat to low. Add the basil, season with salt and pepper and simmer for 5 minutes more. Turn off the heat and swirl in the butter.

To serve, drain the pasta. Place the linguini into the skillet with the sauce. Toss to coat. Place the pasta onto a serving platter. Use a spatula to transfer the cheese-covered chicken and mushrooms to top the pasta. Garnish with additional fresh basil leaves.

Makes 4 servings
Prep Time: 5 minutes
Cook Time: 35 minutes

For the pasta

8 ounces whole wheat linguini
Salt

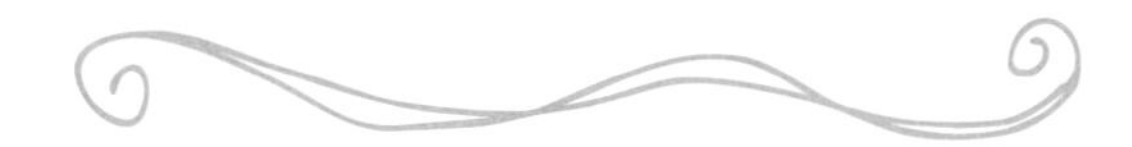

For the chicken

4 4- to 5-ounce skinless, boneless chicken breast cutlets
2 tablespoons olive oil
Unbleached all-purpose flour for dredging
Salt and freshly ground pepper
Juice of 1 medium lemon (about 2 tablespoons)
4 large portobello mushrooms, stem and gills removed
2 ounces shredded reduced-fat mozzarella cheese (about 1/2 cup)

For the sauce

1 cup white wine
2 cups homemade chicken stock or low-sodium chicken broth
2 tablespoons chopped fresh basil
2 tablespoons cold butter

PANCETTA-WRAPPED TURKEY MEDALLIONS

With Broccoli Rabe, Peppers, and Onions

In this dish, pancetta adds the spice and veggies deliver the zip, transforming an everyday supper into a scrumptious turkey entree.

Makes 4 servings
Prep Time: 10 minutes
Cook Time: 15 minutes

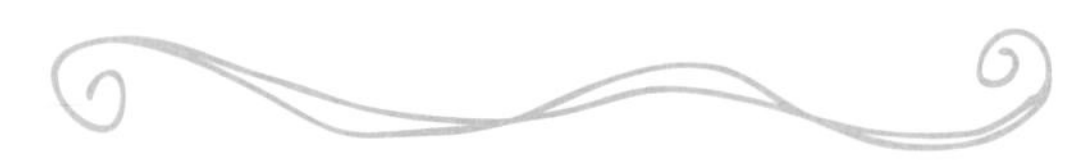

Make sure that the tenderloins are cooked all the way through by using a meat thermometer. The internal temperature should reach 165 to 170 degrees for turkey.

For the turkey medallions

- 2 8- to 10-ounce turkey tenderloins, cut crosswise into 2-inch pieces
- 4 ounces pancetta, thinly sliced
- Salt and freshly ground pepper
- 1 tablespoon olive oil
- 1 cup Madeira wine

For the broccoli rabe

- 1 large bunch broccoli rabe (about 1 pound), sliced into 1-inch pieces
- 1 tablespoon olive oil
- 1 small red onion, peeled and diced (about 1/2 cup)
- 1 large yellow bell pepper, seeded and cut into thin strips

Wrap each turkey medallion with pancetta. Secure with a toothpick. In a skillet heat the olive oil over medium-high heat. Cook the medallions in the skillet until golden on one side, about 3–4 minutes. Turn and continue cooking until golden on the second side, about 3–4 minutes more. Transfer to a platter and keep warm.

Add the Madeira wine to the skillet. Simmer until reduced to 1/2 cup. Reduce the heat to low. Add the turkey medallions back to pan and keep warm.

Blanche the broccoli rabe in boiling (salted) water until crisp-tender, about 3–4 minutes. Drain. In a second skillet heat 1 tablespoon olive oil over medium-high heat. Add the onion and bell pepper and cook until soft, about 3–4 minutes. Toss in the broccoli rabe. Season with salt and pepper.

To serve, spoon the broccoli rabe mixture onto a serving platter. Remove the toothpicks from the turkey medallions. Use tongs to place the medallions on top of the veggies. Pour the reduced Madeira sauce over the turkey.

ROASTED CHIPOTLE SALMON

With Minted Couscous

Roasting the salmon with a spicy paste yields a crusty top and moist center for this salmon dish. The freshness of the mint, infused into the couscous, helps to balance the flavors.

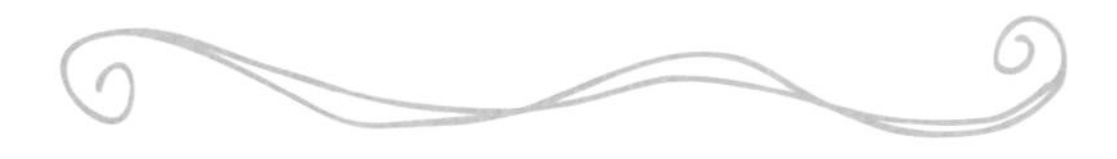

A chipotle is a smoked jalapeno pepper. It adds a smoky, earthy flavor to the dish. Canned chipotles come in a red sauce and are quite spicy. To use, remove 1 pepper from the can. Store the remainder in an airtight container (in the refrigerator) for another use. Open the pepper and scrape the seeds from the center. Cut into pieces and continue with the recipe. Make sure that you wash your hands very well after handling the pepper.

* * *

This recipe is designed to give you more salmon than you need for 4 people. Take advantage of this bounty by creating a tangy salmon salad for tomorrow's lunch. Or flake some into your scrambled eggs.

Preheat the oven to 425 degrees. Place the salmon onto a rimmed baking sheet that has been coated with vegetable oil spray. Drizzle with lemon juice and season with salt and pepper.

Place the brown sugar, chipotle pepper, orange zest, garlic powder, paprika, cumin, and oregano into the bowl of a food processor. Pulse to combine. With the machine running, slowly pour in the 2 tablespoons olive oil. Brush this mixture over the salmon.

Place the salmon into the oven. Roast for 5 minutes. Reduce the heat to 350 degrees and cook until the salmon is still rare in the center, about 20–30 minutes depending on thickness.

Cook the couscous according the directions on the package (usually a ration of 2 parts liquid to 1 part couscous). Fluff with fork. Add 1 tablespoon olive oil and fresh mint.

To serve, transfer the salmon to a serving platter. Spoon couscous alongside the salmon. Garnish with additional lemon slices.

Makes 4 servings
Prep Time: 29 minutes
Cook Time: 30 minutes

For the salmon

- 1 2 1/2-pound center-cut whole salmon fillet
- Juice of 1 medium lemon (about 2 tablespoons)
- Salt and freshly ground pepper
- 1/4 cup brown sugar
- 1 canned chipotle pepper in adobo sauce, seeded
- Zest of 1/2 medium orange (about 1 tablespoon)
- 1 teaspoon garlic powder
- 1 teaspoon paprika
- 1 teaspoon ground cumin
- 1/2 teaspoon ground oregano
- 2 tablespoons olive oil

For the couscous

- 1 cup couscous
- 1 tablespoon olive oil
- 2 tablespoons chopped fresh mint
- Lemon slices (for garnish)

FIVE-SPICE BEEF WRAPS

With Orange Ginger Dipping Sauce

Lean beef and a veggie for wrapping makes this meal a lean, mean, fat-busting machine!

Makes 4 servings
Prep Time: 20 minutes
Cook Time: 20 minutes

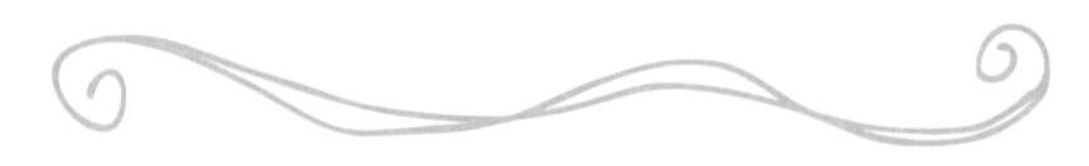

Chinese five-spice is a blend of spices. Look for it in the ethnic section of your grocery store or online.

* * *

This dish can be a bit messy.
Serve it during the week with a roll of paper towels and enjoy the giggles.

For the dipping sauce

- 1/4 cup rice wine vinegar
- Juice of 1 medium orange (about 1/3 cup)
- 2 tablespoons natural sugar
- 1 1-inch piece ginger, peeled and grated (about 1 tablespoon)
- 1 tablespoon prepared chili sauce

For the beef

- 1 1-pound flank steak, cut across the grain into thin slices
- 1 teaspoon Chinese five-spice powder
- 1 teaspoon toasted sesame oil
- 1 tablespoon olive oil
- 1/3 cup dry sherry
- 2 large shallots, minced (about 2 tablespoons)
- Zest of 1/2 medium orange (about 1 tablespoon)
- 1 tablespoon prepared chili sauce
- 1 4-ounce can whole water chestnuts, drained and cut into 24 slices
- 1 bunch (6–8) green onions, thinly sliced on the diagonal (about 1/2 cup)
- Salt and freshly ground pepper

For the wraps

- 8 large Boston lettuce leaves
- 1/2 cup chopped peanuts
- 1 large carrot, shredded (about 1/2 cup)

Pour the rice wine vinegar, orange juice, sugar, ginger and chili sauce into a pan over medium heat. Stir and simmer until reduced and thickened slightly, about 5 minutes. Remove from the heat.

Toss the flank steak with Chinese five-spice powder and sesame oil. In a skillet heat 1 tablespoon olive oil over medium-high heat. Cook until the meat is golden on the edges but still pink in the center, about 5 minutes. Pour in the sherry, shallots, orange zest, and chili sauce. Cook until the sauce thickens slightly, about 3–4 minutes more. Stir in the water chestnuts and green onions. Season with salt and pepper.

To serve, pour the meat into a serving bowl. Place the lettuce leaves and condiments alongside. Pour the dipping sauce into a bowl. Invite your gang to create their own fabulous wrap.

On Shopping Day: Prepare the condiments and dipping sauce. Store in airtight containers in the refrigerator for up to 3 days.

AVOCADO AND GRAPEFRUIT SALAD

A fresh salad is only a couple ingredients away–as shown by this easy recipe!

Makes 4 servings
Prep Time: 10 minutes

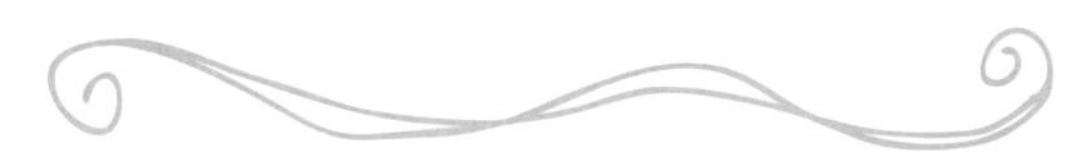

To section the grapefruit, work over a bowl to catch all of the juices. Cut the grapefruit in half horizontally. Use a sharp knife to cut the sections from the membranes. Combine the juice with the sections.

2 large avocados, cut in half and pitted
Juice of 1 medium lime (about 1 tablespoon)
Salt and freshly ground pepper
1 red grapefruit, peeled and cut into segments
2 tablespoons chopped fresh cilantro

Place the avocados onto a platter and sprinkle with lime juice, salt, and pepper.

Toss the grapefruit segments with the cilantro. Spoon this mixture over top of the avocados.

SAUTÉED PEAS

With Mint

Cooking the peas in a bit of butter is reminiscent of the veggies my Grandma served on Sunday nights. The onions and mint bring this dish into the new millennium.

Makes 4 servings
Prep Time: 5 minutes
Cook Time: 5 minutes

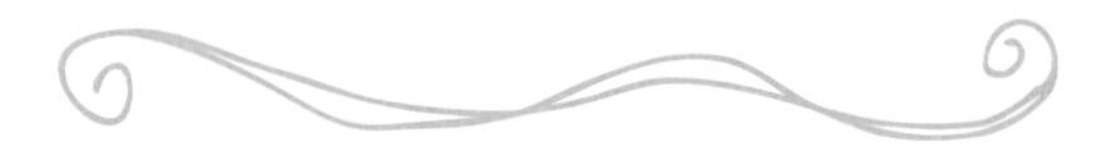

You might find fresh peas already shelled in the produce section of your grocery store. If not, frozen peas are an acceptable substitute.

- 1 tablespoon olive oil
- 1 tablespoon butter
- 2 cups shelled fresh peas or thawed frozen peas
- 1 bunch (6–8) green onions, thinly sliced on the diagonal (about $^1/_2$ cup)
- Salt and freshly ground pepper
- 1 tablespoon chopped fresh mint

In a skillet heat the olive oil and butter over medium heat. Add the peas and onions and cook until the onions are soft, about 5 minutes. Season with salt and pepper. Sprinkle with fresh mint.

GRILLED VEGETABLE SKEWERS

Grilling veggies gives them a crunchy exterior and a velvety smooth interior. Adding fresh herbs and a bit of olive oil adds an extra depth of flavor.

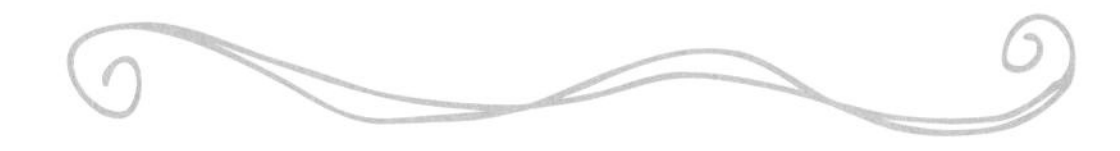

Using similarly sized pieces ensures that your veggies cook in the same time.

* * *

Use LEFTOVER veggies to coarsely chop in your food processor with chicken broth; it'll create a roasted vegetable soup that you'll really, really love!

Place the potatoes into a pot. Cover with water and bring to a boil. Reduce the heat and simmer until the potatoes just begin to soften, about 6–8 minutes. Drain.

Heat a grill pan or outdoor grill over medium heat. Thread the vegetables onto metal skewers, alternating to create interesting patterns such as:

- Yellow squash, green bell pepper, and cherry tomato
- Eggplant, zucchini, and button mushroom
- Potato half with onion chunk

In a small bowl mix together the olive oil with fresh herbs. Season with salt and pepper. Brush this mixture over the vegetables.

Grill until the veggies begin to turn brown and soften, about 12–15 minutes.

To serve, use a fork to gently remove the veggies to a platter.

On Shopping Day: Cut the fresh veggies into pieces and store in an airtight container in the refrigerator for up to 3 days.

Makes 8 servings (reserve half of the veggies for soup!)
Prep Time: 20 minutes
Cook Time: 15 minutes

1 pound small red creamer potatoes, about 6–7, halved
2 medium zucchini, cut into 1-inch pieces
1 pint ripe cherry tomatoes or mixed baby tomatoes
2 medium yellow squash, cut into 1-inch-thick lengths
1 large green bell pepper, seeded and cut into 1-inch pieces
1 large red onion, peeled and cut into 1-inch pieces
4 ounces whole button mushrooms
1 medium eggplant, peeled and cut into 1-inch pieces
2 tablespoons olive oil
2 tablespoons chopped fresh herbs (such as thyme, rosemary, sage, and cilantro)
Salt and freshly ground pepper

SOUTHWESTERN CHOPPED SALAD

With Toasted Peppers and Corn

Whether as a side salad or a hearty main meal, this salad is bursting with flavor and is surely ab-friendly!!

Makes 4 side servings
Prep Time: 15 minutes
Cook Time: 5 minutes

Feel free to vary the veggies with those that are readily available. Summer squash, fresh peas, radishes, and tomatillas are a wonderful addition.

For the vinaigrette

- 2 medium garlic cloves, peeled and chopped (about 1 teaspoon)
- 1 large shallot, peeled and chopped (about 1 tablespoon)
- Juice of 2 medium limes (about 2 tablespoons)
- Juice of 1/2 medium orange (about 2–3 tablespoons)
- 1 tablespoon honey
- 1/2 teaspoon chili powder
- 1/4 teaspoon ground cumin
- 1/4 cup olive oil
- Salt and freshly ground pepper

For the salad

- 1 tablespoon olive oil
- 2 large orange bell peppers, seeded and cut into 1/4-inch dice (about 2 cups)
- 1 medium jalapeño pepper, seeded and diced (about 2 tablespoons)
- 2 ears of fresh corn, kernels sliced from cob (about 1 cup)
- 6 medium plum tomatoes, seeded and diced (about 1 1/2 cups)
- 1 medium zucchini, cut into 1/2-inch dice (about 1 cup)
- 2 large avocados, peeled, pitted and cut into 1/2-inch dice (about 2 cups)
- 1 15-ounce can black beans, drained and rinsed
- 2 tablespoons chopped fresh cilantro
- 2 green onions, thinly sliced (about 2 tablespoons)

Place the garlic cloves, shallot, lime juice, orange juice, honey, chili powder, and ground cumin into the bowl of a food processor. Pulse to emulsify. With the blade running slowly pour in the olive oil. Season with salt and pepper.

In a skillet heat 1 tablespoon olive oil over medium-high heat. Cook the bell pepper and jalapeño pepper in the skillet until just crisp-tender, about 2 minutes. Season with salt and pepper. Transfer to a platter and cool to room temperature. Cook the corn kernels in the skillet until just beginning to turn golden, about 2 minutes. Season with salt and pepper. Transfer to a platter and cool to room temperature.

To serve, assemble the salad by lining up the veggies on a platter. Begin with the sautéed peppers. Place the toasted corn alongside, followed by the tomatoes, zucchini, avocados, and black beans. Sprinkle the cilantro and green onions over the top and drizzle with vinaigrette.

On Shopping Day: Prepare the vinaigrette and store in an airtight container for up to 4 days. Prepare the veggies and store separately in airtight containers for up to 4 days.

ORANGE CAPPUCCINO PARFAITS

The flavors of an afternoon cup of java are just perfect in this creamy, chilled dessert.

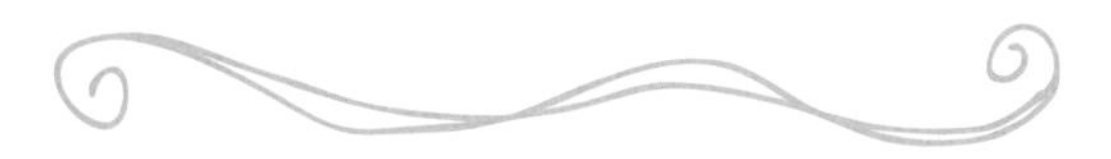

Espresso powder is made from specialty coffee beans that are ground, brewed, then dried. The powder readily dissolves for easy mixing. It is available in specialty markets and online.

* * *

Amoretti cookies are small, crisp rounds that are available in major grocery stores and specialty supermarkets.

Makes 4 servings
Prep Time: 5 minutes plus chilling

2 cups reduced-fat cottage cheese
1/3 cup natural sugar
2 teaspoons instant espresso powder
Zest of 1/2 small orange (about 1 teaspoon)
1 teaspoon pure vanilla extract
4 small amoretti cookies

Place the cottage cheese, sugar, espresso powder, orange zest, and vanilla into the bowl of a food processor. Pulse to purée. Spoon into 4 wine goblets. Cover each goblet with plastic wrap and chill in the refrigerator for at least 1 hour or overnight.

To serve, crush the cookies with a rolling pin. Remove goblets from the refrigerator and sprinkle cookies over the top.

FRESH LIME CAKE

With Warm Blueberry Sauce

Just a hint of citrus adds a burst of something special in this light-as air-cake. The warm blueberry sauce almost melts the cake. What a combo!

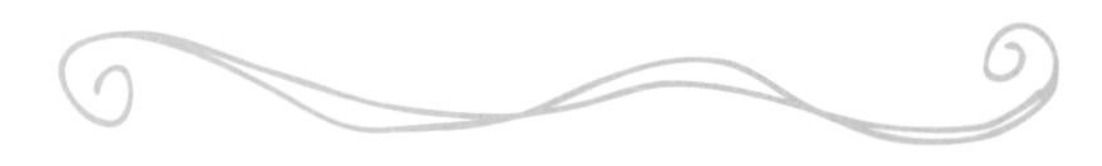

This dessert is all about portion control.
A little bit of something special is just what you need on your path to gorgeous.

Preheat oven to 325 degrees. In a medium bowl wisk together the cake flour, baking powder, and salt.

In a large bowl use an electric mixer to combine the butter and 1½ cups sugar until fluffy. Add the eggs, one at a time. Stir in the flour mixture in 3 additions, alternating with the milk. Stir in the lime juice and the lime zest.

Pour the batter into an 9 x 11 x 2-inch baking dish that has been coated with vegetable oil spray.

Bake until the cake springs back when touched and a tester inserted into the center comes out clean, about 35–40 minutes.

In a pot bring the apple juice, ¼ cup sugar, and lemon juice to a boil over medium heat. Stir until the sugar dissolves. Reduce the heat to medium. Stir in the blueberries. Cook until the berries begin to soften and the sauce is syrupy, about 8–10 minutes. Keep warm.

To serve, remove the cake from the pan. You may have to loosen the cake by running a knife around the edges. Use an angel food cake slicer or two forks to gently slice the cake. Serve with a spoonful of blueberry sauce.

On Shopping Day: Prepare the blueberry sauce and cool to room temperature. Store in an airtight container in the refrigerator for up to 3 days. Reheat to serve.

Makes 12 to 16 servings
Prep Time: 15 minutes
Cook Time: 35 to 40 minutes

For the cake

- 3 cups cake flour
- 3 teaspoons baking powder
- ½ teaspoon salt
- 1 cup unsalted butter, room temperature (2 sticks)
- 1½ cups natural sugar
- 4 large eggs
- 1 cup reduced-fat milk
- Juice of 3 medium limes (about 1/4 cup)
- Zest of 1 medium lime (about 1 tablespoon)

For the sauce

- ½ cup apple juice
- ¼ cup natural sugar
- Juice of 1 medium lemon (about 2 tablespoons)
- 1 pint fresh blueberries (about 2 cups)

TROPICAL BUTTERMILK PANNA COTTA

With Strawberry Sauce

Buttermilk adds a rich, tart taste and texture to this chilled custard. The sweet strawberry sauce is the perfect contrast.

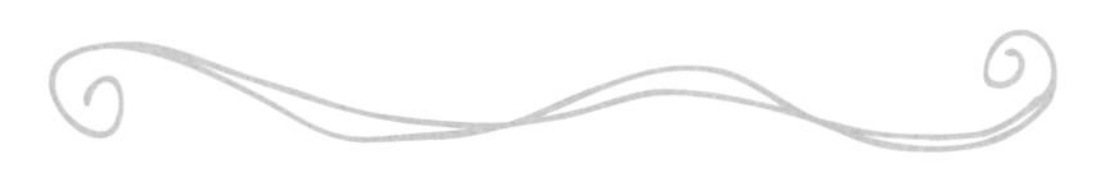

Panna cotta translates to "cooked cream" and is traditionally prepared with cream and whole milk. This lighter version uses reduced-fat buttermilk in place of the cream.

Coat 4 (6-ounce) custard cups with vegetable oil spray. In a saucepan sprinkle the gelatin over the milk. Let stand for 10 minutes. Warm the milk over low heat. Use a whisk to stir until the gelatin dissolves, about 5 minutes. Increase the heat to medium. Whisk in the sugar until dissolved, about 5 minutes more. Remove from the heat. Whisk in the buttermilk, lime zest, vanilla, and coconut. Pour the mixture into the custard cups. Chill for at least 4 hours or overnight.

In a saucepan whisk together the grape juice, sugar, and lime juice over medium-high heat. Bring to a boil and continue whisking until the sugar dissolves, about 3–4 minutes. Stir in the strawberries. Reduce the heat and simmer until the strawberries are soft and the sauce is syrupy, about 15–20 minutes. Cool to room temperature.

To serve, run a knife around the edge of the custard cups to loosen the panna cotta. Place a dessert plate upside down over the custard cup. Turn the cup over so that the panna cotta falls onto the plate. Spoon the sauce around the side and top with toasted coconut and lime slices.

On Shopping Day: Prepare the strawberry sauce and store in an airtight container in the refrigerator for up to 3 days. Prepare the panna cotta and chill for use the next day.

Makes 4 servings
Prep Time: 5 minutes
Cook Time: 15 minutes

For the panna cotta

- 1 teaspoon unflavored gelatin
- 1/2 cup whole milk
- 1/3 cup natural sugar (chose a white variety for the appearance of the final dish)
- 1 1/2 cups reduced-fat buttermilk
- Zest of 1 medium lime (about 1 tablespoon)
- 1 teaspoon pure vanilla extract
- 2 tablespoons shredded coconut

For the sauce

- 1/2 cup white grape juice
- 1/4 cup natural sugar
- Juice of 1 medium lime (about 1 tablespoon)
- 1 pint strawberries hulled and quartered (about 2 cups)
- 2 tablespoons shredded coconut, toasted (for garnish)
- Lime slices (for garnish)

POACHED CHERRY SUNDAES

Rather than place the cherry on top as in a traditional sundae, we make the cherry the center of attention in this dish.

Makes 4 servings
Prep Time: 15 minutes
Cook Time: 20 minutes

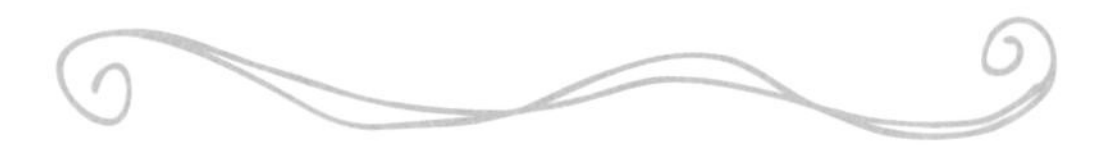

Use your favorite flavor of reduced-fat frozen yogurt for this dish. I like chocolate with cherries—but you get to pick!

- 1 pound cherries, stemmed, pitted and coarsely chopped (about 3 cups)
- 1/2 cup merlot
- 1/2 cup white grape juice
- 1/3 cup natural sugar
- Zest of 1/2 medium orange (about 1 tablespoon)
- Reduced-fat frozen yogurt
- Amoretti cookies, crumbled (for garnish)

In a pot heat the cherries, merlot, grape juice, sugar, and orange zest over medium-high heat. Stir until the sugar dissolves and the mixture begins to boil, about 5 minutes. Reduce the heat and simmer until the cherries are very soft and the liquid is syrupy, about 15–20 minutes.

To serve, divide the cherries into 4 bowls. Garnish with a spoonful of frozen yogurt and a few crumbles of Amoretti cookie.

On Shopping Day: Prepare the cherries. Cool to room temperature and store in an airtight container in the refrigerator for up to 4 days.

Mary Ellen Weighs In

When you begin an exercise routine, start with large muscles and progress to the smaller ones. Work at you own level, performing in varying degrees of intensity and resistance and experimenting with all types of equipment. There are many different exercises that will work the butt (gluteus maximus) and thighs (quadriceps). Here are a few to get you started.

The Squat

Squats are one of the best exercises you can do for your hips, butt, and thighs. There are many different types of squats. Most of these exercises can be performed in your own home, no excuses!

The Wall Squat—Place a large ball against the wall and behind your lower back with your feet shoulder-width apart and your knees slightly bent. Slowly lower your hips and butt, rolling the ball down the wall, so that your knees are directly in line with your toes (like a chair). Keep your chest up and your tummy pulled in. Pause at the bottom of your squat. Use your lower back to push the ball into and back up the wall. Repeat 8 to 12 times and work up to 3 sets.

The Chair Squat—Stand 8 to 10 inches in front of a chair with your feet shoulder-width apart. Keep your chest up and your back straight. Let your butt lightly touch the chair and squeeze your butt to stand up. Repeat for 8 to 12 reps and work up to 3 sets. You can add weights for more intensity. Another trick is to hold your arms out in front of you to help with your balance.

The Lunge

The lunge is a great exercise for your butt and thighs. There are many types of lunges. Here we give you a few to get started.

The Stationary Lunge—Stand tall and reach out with your left hand to touch the wall. Standing on the ball of your foot, move your right foot behind you. Place your left foot flat onto the ground in front of you. Your knee is in line with your ankle. Bend both knees while you lower your body weight straight down. Bend the right leg while sliding the left foot back into a lunge position, keeping the right knee behind the toe, the torso upright, and the tummy in. Slowly slide left foot back to starting position and repeat 8 to 12 times. Switch legs and repeat on each leg, working up to 3 sets.

The Forward Lunge—Is the same as above, but you alternate each leg, lunging forward on a straight path. Remember to hold your tummy in and keep your back straight.

The Backward Lunge—Yeah, just what you think, but this time you are moving backwards. Remember to plant your feet solidly on the floor before you begin to lower your weight.

Plié—Similar to a squat, this move is performed with your feet pointed outward and your legs open about 3 to 4 feet apart. (You can begin using a wall for balance.) Keep your knees in line with your toes.

There's More!!

Hip Extension—Feel the burn in your hamstrings and glutes with this exercise. On a step or platform, lie facedown with hips on the edge of the step, legs straight with toes resting lightly on the floor. Squeeze the glutes and hamstrings and straighten the legs until they are level with the hips. (Make sure not to hyperextend or arch your back.) Hold for 2–3 seconds and slowly lower, letting toes lightly touch the floor. Repeat for 8 to 12 reps, working up to 3 sets.

Side Leg Lift—While lying down on your side and resting on your elbow, keeping your feet side by side, raise the top leg about 2 feet. Keep your hip, knee, and foot in line. Perform 10 repetitions on each leg and work up to 3 sets.

Butt Blaster—Lie on your back with your feet against the wall. Your legs are at a 90 degree right angle to the floor. Place your arms beside your hips. Take one foot off the wall and point it up and forward. Push your right foot against the wall while you lift your butt up and off the floor, pointing the left foot up and forward. Be careful not to strain your weight. Keep your tummy in. Continue the movement until your right hip and thigh are in a straight line. Squeeze, pause, and slowly lower your butt back to the floor. Keep pushing that right foot into the wall for balance. Perform 8 to 10 repetitions, alternating legs, and work up to 3 sets.

Hip Lift (also known as The Bridge)—Lie on your back with your feet flat on the ground, shoulder-width apart, with your knees bent. Place your arms by your hips. Slowly lift your butt off the ground, rolling up one vertebrae at a time, aiming your pelvis towards the ceiling. Come up until your hips and thighs are in a straight line. Pause at the top and slowly lower, rolling your back down to the floor one vertebrae at a time. Perform 15 repetitions and work up to 3 sets.

Calf Raises—Stand tall with your tummy in and your chest forward. Balance on the edge of a step on both feet. Move to the balls of your feet. Slowly raise and lower your toes as you stretch and contract your calves. Repeat 10 to 12 times and work up to 3 sets.

Walk Tall

In addition to working our legs and butts, we can also work our hearts by performing aerobic exercise, essential for overall wellness. There are a lot of varying opinions about just how much aerobic exercise we need on a regular basis, and it is an individual decision. I feel that each of us should perform some aerobic activity (preferably one that we enjoy) for at least 20 minutes every day and up to to 1 hour four to five times a week. If you are trying to lose extra pounds, you need to work out more. If you are maintaining, you won't need to work out as much. The amount of time you spend and the intensity of the workout depends on your personal goals. Here are a few activities that you might enjoy.

Walking—Never underestimate the power of walking. Walking is easy: you can do it anywhere, anytime, with no special equipment. There's no learning curve, and it's something you can incorporate all day long. If you walk up hills, you can really target your butt, and if you pick up the intensity, you'll burn some of that extra flab off your buns! A 140-pound person burns about 300 calories an hour during a brisk walk.

Running—Work up from walking to jogging, and before you know it, you're running. Like walking, running is accessible, easy to learn, reduces stress, helps in weight loss, and it makes you feel good. Plus, it really works your butt, especially when you add a few hills to your regular running route. The most important parts of this exercise are the warm-up and the cooldown.

Hiking—Hiking burns tons of calories because you're typically going up steep mountains and maybe even getting into thin air, which requires lots of energy. Also, walking up an incline automatically gets your glutes more involved, and if you're wearing a backpack, you're really getting a workout. Plus, you get to see nature at its best. A 140-pound person burns about 390 calories in about an hour! It's important to wear the right shoes for this activity.

Biking—Riding a bike is great for your heart, and it also targets almost every muscle in your hips, thighs, and butt. On a stationary bike, alternate 3 minutes at 70–80 rpm with 2 minutes at 100–110 rpm for a calorie-blasting 30-minute workout. You can also try spinning at the gym or riding outside. Gear up to really work your glutes! A 140-pound person burns 335 calories in 45 minutes.

Sprints are another option for folks wanting to both burn more calories and tighten up the old tush. A 140-pound person burns 475 calories during a 45-minute jog.

Swimming—Another lifelong activity that is great for your heart and every muscle in your body. It's often soothing on your joints. Start by floating and moving just your arms and legs and work up to the breaststroke, the backstroke, and the butterfly.

Kickboxing—Kickboxing was a hot item back in the day, but it's still a great workout. Controlled kicks work your hips, thighs, and butt, while complex combinations that include punches will target your abs to make them stronger. A 140-pound woman will burn up to 500 calories with 45 minutes of kickboxing.

Whatever activity you choose, remember to have fun with it and change things up a bit so that you don't get bored and so you use different muscles. Variety in an exercise program is very important.

Down to the Core

We've heard all of the buzzwords about exercising your core—but just exactly what does this mean? Your core is predominantly your abdominal muscles and your lower back. Your core is thought to be a foundation of your strength. There are too many exercises to mention here, but here are a few for you to consider.

Vertical Leg Crunch—Lie flat and press your back into the floor. Clasp your hands behind your neck for support and extend your legs straight up in the air with your knees crossed. Hold in your tummy. Lift your torso up bringing your elbows toward your knees. Raise and lower, crunching your abs. Repeat 10 to 12 times and work up to 3 sets.

Bicycle Sit-ups—Lie flat and press your lower back to the floor. With hands beside head, bring your knees to a 45-degree angle and begin a pedal motion by touching opposite elbow to opposite knee, alternating each side.

Captain's Chair—Stand on chair and grip handholds to stabilize your upper body. Press your back against the pad and slowly lift knees towards your chest. Don't arch the back!

Exercise Ball—Lie face-up on ball and either cross hands over chest or place them behind your head. Contract your abs and lift your torso slightly off the ball, pulling the bottom of your rib cage down toward your hips. For beginners, place the ball under the upper part of the back. For advanced exercises, the ball should be under lower mid-back.

Marathons 'R Us

Marathon training takes a big commitment, but the benefits are well worth the effort. You will experience increased energy, improved health, a sense of accomplishment, increased discipline and organization, and you'll get a pair of great looking gams in the process. Team in Training (www.teamintraining.org) is just one of the many organizations that allow you to compete in a marathon and raise money for a good cause at the same time. Since 1988, more than 295,000 volunteer participants have helped raise more than $660 million. The organization offers personal training for you and a group of supportive teammates for up to 4 or 5 months in advance of your marathon. You are encouraged to walk, jog, or run toward your goal, whether it be a whole or half marathon. What a good way to blend exercise into your *gorgeous* lifestyle.

PART THREE

honor your body

More than just an adjective, *gorgeous* means beauty from the inside out. You emanate it day in, day out, year-round, all the years of your life by shaping and reshaping, fine-tuning and celebrating your appearance. Think about it. You've come this far in your quest for gorgeous, and the healthy lifestyle you subsequently lead feels so "free of charge" it seems like pure instinct. That's because it is! Remember that good physical and mental health bridges the gap between health and happiness, and, at the end of the day, these are what constitute a peaceful state of mind—a place we can't go without enough rest, relaxation, and sexual satisfaction. The chapters in this section talk specifically about sleep, reducing stress, life-affirming relationships, and the powerhouse living behind every femme fatale's smile.

CHAPTER 13

your beauty sleep

"It is better to sleep on things beforehand than lie awake about them afterward."

— Baltasar Gracián

Nothing is worse than a night of unproductive sleep. That's right, I said *unproductive* sleep. While we "rest" during the night, our bodies are actually busier than all get out. Getting some shut-eye means repairing and replacing damaged cells, boosting the immune system, re-energizing muscles and organs, and last but never least, archiving everything we did that day into memory. Sleep is serious business. When we don't get enough, we tempt the blues, hypertension, the early onset of kidney disease and diabetes, and plain old aches and pains. Since we can all agree that these conditions have no place in our *gorgeous* lifestyle, let's read on and differentiate between "the sleepers" and "wakers" in our food groups, what sleep truly (and technically!) entails, and identify the simple things we can do to ensure the sweetest of slumbers.

Ask Dr. Moon

The doctor is in to answer your questions.

The regenerative magic accomplished in the late p.m. relies on so much more than warm glasses of milk and soft feather pillows. In this section, Dr. Moon dishes on sleep, its five stages, what's accomplished in each of those stages, and how to "set the stage" for the best rest possible.

Q: What is insomnia and is there a direct link between it and depression?

A: The American Insomnia Association categorizes insomnia as acute/transient, intermittent, chronic, and psychophysiological (in which bedtime rituals trigger so much anxiety about falling asleep that it doesn't happen at all!). An astonishing 90 percent of people experience transient or short-term insomnia at some point during their lives, and up to 30 percent of Americans struggle with chronic or long-term insomnia.

Yes, insomnia is linked to depression. But take heart: since the public wants more of a solution than herbal and over-the-counter antidepressants, researchers are working on a theory that certain foods containing omega-3 fatty acids, a kind of fat that the body can't make enough of on its own, and uridine can be used to fight depression and help users get more sleep. But we have a long way to go. So far, there is no uridine supplement. It's not found in most foods; however, babies get it daily in the form of formula and/or breast milk.

Q: What can be done to help those who just can't get to sleep?

A: Depression and sleeplessness beg the "chicken or the egg" question. Does depression come first or does insomnia? Most people won't have to address that question if they maintain healthy lifestyles and control certain environmental factors. This means *not delaying* diagnosis and treatment for psychological disorders, illnesses, and diseases; consulting a physician on maintaining harmony during menopause; and regardless of whether you think you are affected by such things, controlling your consumption of caffeine, spicy and acidic foods, herbal or prescribed medications, and ruling out big meals less than 2 to 3 hours before bedtime.

Q: Are smokers and drinkers more at risk for insomnia?

A: Yes! Heavy smokers should be warned that nicotine stimulates the brain and reduces REM (i.e., quality) sleep. Heavy smokers tend to wake up after 3 or

4 hours of sleep due to nicotine withdrawal. Heavy drinkers are issued a similar caveat: while alcohol induces a light sleep, it impairs the more restorative stages of slumber. Reading labels on medications and foods is paramount. You should establish a consistent sleep routine, aiming for no more than an hour's deviation from 6 to 8 consecutive hours of sleep a day.

Q: Are there benefits for people who sleep well?

A: Yes, a Chicago study found that people who don't get enough sleep tend to be fatter than those who do. In fact, experts were so encouraged by their findings that they are seeking to prove a direct link between sufficient sleep and waging (a winning!) war against obesity. Their findings suggest that major extensions of sleep time may not be necessary, as an extra 20 minutes of sleep per night seems to be associated with a lower body mass index.

Q: What are the stages of sleep?

A: Sleep stages are divided between rapid eye movement (REM) and non-REM (NREM). REM is the period of sleep during which most dreaming occurs. Dreams are most consistently recalled if the person is awakened at this time. The average adult spends 20–25 percent of his or her sleep in REM mode, during which he or she experiences a great deal of mental and physical activity—so much so that researchers have found that during REM sleep, a person's heart rate, blood pressure, and breathing patterns are comparable to those found during waking hours.

NREM sleep is much longer than REM sleep and is divided into four stages. **Stage 1** is a transient phase that occurs at the onset of sleep, accounting for up to 75 percent of sleep time. If awakened in this stage, people may claim that they were not really asleep but "only dozing." This stage is generally regarded as the transition stage between wakefulness and actual sleep. **Stage 2** is actual sleep. This stage claims as much as 45 percent of overall sleep time. In this phase, muscle response, along with nervous activity, lowers. Conscious awareness of the external environment disappears, though someone can be easily aroused from this stage. In **Stage 3** delta-waves (large, slow brain waves) develop and transition a person into stage 4 sleep. This stage accounts for a mere 3 to 8 percent of overall sleep time. **Stage 4** is described as true delta sleep or the stage of deepest sleep. This accounts for 10 to 15 percent of total sleep time. If dreams or sleepwalking occur in this phase, we cannot, as a general rule, be expected to remember anything. **Stage 5** is REM. This is the last stage of sleep before waking, in which light and body temperature (circadian rhythms based on the onset of day and night in your given environment) create vivid, random dreams. Stage 5 can be a bit of a wild card, as it is vulnerable to things like jetlag or a sink-or-swim deadline at work.

Q: Can you dispel popular myths regarding sleep?

A: Here are a few of my favorites:

The older you get, the fewer hours sleep you need.

False. No matter your age, doctors recommend between 6 and 8 hours of sleep per day.

Raising the volume on your radio and air conditioner or drinking coffee will help you stay awake while driving.

False. Thirty-one percent of the population reports having fallen asleep while driving. There is nothing that is going to help you stay awake at the wheel. The best thing to do is to pull over and take a nap.

If you have insomnia at night, you should take a long nap during the day.

False. Your daytime sleep, especially if it's longer than 30 minutes, could be causing your nighttime insomnia.

If you exercise early in the morning, you will sleep better at night.

False. The best time to exercise is in the late afternoon or at noontime. Morning exercise has little effect on the quality of sleep that night. If you must exercise in the early morning, do not do so at the expense of needed sleep. Make sure you get to bed in time to fulfill your sleep quotient. Fatigue leads to better sleep. You can exercise to fatigue your muscles.

Q: Can your body adjust to night shift work?

A: No. Our natural sleep-wake cycle, regulated by light and darkness and programmed over thousands of years of evolution, prevents us from easily adjusting to night or rotating shifts and irregular work schedules. In fact, sleep shift workers are 40 percent more likely than day workers to be involved in accidents at work, on the highway, and at home.

Q: What is the science behind foods that help you sleep?

A: An essential key to a restful night's sleep is to get your brain "calmed down" rather than "revved up." Some foods contribute to restful sleep; other foods keep you awake. We can categorize food and drink into two groups: sleepers and wakers. **Sleepers** are tryptophan-containing foods. Tryptophan is an amino acid your body uses to make serotonin, the neurotransmitter that slows down nerve traffic so your brain isn't so busy. Tryptophan is a precursor of the sleep-inducing substances serotonin and melatonin. This means tryptophan is the raw material that the brain uses to build these relaxing neurotransmitters. Eating carbohydrates with tryptophan-containing foods (e.g., turkey, oats and whole grains, soy and dairy products) makes this calming amino acid more available to the brain. A high carbohydrate meal comes highly recommended for release of insulin, which helps your bloodstream clear the amino acids competing with tryptophan. **Wakers** are foods that stimulate neurochemicals (desserts with chocolate, (Ibuprofen for your headache, cough syrups, or anything with caffeine) that perk up the brain.

Q: What are the best bedtime snacks?

A: The best "midnight snacks" contain complex carbohydrates, protein, and calcium. Calcium helps the brain use the tryptophan to manufacture melatonin. This explains why dairy products, which contain both tryptophan and calcium, are one of the top sleep-inducing foods. Foods that are high in carbohydrates and calcium and medium to low in protein make ideal sleep-inducing bedtime snacks.

Q: What are the worst evening meals?

A: Certain foods can acerbate reflux disease and should be avoided, especially before bedtime. Get out your pad and pen and avoid the following litany before cashing in your chips: citrus juices like orange juice and lemonade and foods such as mashed potatoes, French fries, raw onions, ground beef or chuck, marbled sirloin, chicken nuggets, Buffalo wings, sour cream, milk shake, ice cream, regular cottage cheese, macaroni and cheese, spaghetti with sauce, liquor, wine, coffee (even decaffeinated!), salad dressing, oil and vinegar, high-fat butter cookies, brownies, chocolate, doughnuts, corn chips, and potato chips.

Q: Is it true that drinking coffee in the evening will keep you awake at night?

A: As a stimulant, caffeine speeds up the action of not only the nervous system but of other major body systems too. Within fifteen minutes of downing a cup of coffee, the level of adrenaline in your blood rises, which triggers an increase in heart rate, breathing rate, urinary output, and production of stomach acids. Basically, caffeine's effects are the reverse of what you want to happen as you go to sleep. Time your caffeine boost. For most people, the effects of caffeine wear off within six hours, so coffee in the morning will usually not interfere with sleep in the evening. Caffeine-containing beverages at lunch may not affect your sleep, but coffee, tea, or cola in the evening may keep you awake.

Q: What are some non-medical ways to enhance your sleep experience?

A: Keep a sleep diary that records the following info: When did you go to bed?;

How long did it take to drift off?; How long did you sleep before waking?; What, if any, were your dreams?

Keep a regular bedtime. Try a warm bath, relaxation exercises, or whatever calms you. Mentally unwind. Instead of reviewing your daily stressors and anticipating what's to come the following morning, replace your bedtime anxieties with the visual image of a blank sheet of paper with the words "There's nothing I can do about it until morning" written on it. Dim the lights as you prepare for sleep. It is believed that light levels help the brain produce a hormone that regulates sleep.

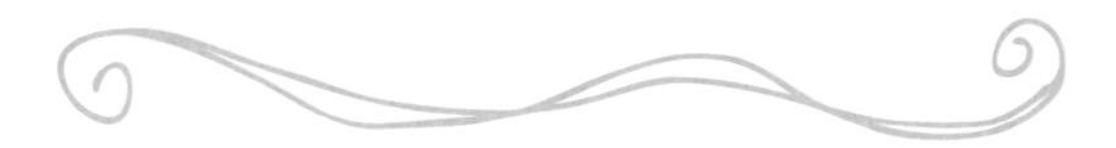

Jorj's "Sweet Dreams" Glam Kitchen

Sweet Dreams are made of these . . . stuffed chicken breasts, blueberry dumplings, sweet potato pancakes, savory turkey breast, just to name a few of the delectable dishes of which Mr. Sandman heartily approves. Just remember to keep your evening meals light, low fat, and reasonably seasoned. That cayenne pepper you've been saving is better spent on a breakfast omelet *after* you've benefited from a full night's rest. Ditto for the garlic, citrus juices, and Vidalia onion that belong in a satisfying lunch or early supper. Most people find it tough, after all, to drift off to sleep when their digestive systems are working overtime—but don't go thinkin' we're anti-midnight snack. This section is happy to dish on snooze foods and night caps.

Feast n' Snooze

Serotonin is a wondrous brain chemical in that it makes us feel contented and calm. When our bodies are in short supply, we crave what we shouldn't and stuff ourselves with sugary, refined, high-carb junk, the effect of which is a short-lived serotonin boost followed by a sugar crash. It doesn't have to be so. We can seek out tryptophan-rich foods (tryptophan is an amino acid that produces serotonin in our bodies at a healthy clip). **Turkey** is the most famous of these foods, but they also include **fish**, **cottage cheese**, **bananas**, **eggs**, **nuts**, **wheat germ**, **avocados**, **milk**, **cheese**, and **legumes**. Smaller amounts of tryptophan are yours for the taking in **breads**, **cereals**, **potatoes**, and **rice**. There's something you should know about tryptophan: because it's a big molecule, other, more easily absorbed amino acids will actively compete with it, lessening its sleep-inducing power. In order to divert them, you'll want to spike your insulin levels by pairing healthy protein foods with good starches like brown rice and whole grain bread.

Heartburn: A Bed Bug Who Bites

Heartburn strikes everybody from time to time. While some might suffer greatly, almost all can experience a small trace of indigestion. Gas and sour stomach are just a few of the symptoms created by fatty foods with high levels of acidity. Cooking technique, like roasting, baking, broiling, poaching, or steaming cut back on bad-fat content, allowing those who are prone to heartburn a better chance of enjoying meals at supper time. Ready your pantry with unrefined foods that require less of your digestive tract than the processed guys. Choose **Basmati** and **wild rice**; **stone ground cornmeal**; **dried spices and herbs** (less offensive to heartburn sufferers than freshly chopped); **reduced-fat peanut butter**, **mayo**, and **salad dressings**; and **angel hair** and **orzo pasta**.

Better Nightcaps

Hot beverages, chiefly coffee, are offered in restaurants after a big meal. Caffeine can stay in a person's system for up to 12 hours. With that in mind, you might consider your consumption of cappuccinos, lattes, espressos, mochas, iced teas, or just plain old cups o' joe and fit them into your schedule during the early part of the day. So what can you drink *before* bedtime? Even if it's grown clichéd in its popularity, a glass of warm milk does the trick. So will a trip to the health food store for melatonin, a hormone made by the pineal gland that helps us know when it's time to sleep. Valerian root is a helpful aid when sleep proves elusive; it possesses some of the same chemical properties found in prescription sleeping pills but doesn't interfere with the sleep stages. For the less adventurous, there's chamomile tea, which has a reputation older than your great-great grandmother for being calming.

Pleasant Dreams

Ideally, at least three hours should elapse between your last meal and going to bed. What will you dream when you get there? How many times have you heard somebody blame their crazy dreams on the Philly cheese steak pizza they ate before turning in? At the risk of sounding cheesy, dreams are like movies: your brain requires the right foods to ensure a high-quality production! At 60 percent fat, your brain needs omega-3s to function properly. Researchers have discovered a link between mood disorders and the presence of low concentrations of omega-3 fatty acids in the body. That's got to wreak havoc with your dreams at night . . . if you manage to get to sleep at all! Some of the foods that contain omega-3s include practically everything from the sea, as well as mixed nuts, edamame (soy), and winter squash.

Snacks for the Night Owl

If you like to stay up past eleven and your last meal was at sunset, that's a long time to go with nothing in the belly. So if you must eat in the p.m., do it right, with miniature doses of tryptophan. Have whole grain toast smeared with reduced-fat peanut butter, a handful of almonds, a piece of 12-grain bread with a slather of all-natural butter and cranberry jam. If you're really hungry, add a slice of lean turkey meat. Wash it down with a glass of soy milk. Your sleep-conscious snack list also includes a bevy of single-serving cheese wedges that include everything but pepper jack and herb-infused feta.

Sleepy-Time Recipes

Start Your Day

Main Plates

On the Side

Snacks & Sweets

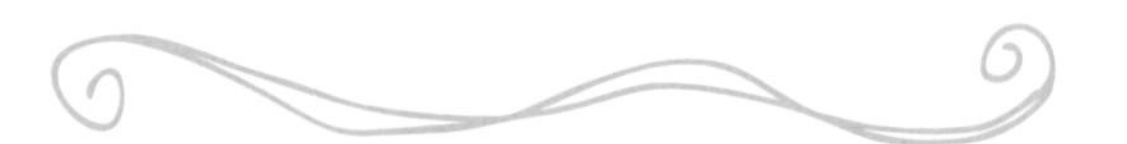

ORANGE BREAKFAST MUFFINS

Citrus flavors abound in this light-as-air muffin, just perfect on a brunch table or as a snack with your afternoon cup of tea.

Makes 10 to 12 muffins
Prep Time: 10 minutes
Cook Time: 25 minutes

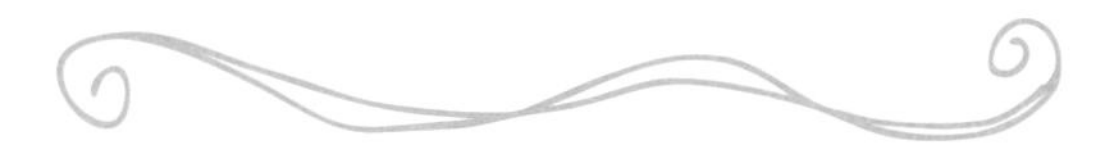

You can easily exchange lemon juice and ZEST for this recipe.

For the muffins

- 1 cup unbleached all-purpose flour
- ½ cup natural sugar
- 1 teaspoon baking powder
- ¼ teaspoon salt
- ½ cup reduced-fat sour cream
- Zest of ½ medium orange (about 1 tablespoon)
- 2 tablespoons canola oil
- 1 tablespoon reduced-fat milk
- Juice of ½ medium orange (about 1½ tablespoons)
- 2 large eggs, beaten

For the glaze

- 1 cup confectioners' sugar
- Juice of ½ medium orange (about 1 tablespoon)
- Zest of ½ medium orange (about 1½ tablespoons)

Preheat the oven to 350 degrees. In a medium bowl whisk together the flour, sugar, baking powder, and salt.

In a separate bowl stir together the sour cream, 1 tablespoon orange zest, canola oil, milk, 1½ tablespoons orange juice, and eggs. Stir this mixture into the flour mixture. Spoon the batter into a muffin tin with paper liners. Bake until the muffins spring back when touched and a tester inserted into the center comes out clean, about 20–25 minutes. Cool on wire racks.

In a bowl stir together the confectioners' sugar, 1 tablespoon orange juice, and 1½ tablespoons orange zest.

To serve, place the muffins onto a serving platter. Drizzle the tops with glaze.

On Shopping Day: Prepare these muffins for an easy breakfast treat during the week. Store in an airtight container for up to 3 days.

SWEET POTATO PANCAKES

With Warm Raspberry Syrup

These hearty pancakes are filled with antioxidants. Why not consider having breakfast for supper? Just remember that you don't want to eat too late in the evening.

You can prepare the sweet potato in advance or use leftover sweet potato. BUTTERNUT SQUASH is a good substitute.

Cook the sweet potato in boiling water until fork-tender, about 8–10 minutes. Drain well and mash with a fork.

Place the raspberries, 1 cup sugar, water, vanilla, orange juice, and orange zest into a saucepan over medium high. Bring to a boil. Reduce the heat to medium and simmer until the sauce reduces by half and is syrupy, about 10–15 minutes. Keep warm.

In a bowl whisk together the flour, cornmeal, baking powder, salt, ground cinnamon, and nutmeg.

Heat a griddle coated with vegetable oil spray to medium high. In a bowl whisk together the sweet potato with the milk. Whisk in the canola oil, brown sugar, and vanilla. Separate the eggs into yolks and whites. Stir the 2 yolks into the batter, reserving the whites. Stir in the pecans.

Use an electric mixer to beat the egg whites to form soft peaks. Fold the egg whites into the batter. Ladle the batter onto the grill. Cook until the top is bubbled, about 3–4 minutes. Turn the pancakes and cook until golden, about 3 minutes more. Repeat until all of the batter has been used.

To serve, place the pancakes on a serving platter. Serve the warm sauce on the side.

On Shopping Day: Prepare the sauce and store in an airtight container in the refrigerator for up to 1 week. Warm before serving.

Makes 4 to 6 servings
Prep Time: 30 minutes
Cook Time: 10 minutes

For the sauce

- 6 cups fresh raspberries (or thawed frozen raspberries)
- 1 cup natural sugar
- 2 cups water
- 1 teaspoon pure vanilla extract
- Juice of 2 medium oranges (about 2/3 cup)
- Zest of 1/2 medium orange (about 1 tablespoon)

For the pancakes

- 1 medium sweet potato, peeled and diced into 1-inch cubes (about 1 cup)
- 1 cup unbleached all-purpose flour
- 1/4 cup yellow cornmeal
- 2 teaspoons baking powder
- 1/2 teaspoon salt
- 1/2 teaspoon ground cinnamon
- 1/4 teaspoon ground nutmeg
- 1 cup reduced-fat milk
- 3 tablespoons brown sugar
- 1 tablespoon canola oil
- 1/2 teaspoon pure vanilla extract
- 2 large eggs, separated
- 1/4 cup chopped pecans

FRUIT 'N SOY MILK DRINKS

Getting more soy into your diet is beneficial. Blending soy milk with frozen fruit is a no-brainer for a quick morning starter or afternoon pick-me-up.

Makes 4 servings
Prep Time: 2 minutes

- 2 cups chilled soy milk
- 2 cups frozen berries (strawberries, blueberries, or raspberries)
- 1 large banana, frozen
- 1 tablespoon honey
- 1/2 teaspoon vanilla

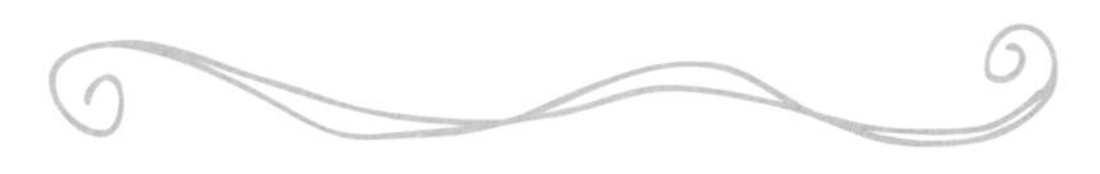

You can add ICE to make this a lighter, frothier beverage.

* * *

Freeze FRESH FRUIT so that you have it on hand for all your quickie drinks.

* * *

Try substituting MAPLE SYRUP for honey for another taste twist. Use 2 tablespoons maple syrup in place of 1 tablespoon honey.

Place the soy milk, fruit, honey, and vanilla into a blender. Pulse to blend.

To serve, pour into 4 glasses.

BREAKFAST TOMATOES WITH SMOKED SALMON

Here's a much *lighter version of bagels with cream cheese and lox. I know there's no bagel in the recipe—that's the "light" part. If you must have a grainy texture to go with the dish, try a triangle of toasted whole grain bread, like pumpernickel or rye.*

Makes 4 servings
Prep Time: 10 minutes

- 2 large beefsteak tomatoes cut into 1/2-inch-thick slices (about 8 slices)
- Salt and freshly ground pepper
- 1 tablespoon capers, drained
- 1/4 small cucumber, seeded and diced (about 1/4 cup)
- 4 ounces smoked salmon
- 1 large egg, hardboiled, peeled, and diced
- 1 tablespoon diced red onion
- Reduced-fat sour cream (for garnish)
- Fresh dill sprigs (for garnish)

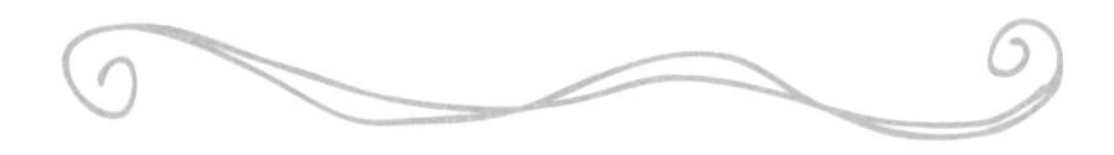

You can substitute leftover SALMON for this dish or experiment with smoked trout or white fish for a different taste.

To serve, lay the tomato slices onto a serving platter. Season with salt and pepper. Top each with capers, diced cucumbers, and smoked salmon. Top with diced hardboiled egg and diced red onion. Garnish with a dollop of sour cream and a sprig of fresh dill.

OPEN-FACED EGGPLANT, TOMATO, AND CHEDDAR GRILLED CHEESE

Upgrade your after-school childhood favorite grilled cheese sandwich with different toppings and gargantuan proportions of flavor! Remember to enjoy this satisfying dish several hours *before cashing in your chips tonight.*

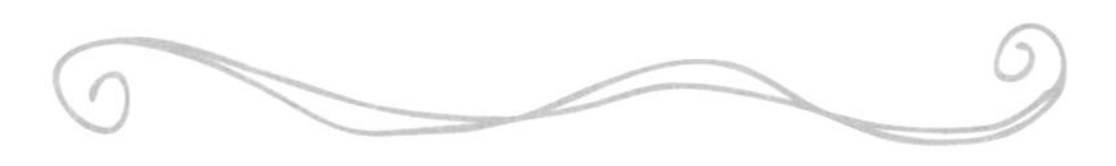

Please, *please* let this recipe be an excuse to use up everything in your refrigerator. Broil bell peppers, hot peppers, red onion, fennel, portabella mushrooms—you name it. ALL CHEESES will work, but my favorites are Swiss, Gorgonzola, and smoked Gouda.

* * *

Use HIGH-QUALITY cheese for your grilled cheese sandwich. Explore artisanal varieties and steer past those resealable bags; it makes all the difference in this dish!

Makes 4 to 6 servings
Prep Time: 10 minutes
Cook Time: 10 minutes

- 3 large heirloom tomatoes, sliced into ½-inch-thick rounds (about 8 slices)
- 1 medium eggplant, sliced into ¼-inch-thick rounds (about 8 slices)
- 3 tablespoons olive oil, divided use
- 1 teaspoon dried oregano leaves
- Salt and freshly ground pepper
- 1 tablespoon unsalted butter
- 1 16-ounce whole grain loaf (French bread–style), cut in half horizontally
- 1 ounce finely grated Parmesan cheese
- 6 ounces grated sharp Cheddar cheese (about 1½ cups)

Preheat the broiler. Lay the tomato and eggplant slices onto a rimmed baking sheet. Drizzle with 1 tablespoon olive oil and season with dried oregano, salt, and pepper. Broil until the vegetables are soft, about 5 minutes. Set aside.

Melt the remaining 2 tablespoons olive oil with 1 tablespoon butter. Remove some of the soft insides of the loaves. Brush each half with the melted butter mixture. Sprinkle with Parmesan cheese. Place onto a baking sheet and broil until just golden, about 1–2 minutes. Remove from the oven.

Lay the eggplant slices into each of the bread loaves. Arrange the tomato slices over top. Generously mound the Cheddar cheese on top of the vegetables. Place the sandwiches back into the oven and broil until the cheese melts, about 2–4 minutes.

To serve, slice the loaves into 3 pieces each and serve warm.

ROAST TURKEY BREAST

With Cornbread-Cranberry Dressing and Madeira Mushroom Gravy

Remember that old wives' tale about sleeping well after eating turkey? Well, it's true! Enjoy this version, blending fresh herbs with cranberries, cornbread, and wonderfully flavored gravy.

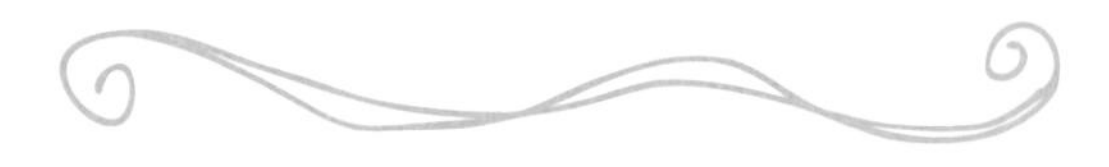

Ask your butcher to remove the bones from a whole turkey breast so that it DRAPES OVER the stuffing in the baking dish. This makes for a beautiful presentation and less cooking time.

Preheat the oven to 375 degrees. Cook the bacon in a skillet over medium-high heat until crisp, about 4–5 minutes. Add the onions and cook until soft, about 4–5 minutes more. Remove from the heat. Put the skillet aside to prepare the gravy.

Place the cornbread and whole grain bread into a large bowl. Pour in the chicken broth and toss to combine. Stir in the bacon/onion mixture, egg, cranberries, sage, thyme, and poultry seasoning. Season with salt and pepper. If the stuffing is too dry, add additional chicken stock. Place the stuffing into a baking dish that has been coated with vegetable oil spray.

Lay the turkey breast over the stuffing, skin-side up. Place whole sage leaves under the skin. Season with salt and pepper, and brush with 2 tablespoons olive oil. Roast until the skin is golden and the internal temperature of the turkey reaches 165 degrees, about 1½ hours.

Heat 1 tablespoon olive oil in the skillet over medium-high heat. Add the mushrooms and cook until soft, about 4–5 minutes. Add the Madeira wine and cook until most of the wine has disappeared, about 5 minutes more. Pour in the chicken broth and bring to a boil. Reduce the heat and simmer. Stir in the thyme and orange zest and season with salt and pepper. Stir in the cornstarch mixture and cook until the gravy has thickened.

To serve, let the turkey rest for at least 15 minutes. Cut down through the center of the turkey breast. Remove one half and cut into 1-inch slices. Serve with a spoonful of dressing and a drizzle of hot gravy.

Makes 8 servings with leftovers
Prep Time: 45 minutes
Cook Time: 1½ hours

For the stuffing

- 6 ounces thick bacon, about 4–6 strips, diced
- 2 medium yellow onions, peeled and diced into ½-inch squares (about 2 cups)
- 8 ounces cornbread, crumbled (about 4 cups)
- 4 ounces whole grain crusty bread cut into 1-inch cubes (about 2 cups)
- 1 cup homemade chicken stock or low-sodium chicken broth
- 1 large egg, slightly beaten
- 1 cup dried cranberries
- 2 tablespoons chopped fresh sage
- 2 tablespoons chopped fresh thyme
- 1 teaspoon dried poultry seasoning

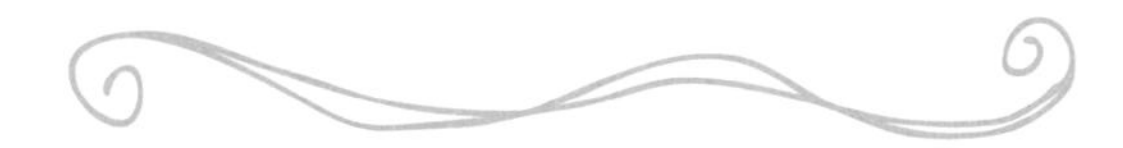

Salt and freshly ground pepper

For the turkey

- 1 5-pound boneless turkey breast
- Fresh sage leaves
- 2 tablespoons olive oil

For the gravy

- 1 tablespoon olive oil
- 8 ounces button mushrooms, sliced (about 2 cups)
- 1/2 cup Madeira wine
- 2 cups homemade chicken stock or low-sodium chicken broth
- 2 tablespoons chopped fresh thyme leaves
- Zest of 1/2 medium orange (about 1 tablespoon)
- 2 teaspoons cornstarch mixed with 3 tablespoons cold water

RACK OF LAMB

With Spinach and Breadcrumb Topping

Here's a novel idea: let's put the stuffing on the outside of the meat. This fast family favorite is also perfect for company.

Makes 4 to 6 servings
Prep Time: 10 minutes
Cook Time: 25 minutes

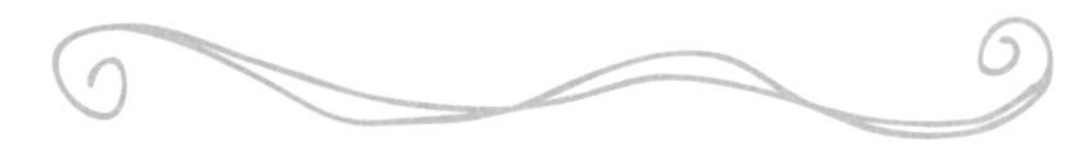

Use a MEAT THERMOMETER to determine doneness. Rare is 125 degrees. Remember the meat will continue to cook (about 5 to 10 degrees more) after you remove it from the oven.

- 6 ounces fresh spinach leaves, washed, dried, and chopped (about 1 cup)
- 1 cup fresh parsley leaves
- 4 medium garlic cloves, minced (about 2 teaspoons)
- 1 cup fresh breadcrumbs
- 1 teaspoon Dijon mustard
- Zest of 2 medium lemons (about 2 tablespoons)
- 3 tablespoons olive oil
- 2 1½-pound racks of lamb (ask the butcher to "french" the bones, which means to trim away the fat)
- Salt and freshly ground pepper

Preheat the oven to 450 degrees. Place the spinach, parsley, garlic, breadcrumbs, mustard, and lemon zest into the bowl of a food processor. Pulse to combine. With the machine running, add the olive oil.

Place the lamb onto a rack sitting in a rimmed baking sheet. Cover the bones with aluminum foil to prevent scorching. Season with salt and pepper. Cover the meat with the spinach mixture. Roast until the topping is golden and the lamb is rare, about 20–25 minutes.

To serve, cut the lamb into chops and place onto a serving platter.

Grilled Coconut Curry Shrimp

With Soba Noodles

Here's a shrimp dish that is easy and fun! The combination of crunchy veggies, coconut, and curry provides an abundance of flavor.

Makes 4 servings
Prep Time: 10 minutes, plus marinating
Cook Time: 4 to 5 minutes

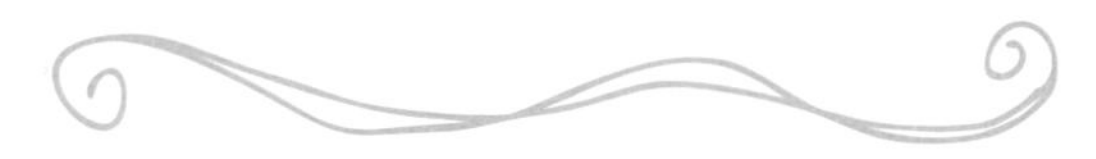

FISH SAUCE is a salty Asian condiment prepared by fermenting fish. Use it as you would soy sauce.

* * *

SOBA NOODLES are found in the Asian section of your grocery store. They are made from buckwheat and wheat flour and are cooked in boiling water.

* * *

If you are not using METAL SKEWERS, soak wooden skewers in cold water for at least 30 minutes.

For the shrimp

- $1\frac{1}{2}$ pounds large uncooked shrimp, peeled and deveined (about 24)
- $\frac{1}{4}$ cup light coconut milk
- $\frac{1}{2}$ medium red bell pepper, seeded and finely diced (about $\frac{1}{3}$ cup)
- 2 tablespoons fish sauce
- Juice of 1 medium lime (about 1 tablespoon)
- 1 tablespoon chopped fresh cilantro
- 1 teaspoon honey
- 1 teaspoon curry powder

For the dish

- 2 large green bell peppers, seeded and cut into 1-inch pieces
- 12 cherry tomatoes
- 4 cups cooked soba noodles
- 2 tablespoons sweetened coconut, toasted (for garnish)

Place the shrimp into a baking dish. Whisk together the coconut milk, red bell pepper, fish sauce, lime juice, cilantro, honey, and curry powder. Pour this mixture over the shrimp. Toss to coat. Cover the dish and marinate in the refrigerator for 20 minutes.

Heat a grill pan over medium-high heat. Thread the shrimp onto skewers, alternating with green bell peppers and tomatoes. Grill the skewers, turning often, until the shrimp are just cooked and the veggies are softened, about 4–5 minutes.

To serve, place the noodles into a shallow pasta bowl. Top with the shrimp-and-veggie skewers. Garnish with toasted coconut.

STUFFED CHICKEN BREASTS

With Mushrooms, Thyme, and Fontina Cheese

A gooey, rich mushroom and cheese filling turns everyday chicken breasts into an extraordinary dish.

Makes 4 servings
Prep Time: 10 minutes
Cook Time: 25 minutes

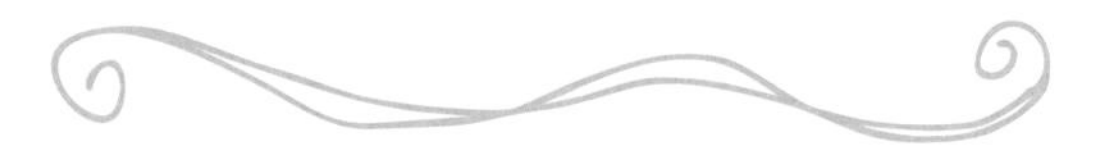

To cut a pocket in the chicken, use a SHARP KNIFE to horizontally cut a one-inch slice through the thickest part of the breast. Continue cutting to create a pocket, being careful not to cut all the way through.

- 1 tablespoon butter
- 2 tablespoons olive oil, divided use
- 8 ounces button mushrooms, finely chopped (about 2 cups)
- Salt and freshly ground pepper
- 2 tablespoons chopped fresh thyme leaves
- 4 large (6- to 8-ounce) skinless, boneless chicken breast halves
- 2 ounces fontina cheese, cut into four pieces

In a skillet heat the butter and 1 tablespoon olive oil over medium-high heat until bubbling. Add the mushrooms. Season with salt and pepper. Cook until the mushrooms are softened and the liquid disappears, about 5 minutes. Stir in the fresh thyme. Cool to room temperature.

Preheat the oven to 350 degrees. Cut a pocket into each breast half. Place 1 piece of cheese into each pocket. Fill each breast with the mushroom mixture. Seal the breast with toothpicks. Season the outside of the chicken with salt and pepper. Lay each breast into a baking dish. Drizzle with the remaining tablespoon olive oil. Bake until the chicken is cooked through and the cheese is melted, about 20–25 minutes.

To serve place the chicken breasts on a serving platter.

On Shopping Day: Prepare and stuff the chicken breasts for baking. Store in an airtight container in the refrigerator for up to 2 days.

BROILED TILAPIA FILLETS

With Arugula Aioli Sauce

Tilapia is a fresh, flakey fish that easily takes on the flavors of your favorite garnishes. This original "fast food" fish is a great dish to serve during a busy workweek. It's also light enough to make sleepy time preparation a breeze.

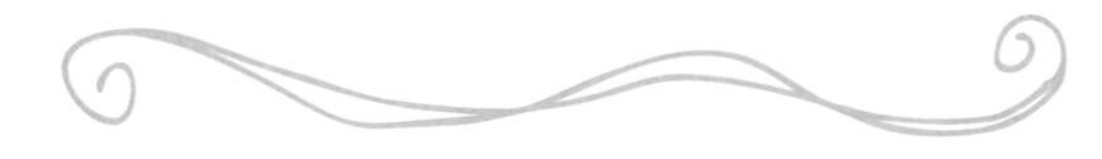

ARUGULA is a peppery green that has a very distinctive taste. Remove the stems before placing into the food processor.

Makes 4 servings
Prep Time: 10 minutes
Cook Time: 10 minutes

For the aioli sauce

- 2 cups arugula leaves, washed and dried
- Juice of 1/2 medium lemon (about 1 tablespoon)
- 1 teaspoon prepared horseradish
- 3/4 cup reduced-fat mayonnaise
- Salt and freshly ground pepper

For the tilapia

- 4 6-ounce tilapia fillets
- 3 tablespoons olive oil
- 1 tablespoon Worcestershire sauce
- Juice of 1/2 medium lemon (about 1 tablespoon)
- 1 teaspoon garlic powder
- 1 teaspoon ground paprika
- Diced tomatoes (for garnish)
- Thinly sliced green onions (for garnish)
- Fresh parsley leaves (for garnish)

Place the arugula leaves into the bowl of a food processor. Add the lemon juice and horseradish. Pulse to combine. Add the mayonnaise and season with salt and pepper. Pulse to form a sauce. Chill until ready to serve.

Preheat the oven to broil. Place the fish into a shallow baking dish. In a medium bowl whisk together the olive oil, Worcestershire sauce, lemon juice, garlic powder, and paprika. Pour this mixture over the fish. Turn the fish to coat both sides. Remove the fish from the marinade and place onto a rimmed baking sheet that has been coated with vegetable oil spray. Place under the broiler (about 4 inches from the heat). Broil, turning once until the fish is cooked though and flakey, about 4–5 minutes per side.

To serve, place the fish onto a plate. Top with a dollop of aioli sauce and garnish with diced tomatoes, green onions, and fresh parsley.

On Shopping Day: Prepare the aioli sauce, store in an airtight container in the refrigerator for up to 3 days.

CRAB CAKE PO' BOYS

Nothing says "take it easy" like down-home food, and these sandwiches have what it takes to make the list. They're huge—so eat early in the afternoon, followed by a game of Frisbee before you chill out for the evening.

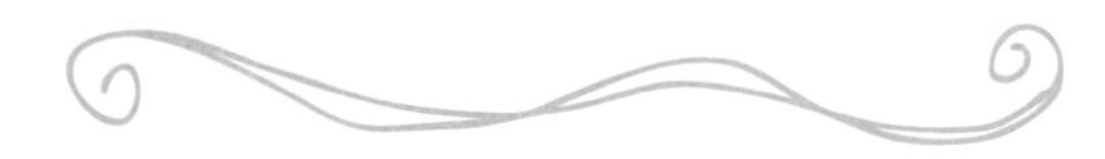

Toast the BUNS (cut-side down) in a skillet over medium-high heat or cut-side up on a baking sheet in a 400-degree oven.

Mix together 1 cup mayonnaise, pickle relish, white onion, and lemon juice. Season with salt and pepper. Chill the tartar sauce until ready to serve.

Heat the olive oil in a skillet over medium heat. Add the red onion, celery, and red and yellow bell peppers to the pan. Stir in the parsley, capers, hot pepper sauce, Worcestershire sauce, and Old Bay seasoning. Season with salt and pepper. Cook until the vegetables are soft, about 15 minutes. Cool to room temperature.

Place the vegetable mixture into a large bowl. Add the crabmeat, breadcrumbs, mayonnaise, mustard, and eggs. Use your hands to gently combine the mixture. Place into the refrigerator for 20 minutes. Form the crab mixture into golf ball–size balls. Flatten to form patties. Place the patties onto a parchment-lined baking sheet.

Heat 2 tablespoons olive oil in a skillet over medium-high heat. Cook the patties (in batches using additional oil as needed) until golden, about 3–5 minutes. Turn and cook on the second side until golden, about 3 minutes more. Transfer to a rack set over paper towels to drain.

To serve, brush the inside of each bun with melted butter and toast until golden. Place 3 crab cakes on each bun. Top with tartar sauce, lettuce, and tomatoes. Place the top half of the bun onto the sandwich.

On Shopping Day: Prepare the tartar sauce and store in an airtight container in the refrigerator for up to 5 days.

Makes 4 servings
Prep Time: 20 minutes, plus chilling time
Cook Time: 25 minutes

For the tartar sauce

- 1 cup reduced-fat mayonnaise
- 1 tablespoon sweet pickle relish
- 1 tablespoon finely diced white onion
- Juice of 1 medium lemon (about 2 tablespoons)
- Salt and freshly ground pepper

For the crab cakes

- 2 tablespoons olive oil
- 1 small red onion, peeled and finely diced (about 3/4 cup)
- 6 medium celery ribs, finely diced (about 1 1/2 cup)
- 1 medium red bell pepper, seeded and finely diced (about 1/2 cup)
- 1 medium yellow bell pepper, seeded and finely diced (about 1/2 cup)
- 1/4 cup chopped fresh parsley

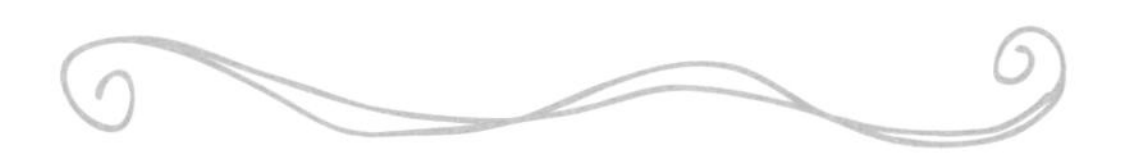

- 1 tablespoon capers, drained
- 4–6 drops hot pepper sauce
- 1 teaspoon Worcestershire sauce
- 1½ teaspoons Old Bay seasoning
- ½ pound lump crabmeat, drained and picked to remove shells
- ½ cup fresh breadcrumbs
- ½ cup reduced-fat mayonnaise
- 2 teaspoons Dijon mustard
- 2 large eggs, lightly beaten
- 2–4 tablespoons olive oil

For the sandwiches

- 4 whole grain hoagie buns
- 1 tablespoon butter, melted
- Shredded lettuce
- Sliced tomatoes

LINGUINI

With Mussels and Snow Peas

Pasta is the star in this dish. Choose a type of noodle that works with your gorgeous lifestyle plan and toss with good stuff—like fresh veggies and shellfish. Mmmmmm—so good!

Makes 4 servings
Prep Time: 5 minutes
Cook Time: 10 minutes

- 6 ounces dried whole wheat linguini
- 2 ounces thick bacon, diced (about 2–3 strips)
- 1 large shallot, minced (about 1 tablespoon)
- 1/2 teaspoon crushed red pepper flakes
- 1/2 cup white wine
- 1/2 cup chicken broth
- 1/4 cup half and half
- Zest of 1 medium lemon (about 1 tablespoon)
- 1 pound mussels, scrubbed, beards removed
- 8 ounces sugar snap peas, trimmed (about 1 cup)
- 1 tablespoon chopped fresh parsley
- Salt and freshly ground pepper
- Parmesan cheese (for garnish)

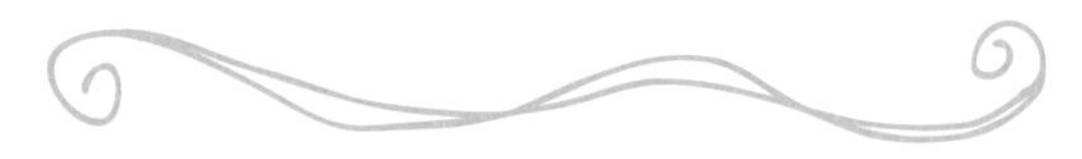

Frozen MUSSELS are a great choice for this dish. Thaw in the refrigerator and discard any that open before cooking.

Bring a pot of water to a boil. Generously salt the water. Cook the linguini according to the directions on the package.

Meanwhile, cook the bacon in a large skillet (with lid) over medium-high heat until crisp, about 3–4 minutes. Use a slotted spoon to transfer to paper toweling. Drain off the bacon drippings. Add the shallot and crushed pepper to the skillet. Cook until soft, about 2 minutes. Stir in the wine. Pour in the chicken broth and half and half. Simmer until the sauce reduces and slightly thickens, about 5 minutes. Stir in the lemon zest and mussels. Cover and cook until the mussels open, about 3–4 minutes. Stir in the snap peas and parsley. Add the bacon back to the skillet. Season with salt and pepper.

Drain the pasta and add to the skillet. Toss well.

To serve, transfer to a shallow pasta dish. Garnish with Parmesan cheese shavings and additional fresh pepper.

PECAN-CRUSTED CHICKEN FINGERS

With Apricot Mustard Dipping Sauce

Way better than those drive-thru chicken bites, these are marinated in buttermilk, baked, and then dipped in a yummy sauce. This recipe offers a vastly superior alternative to fast food!

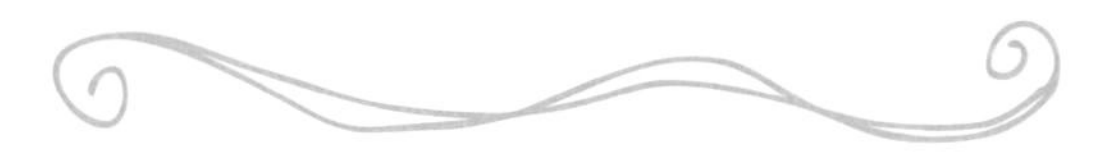

CORN FLAKE CRUMBS can be found in the baking section at your grocery store. A good substitute is prepared breadcrumbs. Remember to take a look at the labels on the package to check out the best product for you.

On Shopping Day: Prepare the sauce and store in an airtight container in the refrigerator for up to 3 days.

Makes 4 servings
Prep Time: 20 minutes, plus marinating time
Cook Time: 20 minutes

For the chicken

- 2 pounds skinless, boneless chicken breasts, cut into 1 1/2-inch-wide strips
- 1/2 cup reduced-fat buttermilk
- 1 teaspoon chili powder
- 1/2 teaspoon ground cinnamon
- 3/4 cup pecan pieces
- 3/4 cup corn flake crumbs
- Salt and freshly ground pepper

For the sauce

- 1/3 cup reduced-fat sour cream
- 1/3 cup Dijon mustard
- 3 tablespoons apricot preserves

Place the chicken into a baking dish. Whisk together the buttermilk, chili powder, and ground cinnamon. Pour this mixture over the chicken. Toss to coat. Cover and place in the refrigerator for at least 30 minutes or up to 4 hours.

Preheat the oven to 350 degrees. Place the pecan pieces into the bowl of a food processor. Pulse to form crumbs. Add the corn flake crumbs and pulse to combine. Pour this mixture into a shallow dish.

Remove the chicken from the buttermilk marinade. Dredge into the pecan crumb mixture. Place onto a rimmed baking sheet that has been coated with vegetable oil spray. Continue until all of the strips have been coated. Season with salt and pepper. Bake until the coating is golden and the chicken is cooked through, about 15–20 minutes.

Mix together the reduced-fat sour cream, mustard, and apricot preserves.

To serve, place the chicken fingers onto a platter. Spoon the sauce into a bowl on the side for dipping.

Sautéed Cauliflower and Spinach Fettuccini Casserole

This is a wonderful casserole—not to mention an interesting twist on everyday fettuccini. Sautéing the cauliflower adds a real depth of flavor. Use this dish as a hearty side or midweek meal.

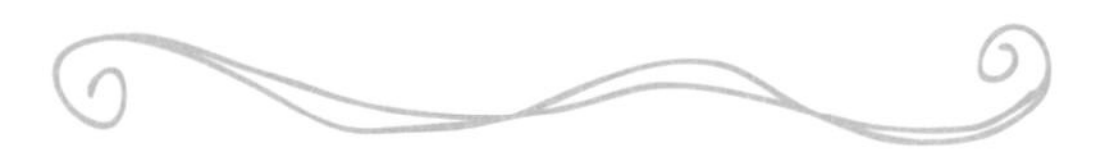

Gruyère is a variety of Swiss cheese that melts easily and has a RICH, SMOKY FLAVOR. It's often used in fondue. You can find Gruyère in the gourmet cheese section of the dairy department.

Heat 2 tablespoons olive oil in a large skillet over medium-high heat. Add the cauliflower. Cook until the cauliflower is golden and browned on the edges, about 8 minutes. Season with salt and pepper. Toss in the thyme leaves. Pour in the chicken stock. Simmer until the cauliflower is crisp-tender and the liquid is reduced, about 5 minutes.

Preheat the oven to 350 degrees. Coat a 9 x 13-inch baking dish with vegetable oil spray. Cut the cheese into cubes and place into the bowl of a food processor. Pour in the half and half. Pulse to combine into a paste.

Cut the fettuccini into 4-inch lengths (roughly into thirds). Cook the fettuccini in salted boiling water until just tender. Drain and return to the pot. Stir in the cheese mixture. Stir in the cauliflower with the liquid. Transfer to the prepared baking dish. Top with fresh breadcrumbs. Drizzle the top of the casserole with olive oil. Bake until the top is golden brown and the casserole is bubbling, about 25–30 minutes.

To serve, let the casserole rest for 5 minutes. Cut into squares and garnish with sprigs of thyme.

Makes 6 side servings
Prep Time: 20 minutes
Cook Time: 25 to 30 minutes

For the cauliflower

- 2 tablespoons olive oil
- 1 small head cauliflower (1 1/2–2 pounds), trimmed and cut into 1-inch florets
- Salt and freshly ground pepper
- 2 tablespoons chopped fresh thyme leaves
- 1 cup homemade chicken stock or low-sodium chicken broth

For the casserole

- 12 ounces Gruyère cheese
- 1 cup fat-free half and half
- 9 ounces fresh spinach fettuccini
- 1/2 cup homemade whole wheat breadcrumbs
- 1 tablespoon olive oil
- Fresh thyme sprigs (for garnish)

BROCCOLI MASH

Better than mashed potatoes, this combination of puréed broccoli and mashed Yukon gold potatoes makes for a side dish that's bound to be a new family favorite. Serve with Roast Turkey Breast (page 310) for a cozy, relaxing meal.

Makes 4 servings
Prep Time: 10 minutes
Cook Time: 30 minutes

- 1 large Yukon Gold potato, peeled and cut into 1-inch chunks (about 2 cups)
- 1 bunch broccoli, stems peeled and sliced, cut into florets (about 2 cups)
- 1/2 cup homemade chicken stock or low-sodium chicken broth
- 4 ounces reduced-fat cream cheese
- 2 tablespoons olive oil
- 1/2 teaspoon ground nutmeg
- Salt and freshly ground pepper

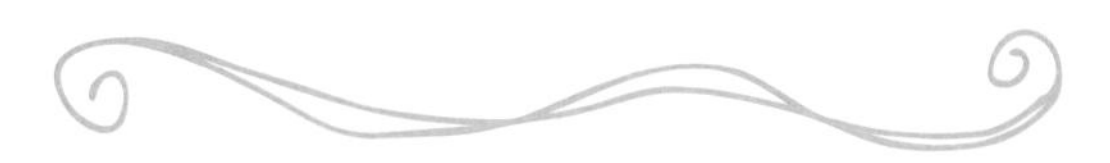

STEAMING the veggies (in place of boiling) reduces the moisture, resulting in a richer tasting dish. You can steam in a microwave or in a pot using a steamer basket.

Steam the potato until fork-tender, about 15 minutes. Transfer to a bowl and mash with the back of a fork or potato masher.

Steam the broccoli until fork-tender, about 15 minutes. Transfer to the bowl of a food processor. Add the chicken stock, cream cheese, olive oil, and nutmeg. Pulse to combine.

Stir the puréed broccoli into the mashed potato. Season with salt and pepper.

To serve, spoon the mashed broccoli and potato into a serving bowl.

STUFFED ZUCCHINI, YELLOW SQUASH, AND EGGPLANT

Sun-dried tomatoes, fresh parsley, and breadcrumbs top sliced veggies in this flavorful side dish.

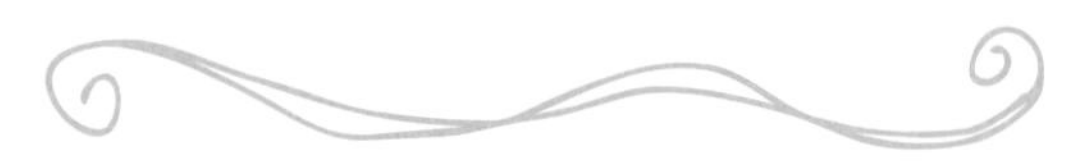

Use the ingredients that you keep in your pantry to top your favorite fresh veggies. Chopped GREEN or BLACK OLIVES or marinated artichoke hearts are fun to experiment with.

Makes 6 servings
Prep Time: 10 minutes
Cook Time: 20 minutes

- 3 baby zucchini, cut in half lengthwise
- 3 small yellow squash, cut in half lengthwise
- 1 medium eggplant cut into 6 (3/4-inch) slices
- 1/2 cup minced oil-packed sun-dried tomatoes, drained with oil reserved
- Salt and freshly ground pepper
- 4 green onions, thinly sliced (about 1/4 cup)
- 1/4 cup seasoned breadcrumbs
- 1/4 cup finely grated Parmesan cheese
- 2 tablespoons chopped fresh parsley

Preheat the oven to 350 degrees. Spray a baking dish with vegetable oil spray. Place the zucchini, squash, and eggplant, cut-side up, into the prepared dish. Use a sharp knife to cut slits into the flesh of the veggies, but not all the way through. Drizzle the veggies with the reserved oil from the sun-dried tomatoes. Season with salt and pepper.

Place the sun-dried tomatoes, onions, breadcrumbs, Parmesan cheese, and parsley into the bowl of a food processor. Pulse to mince. Spread this mixture over the veggies. Bake until the veggies are soft, about 20–25 minutes.

To serve, use a spatula to transfer the veggies to a serving platter. Spoon any extra topping and juice left in the dish over top.

GRILLED RATATOUILLE SALAD

With Tomato Basil Vinaigrette

This dish transforms all the flavors of traditional ratatouille into a gorgeous salad just perfect for an elegant party or simple night at home.

Makes 6 large servings, plus extras for roasted veggie soup later in the week
Prep Time: 20 minutes
Cook Time: 10 minutes

Roasting the veggies is a time-saving alternative for this dish. ROAST the veggies on a rimmed baking sheet at 350 degrees until just beginning to soften, about 15 to 20 minutes.
You can grill the veggies several hours in advance and serve the dish at ROOM TEMPERATURE.
You might as well roast A LOT of veggies. Whatever is not used can be turned into everything from roasted vegetable soup to roasted vegetable dip to roasted veggies on pasta. This recipe is a perfect example of how to cook once and eat a bunch!

For the veggies

- 8 large plum tomatoes, cut in half
- 3 medium carrots (with tops), sliced lengthwise in half
- 2 medium eggplants, cut lengthwise into 1/2-inch thick slices
- 2 medium zucchini, cut lengthwise into 1/2-inch slices
- 2 large yellow squash, cut lengthwise into 1/2-inch slices
- 1 large red bell peppers, stemmed, seeded, and cut into quarters
- 1 yellow bell peppers, stemmed, seeded, and cut into quarters
- 1 large red onions, peeled and cut into 1/2-inch slices
- 1/4 cup olive oil
- 1 teaspoon dried oregano leaves
- Salt and freshly ground pepper

For the vinaigrette

- 3 tablespoons chopped fresh basil , plus garnish
- 2 tablespoons white wine vinegar
- 3 medium garlic cloves
- 1 tablespoon tomato paste
- 1/2 cup olive oil

For the salad

- 6 cups mixed salad greens (romaine, red leaf, Bibb, green leaf, etc.)

Heat an outdoor grill (or grill pan) over medium-high heat. Place all of the veggies onto a rimmed baking sheet. Coat with ¼ cup olive oil. Season with oregano, salt, and freshly ground pepper. Grill the veggies, turning once, until well-marked and beginning to soften, about 6 to 8 minutes (the tomatoes will cook more quickly). Transfer to another baking sheet.

Place the basil, vinegar, garlic, and tomato paste into a food processor. Pulse to combine. With the blade running, slowly add the ½ cup olive oil. Season with salt and pepper.

To serve, place the lettuce onto a serving platter. Drizzle with 2 tablespoons of the dressing. Toss to coat. Arrange the grilled vegetables on top. Drizzle the remaining dressing over top. Garnish with additional fresh basil leaves.

On Shopping Day: Prepare the vinaigrette. Store in an airtight container in the refrigerator for up to 3 days.

SIMMERING BLUEBERRIES

With Cinnamon Dumplings

Think old-fashioned, warm blueberry pie "al a mode," and you know the flavors found in this dish. We focus on the berries in this dessert but don't leave out any of the yum!

Makes 8 servings
Prep Time: 10 minutes
Cook Time: 30 minutes

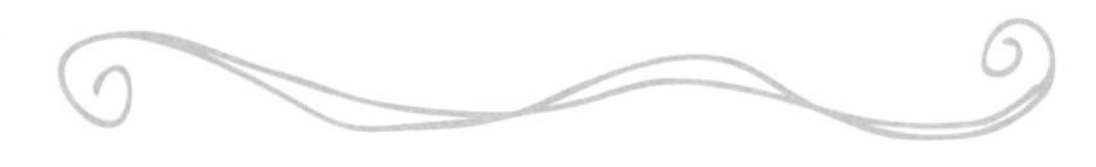

You can substitute FROZEN blueberries or use the freshest berries you can find. If your fruit is very sweet, you can reduce the amount of sugar.

* * *

For LIGHT AND FLUFFY dumplings, make sure you do not overwork the dough. Just bring it together with your hands. It's okay if it is lumpy.

For the berries

- 1 quart fresh blueberries (or thawed frozen berries)
- 1 cup natural sugar
- 2 cups water

For the dumplings

- 1 cup unbleached all-purpose flour
- 2 teaspoons baking powder
- 1/2 teaspoon ground cinnamon
- 1/4 teaspoon salt
- 3/4 cup reduced-fat milk
- Vanilla-flavored reduced-fat frozen yogurt

Place the berries into a deep skillet with lid. Stir in the sugar and pour in the water. Bring to a boil. Reduce the heat to medium and simmer until the berries are soft and syrupy, about 15 minutes.

In a medium bowl stir together the flour, baking powder, ground cinnamon, salt, and milk to form a wet dough. Drop the dough by rounded tablespoonfuls over the simmering berries. Reduce the heat to medium low, cover the skillet, and slowly simmer until the dumplings are set and dry, about 15–20 minutes. Don't peek or you will ruin the dumplings!

To serve, spoon the berries into bowls and top with a dumpling. Top with a spoonful of frozen yogurt.

BUTTERSCOTCH BLONDIES

If you're craving something a little sweet, reach for one of these satisfying cookie bars!

Makes 12 servings
Prep Time: 10 minutes
Cook Time: 35 minutes

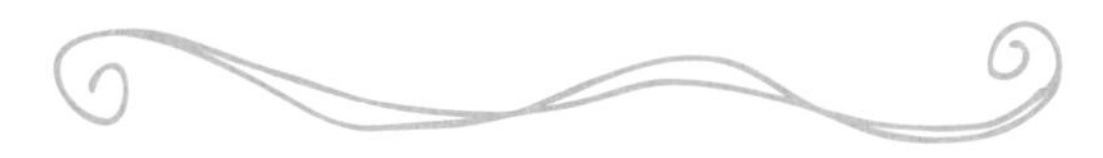

Vary this simple dessert by substituting with any of the FUN chips that are in the marketplace. Try peanut butter chips, double chocolate chips, and even mint chips.

- 1 cup unbleached all-purpose flour
- 1/4 teaspoon baking powder
- 1/8 teaspoon baking soda
- 1/8 teaspoon salt
- 1/2 cup unsalted butter, room temperature (1 stick)
- 1 cup brown sugar
- 1 large egg
- 1 teaspoon pure vanilla extract
- 1/2 cup chopped walnuts
- 1 cup butterscotch chips

Preheat the oven to 350 degrees. In a bowl mix together the flour, baking powder, baking soda, and salt.

In a separate bowl use an electric mixer to combine the butter and brown sugar until fluffy. Stir in the egg. Stir in the vanilla. Stir in the flour mixture, walnuts, and chips.

Spread the batter into a 11 x 9 x 2-inch baking dish that has been coated with vegetable oil spray. Bake until golden, about 30 to 35 minutes. Remove and cool completely.

To serve, cut into 12 bars.

On Shopping Day: Prepare this dessert on shopping day for quick treats during the workweek. Store in an airtight container for up to 4 days.

SIMPLE CHOCOLATE MOUSSE

With Graham Cracker Crumbles

This light, chocolaty snack quells your craving for something sweet yet allows you to nod off without a care in the world. Remember not to partake too late into the evening.

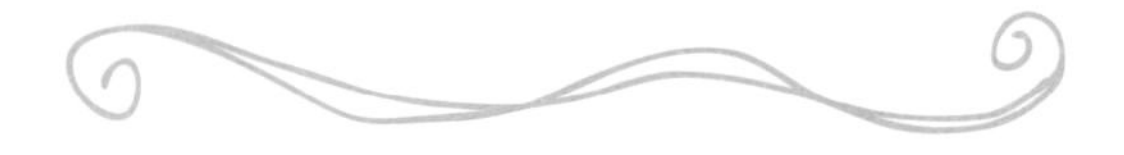

The BETTER the chocolate, the better this dessert will be.

Makes 4 servings
Prep Time: 15 minutes, plus at least 6 hours chilling time

- 6 ounces semisweet chocolate
- 3 large egg whites
- 1/4 cup natural sugar
- 4 graham crackers

Melt the chocolate in a microwave oven or in a double boiler over simmering water. Pour into a large bowl and cool to room temperature.

Use an electric mixer to beat the egg whites to form soft peaks. Add the sugar and whip until just stiff. Pour the egg whites over the chocolate. Use a spatula to gently fold together. Pour into 4 ramekins or champagne glasses. Place in the refrigerator and chill for at least 6 hours or overnight.

To serve, crumble the graham crackers over the mousse and serve.

On Shopping Day: Prepare the mousse and chill for use the next day.

ALMOND COOKIES TWO WAYS

These cookies can be prepared in advance and baked in a hurry—just in time to satisfy your desire for a crisp, nutty treat.

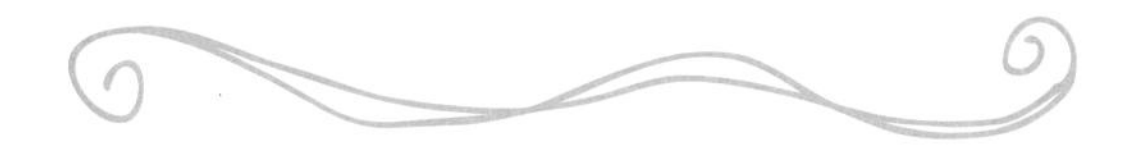

Feel free to use this recipe as a guideline. Choose your favorite CHOPPED NUTS or substitute with dried fruit. In the end, it's still a home-baked cookie!

* * *

Our recipe tester had fun STACKING the cookies. Increase the cooking time if you choose to go this way—and I suggest that you do!

In a medium bowl whisk together the flour, baking powder, and salt in a bowl. In a large bowl use an electric mixer to combine the butter and brown sugar until fluffy. Stir in the almond extract. Stir in the eggs until just combined. Stir in the flour mixture and almonds. Divide the dough in half. Place half of the dough back in the mixing bowl. Stir in the melted chocolate and granulated sugar and beat until the chocolate is mixed throughout.

Form both the plain and chocolate dough into separate logs, about 2 inches in diameter. Wrap each in plastic wrap and place into the refrigerator. Chill for at least 1 hour.

Preheat the oven to 350 degrees. Slice the non-chocolate log into ½-inch slices. Lay each cookie onto a rimmed baking sheet lined with parchment paper or a Silpat liner. Repeat with the chocolate log. Bake for 8–10 minutes. Transfer cookies to a wire rack and cool completely.

On Shopping Day: Prepare the cookie dough and store in plastic in the refrigerator for up to 1 week or freeze for up to 1 month.

Makes about 2½ dozen cookies
Prep Time: 20 minutes
Cook Time: 20 minutes

- 3 cups all-purpose flour
- 1 teaspoon baking powder
- ¼ teaspoon salt
- 1 cup butter, room temperature (2 sticks)
- 2½ cups brown sugar
- 1 teaspoon almond extract
- 2 large eggs
- 1 cup chopped almonds
- 2 ounces unsweetened chocolate, melted but still warm
- 2 tablespoons granulated sugar

Gorgeous Home Spa Secrets . . . for Sweet Dreams

It's estimated that the average person logs more than 50,000 hours of dreams in his or her lifetime. That translates into six solid years—that's a *huge* chunk of our lives spent chasing sweet dreams! This section honors some of the rituals enjoyed before we hit the hay and explores a world beyond aromatherapy that includes Swedish massage and crafting your own "sleep tight" items.

Brought to You by Lavender

In ancient Rome, lavender was the essential bath perfume; it derives its name from the Latin word *lavare*, "to wash." Fast forward to today, where any Sleeping Beauty worth her bath salt recognizes lavender as the star ingredient for creating the ultimate home spa experience. Sweet, pretty lavender has been used for centuries to treat bee stings and repel insects, offering up the fragrant bonus of suppressing mood swings, anxiety, and headaches. The calming effect of lavender has made it a favorite natural sleep aid—even babies enjoy lavender-scented bath soap—so get ready to sleep like one yourself with these pampering lavender secrets.

Tea Cozy

Here's a cozy evening beverage to accompany that book of poetry you're curled up with tonight. You'll be "going gentle into that good night" by whipping up the following ingredients: 1 teaspoon dried lavender, 2 tablespoons fresh mint leaves, and 1 cup boiling water. In a teapot or saucepan combine the lavender and mint (either loose or using a tea infuser). Pour boiling water over the mixture and steep 5 minutes. Take out the infuser or use a strainer to remove the leaves. Pour into a mug and sip.

A Sachet by Any Other Name

Because we're concerned here with rest and relaxation, this sachet is naturally chock-full of lavender. To get started, gather lavender stems, leaves, or buds (it's totally up to you), lavender essential oil, a clean handkerchief, 2 needles (1 large, 1 small), thread, and a ¼"-wide ribbon that color-complements the handkerchief. Fold your handkerchief in half, and then fold it in half again. Sew three sides together using needle and thread. Open one side of the handkerchief and stuff it, generously, with lavender plant pieces and/or buds. Sprinkle the pieces with no more than 10 drops lavender essential oil. Thread your large needle with the ¼" ribbon and loosely thread to keep the plant materials inside your homemade sachet. Tie the whole thing off with a knot and, violà, you're done!

The Ultimate Elixir

If you're finding sleep elusive, a hot bath may be just the answer you're looking for to conquer restlessness at last. Heat brings down the body's internal temperature, allowing for natural relaxation that's so much better than what you're likely to find in a sedative capsule. The best fragrances to mingle with your tub water are ginger, rosemary, Bergamot, Balsam Fir, and, of course, lavender. Add a touch of olive and canola oils and beeswax as a special favor to your skin. A last-minute addition of cinnamon and eucalyptus only benefits this soothing elixir of fragrances. Set aside a potpourri of these guys for inclusion in a homemade pillow.

Get a Swedish Massage

The most likely place to fall asleep when you really hadn't planned on it is the massage table. Because its firm but gentle pressure improves circulation, eases muscle aches and tension, and promotes flexibility and creates relaxation, the Swedish massage is a surefire way to get on the fast track to Dream Land. It's the best known type of massage and comes highly recommended for first-timers. Its techniques can be mimicked by the amateur more easily than shiatsu, tantric, or deep tissue massages—better yet, the Swedish massage is the most affordable thing at the spa. An hour's worth of its characteristic long gliding strokes, kneading of individual muscle groups, friction, hacking, tapping, and vibration run between $75 to $100 per hour at most American salons and resorts. Swedish massage was developed by Swedish physiologist Henri Peter Ling at the University of Stockholm in 1812 and serves as the foundation for all other types of Western massage, including sports, deep tissue, and aromatherapy. The therapist generally uses massage oil to facilitate making long, smooth strokes over the body. The customer is covered by a sheet, a technique called "draping." One part of the body is uncovered, massaged, and then covered up again before moving on to another part; so if modesty is what is keeping you from having your kinks worked out by a professional, Swedish massage may be just the thing for you. Tell 'em Mr. Sandman sent ya!

Sleepy Time Mantra

What about that old wives' tale about counting sheep as a way to dose off? *Yes*, Virginia, it will work. Counting sheep, like other mantras, is one way to clear your mind of those things that are keeping you awake at night. Try counting backward the next time you can't get to sleep. What you'll find is that your mind will keep drifting back to that unpleasant telephone call or conversation with your coworker. Get back on track and start again. It might take a time or two, but eventually you will concentrate so hard on counting backward that the other scenarios will take a backseat. Here's another idea. The next time you have trouble drifting off, try my "toes to nose" technique. Start with your feet. Think about relaxing every toe. Concentrate on the soles of your feet—are they loose and unwound? Work up to your ankles, attempting to relax every muscle. Continue upward to your calves, legs, lower back, and finally up to your shoulders, head, and nose. You will have consciously relaxed your body and cleared your mind at the same time.

Your Best Night-Time Pal

Remember your favorite stuffed animal, the one you couldn't go to bed without? You wrapped your arms around that stuffed teddy (or giraffe or tiger) and clung to him all night long. Heaven forbid he was missing at bedtime—the whole family would be on safari hunting him down. While he's probably been abandoned on your path to adulthood, no doubt you've found other comforts. You can help a child sleep a little easier by making sure he has a nighttime companion. Consider volunteering with the Marine Toys for Tots Foundation at www.ToysforTots.org. They round up stuffed animals and toys for distribution to needy children. You'll be amazed at how well you can sleep at night when you've spent the day making others feel good.

CHAPTER 14

living without stress

"There is more to life than increasing its speed." —*Mahatma Gandhi*

If your daily stressors are so insignificant that sleep, diet, relationships, and "all your glorious parts" go unaffected, count yourself lucky and keep up the good work. But for most of us, stress is a daily part of our lives. Why should you worry about stress? Because it just may be killing you softly. Stress ages you by increasing the production of free radicals in your body. Some studies propose that stress releases fat into the bloodstream and raises cholesterol levels. Acute stress can constrict the arteries in your heart by demanding more pump action. And if that's not bad enough, unchecked stress is no friend of the digestive tract either. When the going gets tough, the tough get heartburn! In light of all this potential damage, there is an antidote. Balancing everyday stress with much-needed comfort is a milestone on the path toward gorgeous. Here we talk about the role of *honest to goodness* comfort food, unveiling (God bless us!) sinful snacks that really ain't so sinful! We'll dish on what the Dalai Lama himself drinks to calm down and what exercises Mary Ellen does to get back up. The end result is a massive slow down in the production of stress hormones.

Ask Dr. Moon

The doctor is in to answer your questions.

In the cave dweller's day, physical changes in response to stress were critical to survival. In the modern world, the stress response is still invaluable (it raises our performance level when we need to "step up to the plate" or otherwise excel in life), but too much stress, just like too much of anything, poses a threat to our overall health and well-being. Long-term stress compromises all parts of the body's stress apparatus (i.e., brain, lungs, heart vessels, and muscles), and over time these can become chronically over-activated. Read on and discover how learning not to sweat "the small stuff" helps prevent *big* health problems.

Q: Can stress *really* cause medical problems?

A: It's hard to assign 100 percent of the blame on stress for creating an illness. Certainly stress compromises immunity and increases susceptibility, but genetic disposition, and sometimes environmental factors, have to be there first. Still, we have a lot to learn from the old saying "Your body is your mind, your mind is your body." There has never been a truer statement—otherwise, psychosomatic illnesses and the placebo effect would not have influence over our health. Unfortunately, living stress free has a lot to do with our environment—a separate entity that can't always be predicted, much less controlled. Just a few items from the *long* list of diseases exacerbated by stress are: irritable bowel syndrome (IBS), chronic fatigue syndrome (CFS), fibromyalgia, acid reflux, skin conditions (eczema, especially), heart disease, backaches, and headaches.

Q: Does stress discriminate by gender?

A: Well . . . sort of. Women are particularly susceptible to stress and the disorders it feeds on. From puberty through menopause, hormone fluctuations are a primary stress trigger and play a role in delaying menses or causing abnormal bleeding. Disorders like these aggravate the presence (or potential presence) of endometriosis or fibroids. And yet the world has its share of frazzled men too. Extreme heat, cold, altitude, and other environmental factors, like toxins, create stress for everybody.

Q: Is it true that stress can impact the health of your heart?

A: "Stress and Your Heart" is likely to be a symposium title in the medical community, which, when it talks about stress and heart disease, is mostly referring to *physical* (*not* emotional) stress. If your heart is normal, cardiovascular exercise can only do it good. However, if you're straining diseased heart muscle with extreme physical activity that your coronary arteries can't accommodate, you're running a risk of heart attack. Unlike the scientific evidence that proves the above, the idea that emotional stress can contribute to a coronary event is not as definitively agreed upon. The fight/flight response does call on the organs in the human body to work much, much harder than they do in a relaxed state and will increase heart rate, constrict arteries, and pose a slight risk of blocking coronary blood flow. There is, too, research claiming that mental stress can alter heart rhythm and create arrhythmias in people with existing disturbances. In women, chronic stress may reduce estrogen levels, which are important for cardiac health. Some studies submit that mental stress poses the same threat of angina as physical stress. Fight or flight stress may be countered by the relaxation response, a physical state of deep rest that changes the physical and emotional responses to stress, according to Dr. Herbert Benson of Harvard. These debates aside, *one thing is for certain*: victims of too much stress are *far* more likely to smoke, drink, and/or eat poorly—*incontestable* catalysts in heart disease!

Q: Does stress cause gastrointestinal problems and ultimately lead to weight gain?

A: Stress hormones slow the release of stomach acid and the emptying of the stomach into the small intestine—factors that can cause diarrhea and the tummy ache that goes along with it. Beyond its role in causing peptic ulcers, chronic and prolonged stress can produce high levels of cortisol in your body, a hormone that increases your appetite and can cause weight gain.

Q: Is there a flip side of the coin, like a relationship between stress and weight *loss*?

A: The key to fast, permanent weight loss is in keeping your stress hormone production low. In recent scientific studies, researchers have heavily investigated the world of "comfort foods" and have focused on the temporary effects of lessening stress. Scientists have found that those people who eventually give in to temptation and allow all their stresses to be eased with these indulgent comfort foods find an effective way to lower escalating stress levels in everyday life. The University of California at San Francisco has been diligently conducting experiments to uncover the truth about "sinful snacking." The researchers at UCSF have said that by eating that random package of Twinkies, a plateful of nachos and cheese, or that 500-calorie Frappuccino®, one is likely to alleviate stressful symptoms. In a recent excerpt from an article in the *New York Times*, scientists reported that comfort foods like chocolate cake and ice cream literally blunt the body's response to chronic stress, and because that cuts back on cortisol production, it doesn't inhibit weight loss—*provided* the sinful snacking is balanced with an overall healthy diet.

Q: Are there other studies that illustrate the effects of stress reduction and good health?

A: Yes. A 2001 study reported that treatments that reduce psychological distress after a heart attack appeared to improve long-term outlook. Some evidence exists that stress management programs may reduce the risk of heart events by up to 75 percent in people with heart disease. One study found that stress management programs are more effective than exercise in reducing heart risks (although exercise is also protective). The study also reported that stress management techniques, along with methods for coping with anger, were associated with lower blood pressure.

Q: What nutrients found in what foods are associated with stress reduction?

A: L-theanine reduces stress and anxiety without the tranquilizing effects found in many other calming supplements. This amino acid comes from tea leaves (*Camellia sinensis*) which contain L-theanine in tiny amounts. The Japanese use an extract form of L-theanine to relax. They consume foods or chewing gums that have L-theanine added, which are marketed to calm jitters. They may take it as a dietary supplement. The good news for us is that this supplement has recently begun to appear in American stores!

Q: What else should I know about L-theanine?

A: You should know that it's a great thing but not the entire solution to feeling calm. It needs a little help. As it is digested in your small intestine, L-theanine stimulates your brain's production of alpha waves, which make you feel relaxed and alert, but not drowsy. L-theanine also helps you stay relaxed by stimulating your body to produce other calming amino acids, such as dopamine, GABA, and tryptophan. It happens that serotonin, an invaluable hormonal component to healthy sleep, is synthesized from the amino acid tryptophan. Thus to produce serotonin, you need tryptophan. Tryptophan is an amino acid that can be obtained *by consumption only*. Therefore, you want to consider eating foods containing sufficient levels of tryptophan to help replenish your serotonin levels each day. The bottom line is that while the Japanese may be on to something with their use of L-theanine, that alone isn't enough to produce the healthy and enduring calm our bodies need.

Q: Is there a recommendation for keeping us calm and making us healthier?

A: Leading a healthy lifestyle that includes a healthy diet is an essential companion to any stress-reduction program. General health and stress resistance can be enhanced by a regular exercise; a diet rich in a variety of whole grains, vegetables, and fruits; and the avoidance of excessive alcohol, caffeine, and tobacco.

Jorj's Comfort Food Glam Kitchen

Unhealthy cuisine (an oxymoron!) carries with it a vicious cycle of more body fat, lethargy, malnourishment, and in the end, *stress*. By contrast, a healthful meal plan filled with appealing omega-rich goodies and complex carbohydrates offers dual incentives for the reluctant chef.

The first incentive is that cooking is cathartic because it allows you to improvise, experiment, and express yourself. Cooking can be as flavorful as it is creative, featuring the likes of brown butter and pineapple-infused cilantro. Once you start discussing the menu with folks at home, collecting ingredients, and slicing and dicing with ambient music playing and a little red wine at your side, you're more likely to make culinary history with twists and turns on ordinary meatloaf. The second incentive is that gourmet cooking provides a catharsis in its preparation. It's easy to lose yourself in bringing fruit compote to fruition—so much so, you'll momentarily forget about daily stresses and actually find that you enjoy yourself in the kitchen.

Dressing up the Classics

The recipes in this chapter *beg* to be chopped, sliced, stirred, and whisked because they feature creamy sauces and full-bodied marinades. Don't despair over how to stock your pantry for this; we're ready to dish on what the more specific ingredients of healthy, cathartic cooking are so that your pantry is perpetually armed and gorgeous. It may surprise you to find, after a colorful and aromatic hour spent as a gourmet chef, that you're a tad reluctant to shift focus from whisking and puréeing to everyday grievances. Start your savory adventure by dressing up American classics, like PBJ and BLT sandwiches. Use easy gourmet flourishes that make mealtime an occasion rather than just another meal.

Slow Down and Smell the Sausage

For whatever the reason—maybe it's because you want to save money, monitor portion control, or just talk during mealtime without your server interrupting—opting to stay in and cook adds up to be more pro than con. It gets your mind off everything *but good food*, burns a fair amount of calories, and does so all for the greater gustatory good of family and friends. Here's a gorgeous fact: by the time you've lugged in groceries for a week's worth of good eats and washed and readied the dishes, not to mention engaged in standard food prep activity, you've burned more than 100 calories!

A Pantry Up to Par

If you're going to take the time to make something special, creative augmentation is in order: add **thyme**, **sage**, **parsley**, **curry**, **cilantro**, **tarragon**, **wasabi**, **ginger**, **citrus**, **avocados**, and **hoisin** sauce to your salsas and marinades. When you're making something like . . . let's say, stew . . . identify those adjectives you want to describe the dish's flavor. If you want a hearty beef stew, *really think* about what's filling, robust, and darn good. It's now more than ever that last-minute additions are welcome. For full-bodied flavor, your pantry should never be without **red wine**, **bay leaves**, **garlic cloves**, **tomato sauce**, and **tomato paste**. You never know when any of the entrees in your repertoire of comfort foods will need fattening up (to go a little further), so the following should be available at a moments' notice: **Yukon potatoes**, **Worcestershire** sauce, **rice wine vinegar**, **brown rice**, **cooking sherry**, and **chicken stock**.

Toppings that Heal

A pinch or dash of the following can make a dish unique, fresh-tasting and even award-winning—better yet, these spices contain age-fighting, healthy antioxidants, so stock your spice rack! Get **black** and **red pepper**, **chili peppers**, **cloves**, and **marjoram**. While you're at it, sweeten things with **honey**; it too, contains antioxidants (better yet, honey may offer some protection against heart disease). Spreading honey on ham or turkey helps prolong the freshness of the meat, protects it from bad aftertastes, and guards against harmful byproducts of meat oxidation that may increase the risk of heart disease. A teaspoon a day of local, unpastuerized honey may offer the additional benefit of lessening symptoms in the allergy suffer. The range of antioxidants in honey is comparable to that of **bananas**, **oranges**, and **strawberries**—funny how all these aforementioned foods taste great with a little honey! **Turmeric**, **licorice**, **rosemary**, and **oregano** should round out your free radical-fighting arsenal.

Groceries to Soothe the Savage Beast

What could be more synonymous with chillin' out than benefiting from a good night's sleep? Tryptophan is found in the following foods: **cottage cheese**, **brown rice**, **avocados**, **bananas**, **walnuts**, **tomatoes**, and **soy protein**. **Turkey** is probably the highest serotonin-containing food. Eat turkey to help increase serotonin levels. Rest easy and dream guilt-free in remembering that, at least in the interest of healthy eating, it's (actually) preferable to be unrefined! Choose *all* **unrefined**, **unbleached** foods. Don't scorch your olive, sesame, and canola cooking oils by overheating the pan. Remember to store oils properly so as to retain all their healthy goodness. Reduce your intake of red meats and make all your cookies at home—*just say no* to the prepackaged, preservative-packed, and massed-produced foods.

Quit Stressing Over Your Food

Which is the best diet to follow to prevent weight gain? Is it low-fat, low-carb, low-calorie, fat-free, sugar-free, low-sodium, no red meat, all-veggie, or what? Modern science and conventional wisdom suggest that a balanced diet that includes fresh, nonprocessed ingredients is a precursor for good health. So why do we stress over all of the "diet plans" that are marketed to us instead of utilizing common sense?

Researchers are looking into just what makes us fat. Some early results suggest that stressing over food just may lead to weight gain.

If you are an empty-calorie eater, your chance of getting fat over the next ten years is a stunning 41 percent. You are in trouble, baby. You need to change your eating patterns. You must replace simple sugars and carbs with complex ones such as whole grain bread. Remember, these simple sugars and carbs can cause a spike in blood sugar that disappears as soon as it peaks, making you reach for more and more sugar. Now that *is* something to stress about! Instead, you need to slash fat, replacing bad fat with good. Also, make sure some of your sweets have nutrients. Try dried fruit such as mangoes and raisins or spoon out a fruity sorbet in place of a candy bar.

Or perhaps you are a "light" eater—a person who eats little or no fat and a reduced-calorie diet—who happily counts calories in a daily journal. Often, you are so pleased with your ability to control your calorie intake that you splurge on bad foods as a reward. A diet that is very low in calories can slow down your metabolism, putting your risk for weight gain over the next ten years at 30 percent. In order to change this forecast, the light eater (with the splurging habits) needs to stop thinking of food as either "good" or "bad." Instead, balance your food choices and realize that eating is good for you—go ahead and live a little!

If you are a high-fat eater, you have a 28 percent risk of becoming overweight over the next 10 years, which isn't far from the other eaters, but your high saturated fat intake is bad news for your heart. You have probably been influenced by the low-carb diet craze and think a cheeseburger topped with bacon and cheese sans bun is the way to go. The good news is that you keep your calories somewhat under control, but you need to replace saturated fats with unsaturated fats.

A heart-healthy eater has only a 24 percent chance of becoming overweight. If your habits include a meal plan that is heavy on veggies and includes low-fat dairy, you probably cover most of your vitamin and mineral needs. You are able to say "no thanks" to most desserts because just a bite of something special does the trick. Your Achilles heel is that because your diet is so darn good, you are often tempted to overlook exercise as an important component in your gorgeous lifestyle plan.

Now here are the most interesting findings. If you are a moderate eater, you have the lowest percentage—at only a 22 percent chance—of becoming fat over the next ten years. Why? Because, you balance indulgence and common sense. Adults on a moderate-fat diet lost significantly more weight than adults on a lower-fat diet, a study at Brigham and Women's Hospital and Harvard Medical School in Boston shows. So relax and enjoy your meals. There is no need to stress over good food when you learn to balance.

Start Your Day

Main Plates

On the Side

Snacks & Sweets

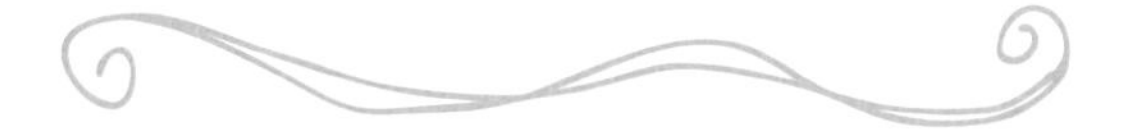

OPEN-FACED BLT BREAKFAST SANDWICH

I am a sucker for breakfast. Just the thought of bacon frying on a grill sets my mouth watering. I could eat eggs every day—but I don't. When I do, I make sure that I pair the egg with good stuff and try to cut done on fattening side dishes.

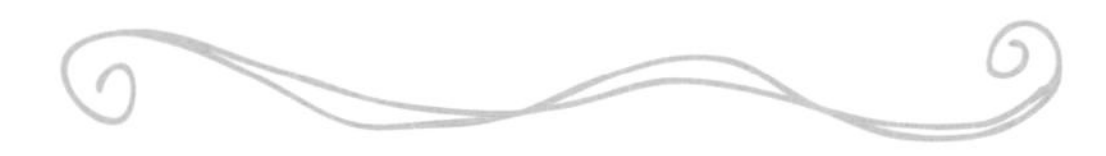

By choosing Canadian bacon and reduced-fat cheese in this dish, you create a LEANER alternative to the traditional fried-egg breakfast sandwich.

* * *

You can make this sandwich at home in under 10 minutes, which is probably less time than you would spend in a fast food drive-through lane during rush hour. Now this is STRESS REDUCING!

Makes 2 servings
Prep Time: 10 minutes
Cook Time: 6 to 8 minutes

- 2 large eggs
- 1 whole wheat muffin, split into 2 halves
- 2 slices Canadian bacon
- 2 romaine lettuce leaves
- 2 slices tomato
- 2 1-ounce slices reduced-fat white Cheddar cheese
- 1 tablespoon chopped fresh basil

Preheat the oven to 400 degrees.

Coat a small pan with vegetable oil spray. Cook the eggs in the pan over medium heat for 3–4 minutes until the yolks are just beginning to set up.

Toast the muffin halves and place onto a baking sheet. Heat the Canadian bacon in a skillet (or microwave oven) to warm through.

Place a lettuce leaf on top of each muffin half. Top with a Canadian bacon slice and a slice of tomato. Top the tomato with an egg and top the egg with a slice of cheese.

Cook the sandwiches in the oven until the cheese melts and the eggs are firm, about 3 to 4 minutes.

To serve, place an open-faced sandwich onto a plate and sprinkle with fresh basil.

HAM AND CHEESE SCRAMBLE

This hearty breakfast will get your weekend off to a great start. Follow up with a brisk morning walk with your favorite walking buddy. Bet you win the race!

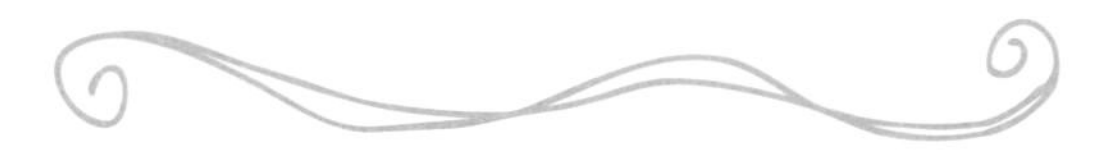

EGG SUBSTITUTE is an appropriate ingredient switch in this recipe.

Makes 2 servings
Prep Time: 5 minutes
Cook Time: 8 to 10 minutes

- 4 large eggs
- 1 tablespoon chopped chives, plus garnish
- 1 tablespoon unsalted butter
- 2 ounces Gruyère cheese, shredded (about 1/2 cup)
- 1/4 pound deli-baked Tavern ham, cut into 1/4-inch dice
- Salt and freshly ground pepper

Whisk the egg and chives in a bowl. Heat the butter in a skillet over medium heat. Pour in the eggs. Gently stir the eggs with a wooden spoon until they just begin to set, about 4 minutes. Reduce the heat to medium. Arrange the cheese and ham on top of the eggs. Season with salt and pepper. Continue cooking until the eggs are set and the cheese has melted, about 4–6 minutes more.

To serve, divide the eggs onto two plates. Garnish with lengths of fresh chives.

BACON AND ASPARAGUS QUICHE

Creamy, rich, filled with crisp bacon and savory asparagus, this dish is as good for breakfast as it is for lunch and dinner. In fact, it is an all-day stress-free treat for your mouth.

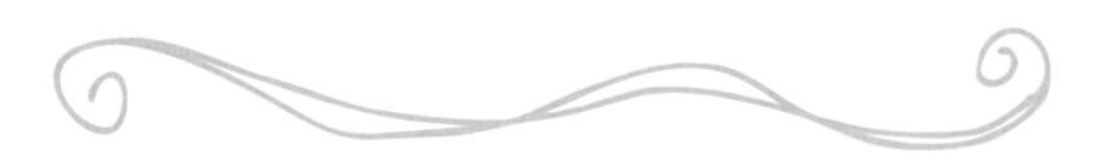

Don't stress out over the ingredients in this recipe. Fill your quiche with any VEGGIE AND HERB you have on hand. Don't have bacon? No sweat—try slivered ham or slices of prosciutto.

Preheat the oven to 400 degrees. Place the flour, salt and chilled butter in the bowl of a food processor. Pulse until the mixture resembles course crumbs. Add 1 tablespoon ice water and pulse again. Continue adding water and pulsing until the mixture forms a ball. Transfer the dough to a lightly floured surface and shape into a flat disc. Refrigerate for at least 1 hour or overnight.

Remove the dough from the refrigerator. Transfer to a lightly floured surface. Roll out the dough to ¼-inch thickness. Place the dough into a pie plate. Refrigerate for 30 minutes more. Place a sheet of parchment paper over the shell. Fill the tart shell with pie weights. Bake for 12–15 minutes or until lightly golden. Remove from the oven. Remove the pie weights and foil. Bake for another 3–5 minutes. Remove from the oven and brush with beaten egg white.

Cook the bacon in a skillet over medium-high heat until just beginning to crisp. Remove with a slotted spoon and drain on paper towels.

Blanch the asparagus in salted, boiling water until crisp-tender, about 3–5 minutes. Submerge into an ice water bath to stop the cooking process. Drain well.

Heat the half and half in a sauce pan over medium-high heat, just to the boiling point. Remove from heat and cool slightly.

Beat the eggs with nutmeg, salt and pepper. Slowly whisk the egg mixture into the warm milk. Stir in the chives.

Sprinkle the cheese and bacon into the bottom of the prebaked tart shell. Pour the custard into the tart shell. Reduce the oven temperature to 375 degrees. Bake the quiche until the top is golden brown and the center is set, about for 35–40 minutes. Cool to room temperature.

To serve, cut the quiche into wedges and serve with a green salad.

On Shopping Day: Prebake the tart shell so that it is ready when you are. Store in plastic wrap in the refrigerator for up to 5 days or in the freezer for up to 1 month.

Makes 8 servings
Prep Time: 20 minutes, plus chilling crust
Cook Time: 35 minutes

For the crust

- 1¼ cups unbleached all-purpose flour
- ¼ teaspoon salt
- ½ cup butter, chilled and cut into pieces (1 stick)
- 3–4 tablespoons ice water
- 1 large egg white, beaten

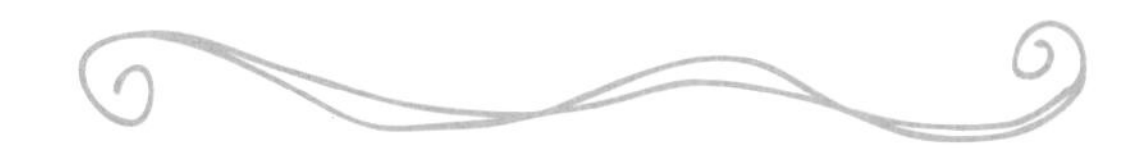

For the filling

- 1/4 pound bacon, cut into 1-inch pieces
- 8 ounces fresh thin asparagus spears, ends trimmed, cut diagonally into 1/2-inch lengths (about 1 cup)
- 2 cups reduced-fat half and half
- 3 large eggs
- 1/8 teaspoon nutmeg
- Salt and freshly ground pepper
- 1 tablespoon chopped fresh chives
- 4 ounces grated Gruyère cheese

GRILLED PEANUT BUTTER AND BANANA SANDWICHES

With Just A Touch of Honey

Move over, Elvis. Let everyone have a bite of this delicious combo, and we'll be groovin' all day long.

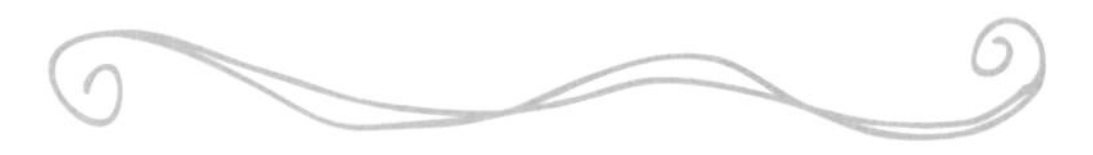

Peanut butter is high in calories and in fat, but it is also full of PROTEIN and contains the GOOD FAT that may be needed to reduce the risk of coronary disease. As with all things wonderful, a little goes along way. That's why a half a sandwich in the morning is a perfect grab-and-go breakfast.

Makes 4 servings
Prep Time: 5 minutes
Cook Time: 5 minutes

- 4 slices whole grain bread
- 2 tablespoons peanut butter
- 2 ripe bananas, peeled and sliced into $^1/_2$-inch rounds
- 2 tablespoons honey

Spread the peanut butter on 2 slices of bread. Top with bananas and drizzle with honey. Place the remaining bread on top.

Heat a nonstick skillet coated with vegetable spray over medium heat. Place the sandwiches into the skillet. Cover with a lid. Heat until golden on one side, about 3–4 minutes. Remove the lid, turn and cook until golden on the second side, about 3–4 minutes more.

To serve, cut each sandwich diagonally into halves.

OLD-FASHIONED TURKEYLOAF

With Hidden Mushrooms

Eating healthful is all about updating comfort food. This recipe reminds me of my grandmother's meatloaf, but I sneak in a few veggies, which keeps the loaf moist and the kids guessing!

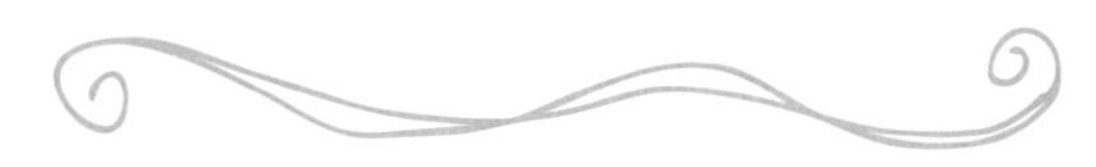

I use ground turkey in this recipe because it is a good source of LEAN PROTEIN. You can easily substitute ground beef or a combination of ground beef, pork, and veal.

* * *

Diced SQUASH OR EGGPLANT works well in this recipe in place of (or in addition to) mushrooms of any variety.

Heat the olive oil in a skillet over medium-high heat. Chop the mushrooms into very small pieces. Place them into the skillet. Season with salt, pepper, and rosemary. Cook, stirring with a spatula, until the mushrooms are golden brown, about 3–4 minutes. Remove the pan from the heat and cool to room temperature.

Preheat the oven to 350 degrees. Place the ground turkey into a large bowl. Add the breadcrumbs, shallots, egg, and cooked mushrooms. Pour in half of the marinara sauce. Season with salt and pepper. Use your hands to combine the mixture. Shape into a loaf and place into a large loaf pan. Place the loaf pan onto a baking sheet with lip.

Cook for 30–40 minutes. Pour the remaining marinara sauce over the top and continue cooking for 10 minutes more. Cook the turkeyloaf until a thermometer inserted into the center of the loaf reads 175 degrees.

To serve, allow the loaf to rest for 15 minutes. Cut into ½-inch slices and arrange on a platter. Use extras later in the week for turkeyloaf sandwiches.

Makes 4 servings (reserving half of the turkey loaf for another use)
Prep Time: 10 minutes
Cook Time: 40 to 50 minutes

For the sneaky veggies

- 1 tablespoon olive oil
- 8 ounces button mushrooms, sliced (about 2 cups)
- Salt and freshly ground pepper
- 1 teaspoon dried rosemary

For the loaf

- 2 pounds ground turkey
- 4 slices whole wheat bread, processed into crumbs
- 2 large shallots, minced (about 2 tablespoons)
- 1 large egg
- 1 cup marinara sauce, divided use

SHRIMP SCAMPI

With Angel Hair Pasta

This version of shrimp scampi replaces lots of butter with tongue tangy spices. A couple of bites of this spirited dish will take your mind away from anything stressful.

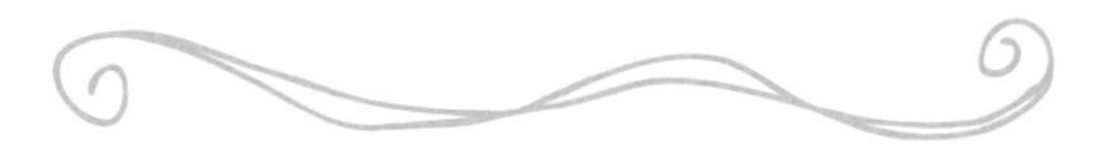

Purchase FROZEN SHRIMP and THAW under running water. It's one of those shortcuts that just makes life a little easier.

Makes 4 servings
Prep Time: 10 minutes
Cook Time: 10 minutes

- 6 ounces whole wheat angel hair pasta
- 3 tablespoons olive oil, divided use
- 1 pound large uncooked fresh shrimp, peeled and deveined (about 20)
- Salt and freshly ground pepper
- 1 tablespoon butter
- 1 2-ounce tin anchovies, packed in oil, drained
- 4 medium garlic cloves, thinly sliced (about 2 teaspoons)
- 1 bunch (6–8) green onions, chopped (about 1/2 cup)
- 1 pint ripe cherry tomatoes or mixed baby tomatoes
- Juice of 1/2 medium lemon (about 1 tablespoon)
- 2 tablespoons chopped fresh parsley
- 1 tablespoon chopped fresh basil
- Zest of 1/2 medium lemon (about 2 teaspoons)
- Parmesan cheese shavings (for garnish)

Bring a pot of water to boil. Generously season with salt. Cook the pasta according to the directions on the package.

Meanwhile, heat 1 tablespoon olive oil in a skillet over medium high heat. Season the shrimp with salt and pepper. Cook the shrimp in the oil until just pink, about 4 minutes. Use a slotted spoon to transfer the shrimp to a platter.

Add the remaining 2 tablespoons olive oil and butter to the skillet. Reduce the heat to medium. Add the anchovies and garlic and cook until the garlic is soft and the anchovies disappear, about 2 minutes. Add the shrimp back to the skillet. Stir in the green onions, tomatoes, and lemon juice and simmer.

Drain the pasta. Toss the pasta with the shrimp in the skillet to coat. Toss in the parsley, basil, and lemon zest.

To serve, place the pasta into a serving dish. Garnish with Parmesan cheese shavings and additional ground pepper.

GINGER-MARINATED TUNA STEAKS

With Dill-Lime Butter

Seasoned butter melting over flavorful, rare tuna is a mouth-watering temptation. The best news is that it is ready in just minutes.

Makes 4 servings
Prep Time: 20 minutes, plus marinating time
Cook Time: 6 minutes

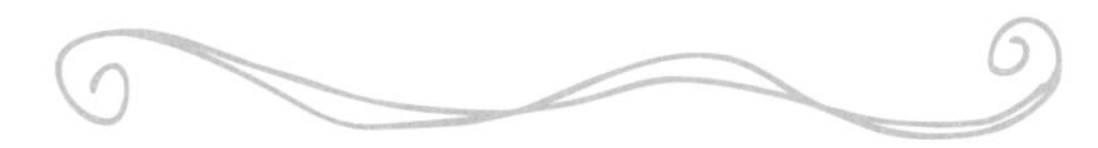

To prevent the tuna from sticking to your GRILL PAN, coat it with vegetable oil spray before heating. Watch for smoking and remember to turn on the exhaust fan!

For the butter

- 4 tablespoons unsalted butter, room temperature (1/2 stick)
- 1 tablespoon chopped fresh dill
- Juice of 1 medium lime (about 1 tablespoon)
- Zest of 1 medium lime (about 1 tablespoon)

For the tuna

- 1/3 cup rice wine vinegar
- 3 tablespoons honey
- 2 tablespoons soy sauce
- 1 tablespoon chili sauce
- 1 tablespoon sesame oil
- 4 green onions, thinly sliced (about 1/4 cup)
- 4 medium garlic cloves, minced (about 2 teaspoons)
- 1 1-inch piece ginger, peeled and grated (about 1 tablespoon)
- 4 6- to 8-ounce tuna steaks
- Salt and freshly ground pepper

Place the butter into the bowl of a food processor. Add the dill, lime juice, and lime zest. Pulse to combine. Transfer to parchment paper. Form into a log, wrap, and refrigerate for at least 30 minutes.

In a small bowl whisk together the rice wine vinegar, honey, soy sauce, chili sauce, and sesame oil. Stir in the green onions, garlic, and ginger. Place the tuna steaks into a shallow baking dish. Pour the marinade over top and turn the steaks to coat. Cover and chill for at least 20 minutes and up to 1 hour.

Heat a grill pan over medium-high heat. Remove the tuna from the marinade. Season with salt and pepper. Sear the tuna on one side, about 2–3 minutes. Turn and sear on the second side for 2–3 minutes more for rare.

To serve, place the tuna steaks onto a serving platter. Top with a pat of dill-lime butter.

On Shopping Day: Prepare the dill-lime butter and store in an airtight container in the refrigerator for up to 5 days.

HEARTY BEEF STEW

This is a fabulous dish, perfect to serve on a cold day. This recipe makes plenty, so serve your family on the day you prepare the dish and freeze any extras to use on your next "day off."

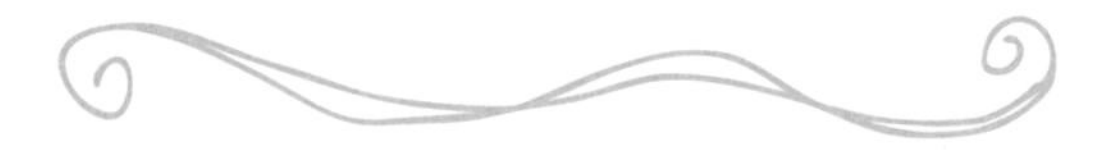

This recipe is PURRfect for your slow cooker. Follow the recipe, browning the beef and veggies. At this point, place the ingredients into your slow cooker. Add the rest of the ingredients, set the cooker, and come back later for the finished dish. If the sauce is not as thick as you like it, simply pour the stew back into the Dutch oven, heat to boiling, reduce heat, and simmer until desired consistency—usually about 20 minutes. The flour and tomato paste are natural thickeners.

* * *

Leave the SKIN on the potato for an added boost of good-for you nutrients.

Preheat oven to 350 degrees. Place the beef cubes in a bowl. Toss with flour and season with salt and pepper. Heat a Dutch oven (or large deep pan with cover) over medium-high heat. Add the diced bacon. Cook until crisp. Remove the bacon from the pan with a slotted spoon. Drain on paper towels. Pour off excess drippings.

Cook the beef cubes in the Dutch oven until brown on all sides. Remove the beef from the pan and place in a bowl. Cook the potatoes, carrots, onions, and garlic in the pan for 5–8 minutes, stirring often until the vegetables just begin to brown. Add the beef cubes and bacon back to the pan. Pour the wine and beef stock into the pan. Stir in the tomato paste. Tuck the bay leaves into the mixture. Season with thyme and additional salt and pepper.

Bring the sauce to a boil. Cover and place into the oven. Cook for 45 minutes to 1 hour or until the meat is tender.

To serve, ladle the stew into crocks and garnish with fresh parsley.

On Shopping Day: Prepare the beef by cutting into cubes and storing in an airtight container in the refrigerator for up to 5 days. Prepare the carrots and onions and store in an airtight container for up to 5 days.

Makes 4 to 6 servings, reserving half of the stew for another day
Prep Time: 30 minutes
Cook Time: 45 minutes to 1 hour in the oven or all day in the slow cooker

- 3 pounds beef chuck roast, trimmed of all but 15 to 20 percent of fat, cut into 1 1/2-inch cubes
- 1/2 cup unbleached all-purpose flour
- Salt and freshly ground pepper
- 6 ounces lean bacon, about 4–6 strips, diced
- 4 medium Yukon gold potatoes, cut into 2-inch pieces, about 3 cups
- 6 large carrots, peeled, cut into 1-inch pieces (about 3 cups)
- 2 large yellow onions, peeled, sliced into wedges, (about 2 cups)
- 4 –6 garlic cloves, chopped
- 2 cups red wine

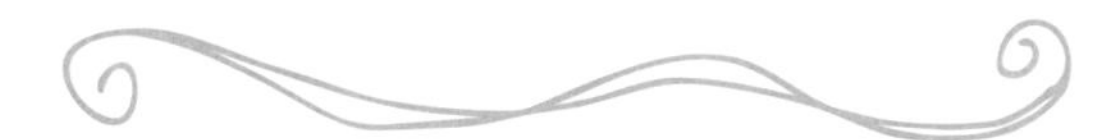

2 cups beef stock
1 6-ounce can tomato paste
2 bay leaves
2 teaspoons dried thyme
Chopped fresh parsley (for garnish)

BUTTERNUT SQUASH AND SWISH CHARD ROLL-UPS

With Sun-Dried Tomato Basil Sauce

Bring out the smiles and gather everyone to the table for this veggie-filled simple supper that can be prepared in advance and baked in just minutes.

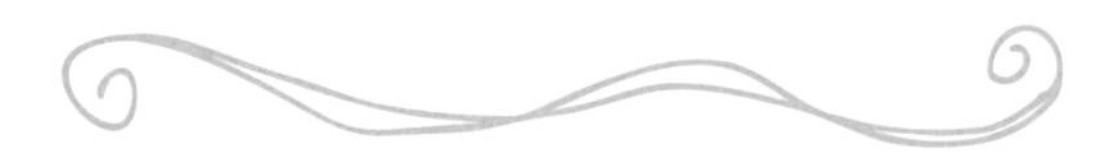

If you have been very, very good,
a light Béchamel sauce on top of these roll-ups
is a DECADENT touch!

Makes 4 servings
Prep Time: 30 minutes
Cook Time: 30 minutes

For the sauce

- 1 tablespoon olive oil
- 1 medium yellow onion, diced (about 1 cup)
- 2 medium cloves garlic, minced (about 1 teaspoon)
- 6 plum medium tomatoes, seeded and chopped
- 1 cup minced oil-packed sun-dried tomatoes, drained
- $\frac{1}{2}$ cup dry white wine
- 1 cup homemade chicken stock or low-sodium chicken broth
- 3 tablespoons chopped fresh basil
- Salt and freshly ground pepper

For the lasagna

- 8 lasagna noodles
- 1 tablespoon olive oil

Heat 1 tablespoon olive oil in a pan over medium-high heat. Add the onion and garlic and cook until soft, about 3 minutes. Stir in the tomatoes, wine, and 1 cup chicken broth and reduce the heat. Simmer the sauce for 20–25 minutes, stirring often. Stir in the basil and season with salt and pepper. Use a hand held blender or food processor to emulsify the sauce. Keep warm.

Cook the noodles in salted, boiling water until just al dente. Drain and place on a baking sheet that has been coated with vegetable oil spray.

Heat 1 tablespoon olive oil in a deep skillet over medium-high heat. Add the squash and onion and cook until soft, about 5 minutes. Stir in $\frac{1}{4}$ cup chicken broth and Swiss chard. Season with salt and pepper. Cook until the chard is wilted and the squash is soft, about 5 minutes. Remove the pan from the heat and cool slightly. Stir in the Gruyère cheese, ricotta, $\frac{1}{3}$ cup Parmesan, and egg.

Preheat the oven to 350 degrees. Pour 1 ladle of the sauce into a baking dish. Lay out 1 lasagna noodle on your work surface. Spread 2 tablespoons of the filling over top. Roll up the noodle and place, seam-side down, into the baking dish. Repeat with all of the noodles and all of the filling. Spoon the remaining sauce over the top. Sprinkle with remaining 2 tablespoons Parmesan cheese. Bake the roll-ups until the top is golden and the sauce is bubbling.

On Shopping Day: Prepare the sauce and filling. Store both, separately, in airtight containers in the refrigerator for up to 4 days.

- 1 medium butternut squash, peeled and diced into 1-inch squares (about 2 cups)
- 1 medium yellow onion, diced (about 1 cup)
- 1/4 cup homemade chicken stock or low-sodium chicken broth
- 4 ounces Swiss chard, washed, dried, stems removed, leaves torn (about 2 cups)
- 4 ounces Gruyère cheese, shredded (about 1 cup)
- 1/2 cup reduced-fat ricotta cheese
- 1/3 cup finely grated Parmesan cheese, plus 2 tablespoons for topping
- 1 large egg, beaten

HUNTER'S-STYLE CHICKEN STEW

With Yellow Rice

The fragrance of this simple, peasant dish will fill your kitchen and bring the troops to the table for a meal that is fit for royalty. Reminiscent of chicken cacciatore, it is packed full of yummy veggies.

Makes 6 servings
Prep Time: 20 minutes
Cook Time: 60 minutes

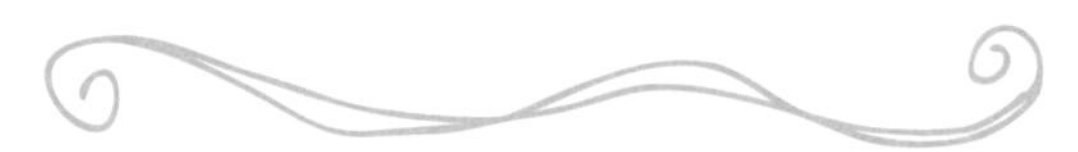

Make this dish even LESS STRESSFUL by preparing it using a slow cooker. Brown the chicken in the skillet and then place the pieces into the slow cooker. Brown the veggies in the skillet and deglaze with wine. Pour these into the slow cooker. Add the remaining ingredients and cover with the lid. Set the slow cooker and walk away for the day. Supper will be ready when you are.

- 1 4-pound chicken, rinsed and patted dry, cut into 8 pieces
- Salt and freshly ground pepper
- 2 tablespoons olive oil
- 1 large red onion, peeled and thinly sliced (about 1 cup)
- 1 large green bell pepper, seeded and thinly sliced (about 1 cup)
- 1 large red bell pepper, seeded and thinly sliced (about 1 cup)
- 1 large yellow bell pepper, seeded and thinly sliced (about 1 cup)
- 4 ounces button mushrooms, sliced (about 1 cup)
- 4 medium garlic cloves, thinly sliced (about 2 teaspoons)
- 1 cup red wine
- 1 28-ounce can diced tomatoes
- 2 tablespoons tomato paste
- 1 teaspoon dried oregano
- 1 teaspoon dried rosemary
- ½ teaspoon crushed red pepper
- 3 cups cooked yellow rice
- 2 tablespoons chopped fresh parsley (for garnish)

Season the chicken with salt and pepper. Heat the olive oil in a deep skillet (with lid) over medium-high heat. Brown the chicken pieces on all sides until golden, about 8 minutes. Remove the chicken to a platter.

Add the onion, the three bell peppers, mushrooms, and garlic to the pan. Cook until the veggies are soft and begin to brown, about 8 minutes. Pour in the wine and cook until much of the liquid has disappeared, about 5 minutes more.

Pour in the tomatoes. Stir in the tomato paste, oregano, rosemary, and crushed red pepper. Add the chicken back to the pan. Reduce the heat to medium low and simmer until the chicken is cooked through, about 1 hour.

To serve, divide the rice among 6 plates. Place chicken pieces on top of the rice. Ladle the sauce over top. Garnish with fresh parsley.

SPICY FLANK STEAK SANDWICH

With Roasted Pepper Blue Cheese Sauce

Marinate the flank steak in the morning before you start your day. In the evening, all you have left to do is grill the steak and assemble the sandwiches. Not only stress free—but totally comforting as well!

You will have extra flank steak—which is just what you want. Use the remainder later in the week for flank steak QUESADILLAS or flank steak salad.

* * *

Chipotle chili in adobo sauce is SPICY. If it is too spicy for your family, substitute ½ teaspoon crushed red pepper or 1 tablespoon chili powder.

Place the steak into a shallow baking dish. In a small bowl whisk together the tomato juice, Worcestershire sauce, and diced chipotle pepper. Stir in the onions. Pour this mixture over the steak, turning to coat. Cover and refrigerate for at least 1 hour or overnight.

Place the mayonnaise, red pepper, blue cheese, shallot, and cilantro into the bowl of a food processor. Season with salt and pepper. Pulse to combine. Transfer to an airtight container and store in the refrigerator until ready to use.

Heat a grill pan over medium-high heat. Remove the steak from the marinade. Season with salt and pepper. Grill the steak until browned, about 8–10 minutes. Turn and grill until medium rare, about 8 minutes more (depending on thickness). Transfer to a cutting board and let rest for 10 minutes.

Brush the cut side of the rolls with olive oil. Grill, cut-side down, in the grill pan, over medium heat until golden, about 4–5 minutes.

To serve, slice the flank steak across the grain into thin pieces. Divide the arugula leaves among the bottom halves of the 4 rolls. Top with flank steak slices. Spoon the sauce over the steak. Place the top half of the roll on top.

On Shopping Day: Prepare the sauce and store in an airtight container in the refrigerator for up to 3 days.

Makes 4 servings
Prep Time: 15 minutes, plus marinating
Cook Time: 15 to 20 minutes

For the steak

- 1 large (about 1½ pound) flank steak
- 1 cup tomato juice
- 1 tablespoon Worcestershire sauce
- 1 canned chipotle pepper in adobo sauce, seeded and finely diced (about 1 tablespoon)
- 4 green onions, thinly sliced (about ¼ cup)

For the sauce

- ½ cup reduced-fat mayonnaise
- ½ cup jarred roasted red pepper
- 1 ounce blue cheese, crumbled (about ¼ cup)
- 1 large shallot, chopped (about 1 tablespoon)
- 2 tablespoons chopped fresh cilantro
- Salt and freshly ground pepper

For the sandwich

- 4 ciabatta rolls, cut in half
- 1 tablespoon olive oil
- 2 cups arugula leaves, washed and dried

REALLY GOOD TURKEY BURGERS

With Cheddar Cheese and Horseradish Sauce

Baby, if you want a burger, you've come to the right recipe. Use really good Cheddar cheese and enjoy a generous slathering of sauce. There's no secret sauce going on here—it's an open book—all for you!

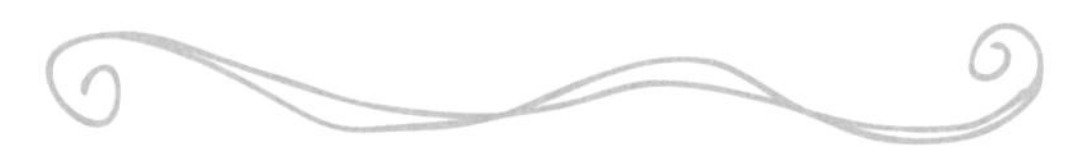

Because we're using GROUND TURKEY in place of ground beef, make sure that the burger reaches an internal temperature of 165 to 170 degrees. You can turn the grill pan to low and continue cooking in the foil tent to bring up the temperature. Watch carefully so that you do not dry out the burger.

Place the ground turkey into a large bowl. Add the olive oil and Worcestershire sauce. Generously season with salt and pepper. Use your hands to gently combine and form into 4 patties.

Heat a grill pan over medium-high heat. Place the burgers onto the grill pan, cook until seared, about 4–5 minutes. Carefully flip the burgers and cook until seared on the second side, about 5 minutes more. Turn off the heat. Divide the Cheddar cheese over the burgers. Tent the grill pan with aluminum foil. Allow the burgers to rest for 5 minutes.

Toast the buns in a toaster oven or on a baking sheet in the oven.

Whisk together the mayonnaise, horseradish, lemon juice, and paprika.

To serve, place the burger onto the bottom half of the bun. Top with a slice of tomato and a spoonful of the horseradish sauce. Place the top half of the bun onto the burger.

On Shopping Day: Prepare the sauce. Store in an airtight container in the refrigerator for up to 4 days.

Makes 4 servings
Prep Time: 15 minutes
Cook Time: 10 minutes

For the burger

- 2 pounds ground turkey
- 1/4 cup olive oil
- 1 tablespoon Worcestershire sauce
- Salt and freshly ground pepper
- 2 ounces grated Cheddar cheese
- 4 whole wheat hamburger buns
- 4 1/2-inch slices beefsteak tomato

For the sauce

- 1/2 cup reduced-fat mayonnaise
- 1 tablespoon prepared horseradish
- Juice of 1/2 medium lemon (about 1 tablespoon)
- 1/4 teaspoon paprika

PAN-SAUTÉED GNOCCHI

With Sun-Dried Tomato and Sage

It's not as complicated as you think. Delight your friends with an authentic rustic Italian treat. Now this is de-stressing. . . .

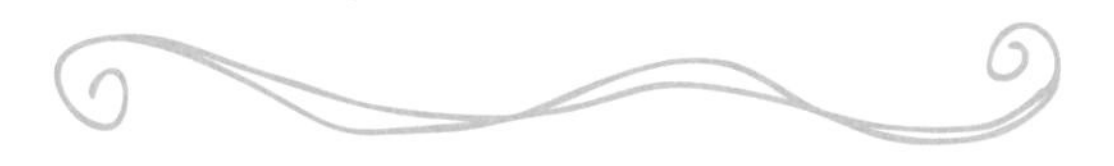

You can prepare the gnocchi in ADVANCE for later use by plunging the cooked gnocchi into a bowl of ice water. Drain and place onto the coated baking sheet to prevent sticking. When ready, warm up the gnocchi in a pot of boiling water for 1 minute.

Cover the potatoes with water in a deep pot. Bring to a boil and cook until the potatoes are fork-tender, about 10–15 minutes.

Preheat the oven to 350 degrees. Drain the potatoes and place onto a baking sheet. Bake the potatoes in the oven to release the moisture, about 5–7 minutes. Press warm potatoes through a potato ricer onto your work surface. Sprinkle the flour, Parmesan cheese, salt, and nutmeg over the potatoes. Make a well in the center. Place the egg and olive oil into the well. Use a pastry scraper to combine the ingredients until the mixture resembles course crumbs. Use your hands to bring the crumbs together into a soft and slightly sticky dough. Dust your work surface with additional flour. Divide the dough into 4 sections. Roll each section into a 1-inch-diameter logs. Cut the logs into 1-inch pieces. Roll each piece over the back of the tines of a fork to create ridges. Place gnocchi onto a baking sheet.

Bring a deep pot of water to a boil. Season generously with salt. Drop the gnocchi into the boiling water. When the gnocchi float to the top, use a slotted spoon to transfer to a rimmed baking sheet that has been coated with vegetable oil spray.

Heat the butter in a large skillet over medium heat. Stir in the sun-dried tomatoes with their oil. Stir in the sage. Add the gnocchi and cook until golden.

To serve, transfer the gnocchi and sauce to a serving bowl. Season with grated cheese.

Makes 4 to 6 servings
Prep Time: 30 minutes
Cook Time: 10 minutes

For the gnocchi

- 4 medium russet potatoes, about 2 pounds, peeled and cut into 1-inch pieces
- 1 cup unbleached all-purpose flour, plus some for dusting
- 2 ounces finely grated Parmesan cheese (about 1/2 cup)
- 1 teaspoon kosher salt
- 1/4 teaspoon nutmeg
- 1 large egg
- 1 tablespoon olive oil

For the sauce

- 2 tablespoons butter
- 2 tablespoons minced oil-packed sun-dried tomatoes
- 2 tablespoons chopped fresh sage
- 2 tablespoons grated Asiago cheese

FRESH VEGGIE MINESTRONE SOUP

With Chickpeas

There's nothing better than a steaming bowl of savory soup to satisfy your craving for comfort food. This one is loaded with lots and lots of veggies.

Makes 8 servings
Prep Time: 20 minutes
Cook Time: at least 45 minutes or up to several hours

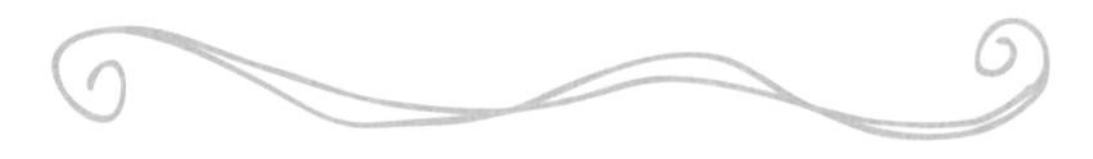

You can use ANY vegetable that you have in your refrigerator for this soup. You can also substitute with chicken or vegetable broth in place of beef. The additions of pasta, rice, or barley will add a heartier dimension—and don't hesitate to add cheese tortellini for a truly authentic dish.

- 1 tablespoon olive oil
- 1 leek, white part only, rinsed well and sliced
- 2 large zucchini, diced into 1/2-inch pieces (about 1 cup)
- 2 large yellow squash, cut into 1/2-inch dice (about 1 cup)
- 1/2 1-pound head green cabbage, sliced (about 3 cups)
- 1/2 pound fresh green beans, cut into 1-inch pieces (about 1 cup)
- 2 ears of fresh corn, kernels sliced from cob (about 1 cup)
- 4 medium garlic cloves, minced (about 2 teaspoons)
- 1 28-ounce can diced tomatoes
- 1 quart homemade beef stock or low-sodium beef broth
- 2 bay leaves
- 2 teaspoons dried oregano
- 1 15.5-ounce can chickpeas, drained
- 2 tablespoons chopped fresh parsley
- Salt and freshly ground pepper

Heat the olive oil in a soup pot over medium-high heat. Add the leek, zucchini, yellow squash, and cabbage. Cook until the veggies begin to soften, about 15–20 minutes. Stir in the green beans, corn, and garlic. Cook for 5 minutes more.

Pour in the tomatoes and beef stock. Stir in the bay leaves and oregano. Bring the soup to a boil. Reduce the heat to medium low and simmer to allow the flavors to blend, at least 30 minutes. Stir in the chickpeas and parsley. Season with salt and pepper and continue simmering, covered, until ready to serve.

To serve, ladle the soup into bowls. Serve with cheese toast or whole grain crackers.

On Shopping Day: Prepare all of the veggies for the soup. Store separately, in airtight containers in the refrigerator for up to 4 days.

CREAMY WILD MUSHROOM SOUP

With Sherry and Fresh Thyme

Had a stressful day? Warm up a bowl full of this deliciously comforting soup, take off your shoes, and sip slowly while you unwind.

Makes 4 servings
Prep Time: 15 minutes
Cook Time: 20 minutes

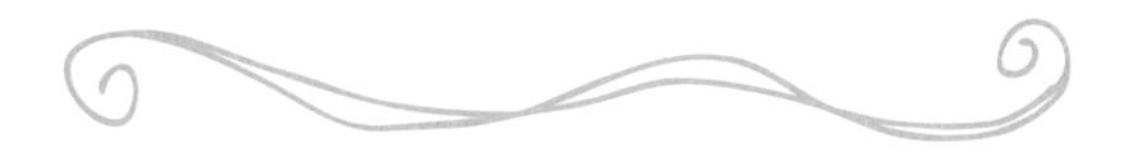

I use the TECHNIQUE of removing 1 cup of the cooked mushrooms before blending the soup to produce a rustic texture. You can skip this step for a smoother soup.

- 2 tablespoons olive oil
- 1 medium yellow onion, peeled and diced into ½-inch squares (about 1 cup)
- 4 tablespoons butter
- 8 ounces button mushrooms, sliced (about 2 cups)
- 8 ounces baby portobello mushrooms, sliced (about 2 cups)
- 4 ounces shiitake mushrooms, stems removed, chopped (about 1 cup)
- 4 ounces oyster mushrooms (about 1 cup)
- Salt and freshly ground pepper
- ¼ cup dry sherry
- 3 tablespoons chopped fresh thyme, plus garnish
- 1 quart homemade chicken stock or low-sodium chicken broth
- 1 cup reduced-fat half and half
- Juice of ½ lemon (about 1 tablespoon)

Heat the olive oil in a deep pot over medium-high heat. Cook the onion in the oil until soft, about 5 minutes. Add the butter to the pot. Reduce the heat to medium and add the four varieties of mushrooms. Cook until soft, about 4–5 minutes more. Season with salt and pepper. Add the sherry and cook until most of the liquid is absorbed. Stir in the fresh thyme.

Remove 1 cup of the mushrooms to a bowl. Pour in the chicken stock. Bring to a boil. Reduce the heat and simmer until the mushrooms are tender, about 8–10 minutes.

Use a handheld blender or food processor to emulsify the soup. Pour in the half and half and the lemon juice. Add back in the reserved mushrooms. Continue to simmer the soup for at least 10 minutes.

To serve, ladle the soup into bowls. Garnish with additional chopped fresh thyme.

On Shopping Day: Prepare this soup so that it's ready for you during the week. Cool to room temperature. Store in an airtight container in the refrigerator for up to 5 days or in the freezer for up to 1 month.

THE REAL DEAL FRIES

With Ketchup of Course!

Okay, sometimes you just gotta eat fries. But, don't waste calories on the greasy cardboard variety. Grab a knife and a spud and prepare the best fries you're ever gonna eat. Oh, and don't forget the ketchup!

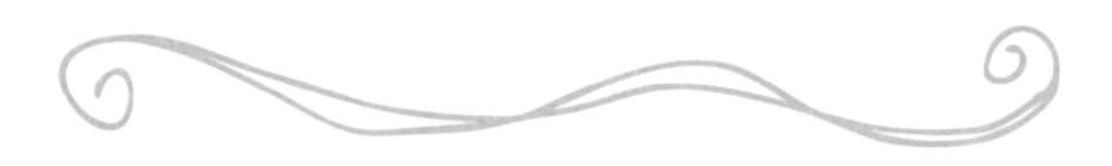

Cooking the fries TWICE makes sure that the center is soft and the outside is crisp. You'll need a deep pan and a bunch of oil. To save the oil, cool to room temperature and strain into an airtight container. Store in the refrigerator for up to 2 weeks.

Heat the olive oil in a saucepan over medium-high heat. Stir in the tomatoes, onions, bell pepper, and garlic. Cook until the veggies are soft, about 20 minutes. Use a handheld blender or food processor to emulsify the veggies. Return to the pot. Stir in the tomato paste, sugar, bay leaf, cloves, allspice, mace, pepper, cinnamon, mustard, and vinegar. Bring to a boil. Reduce the heat and simmer for 10–15 minutes. Remove the bay leaf and strain through a sieve (or blend again with a handheld blender or food processor).

Pour in enough canola oil to come one-third of the way up the sides of a deep pot. Heat the oil to 325 degrees. Peel the potatoes. Cut into ¼-inch slices. Stack and slice lengthwise into ¼-inch strips. Rinse and pat dry with paper towels. Cook the fries in the oil, in batches, until soft, but not golden, about 4–5 minutes. Use a slotted spoon or wire basket to transfer the fries to a rack placed onto a rimmed baking sheet lined with paper towels. Chill the fries, in the refrigerator for at least 15 minutes.

Stir together the salt, pepper, and paprika.

Reheat the oil to 375 degrees. Cook the cold fries in oil, in batches, until crisp and golden, about 2–3 minutes. Use a slotted spoon or wire basket to transfer to the rack. Sprinkle with seasoned salt.

To serve, mound the fries into a basket and ladle the ketchup into a dipping bowl.

On Shopping Day: Prepare the ketchup. Store in an airtight container in the refrigerator for up to 5 days.

Makes 4 servings with extra ketchup
Prep Time: 15 minutes
Cook Time: 15 minutes for fries, 30 minutes for ketchup

For the ketchup

- 1 tablespoon olive oil
- 8 large plum tomatoes, seeded and diced (about 4 cups)
- 2 medium yellow onions, peeled and diced (about 2 cups)
- 1 large red bell pepper, seeded and diced (about 2 cups)
- 2 medium garlic cloves, minced (about 1 teaspoon)
- ¾ cup tomato paste
- ¼ cup brown sugar
- 1 bay leaf
- ¼ teaspoon ground cloves
- ¼ teaspoon ground allspice

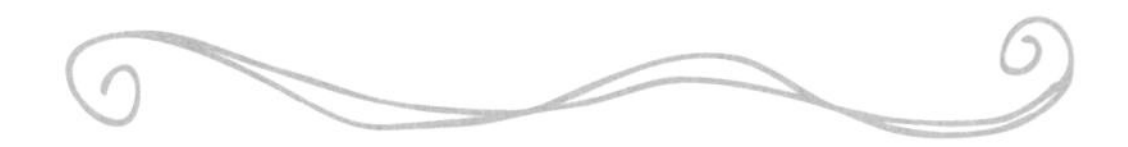

- 1/4 teaspoon ground mace
- 1/4 teaspoon freshly ground pepper
- 1/8 teaspoon ground cinnamon
- 1/4 teaspoon dry mustard
- 1/4 cup red wine vinegar

For the fries

- 1 quart canola oil
- 2 large russet potatoes (about 2 pounds)
- 2 teaspoons salt
- 1/2 teaspoon freshly ground pepper
- 1/4 teaspoon paprika

KEY LIME POUND CAKE

Tart lime juice flavors an otherwise decadent cake for a refreshing dessert treat that is perfect for unwinding.

Makes 12 servings
Prep Time: 20 minutes
Cook Time: 1 hour 10 minutes

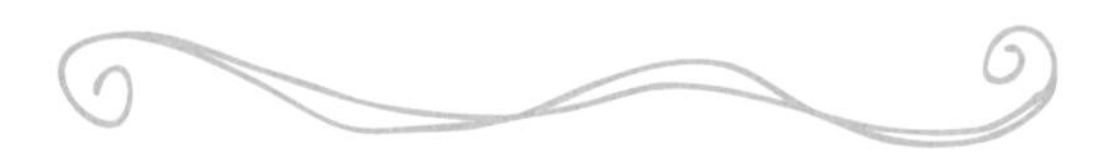

Purchase KEY LIME JUICE for this recipe if fresh key limes are not available.

For the cake

- 1 1/2 cups cake flour
- 1/4 teaspoon baking soda
- 1/8 teaspoon salt
- 1/2 cup unsalted butter, room temperature (1 stick)
- 4 ounces reduced-fat cream cheese
- 1 1/2 cups natural sugar
- 3 eggs
- 1 teaspoon pure vanilla extract
- 1/4 cup key lime juice
- Zest of 1 medium lime (about 1 tablespoon)

For the glaze

- 1/2 cup confectioners' sugar
- 1 tablespoon key lime juice
- Mixed fresh berries

Preheat the oven to 325 degrees. Coat a Bundt pan with vegetable oil spray and dust with flour. Set aside.

In a small bowl whisk together the flour, baking soda, and salt. In a separate bowl use an electric mixer to combine the butter and cream cheese. Add the sugar and beat until fluffy. Stir in the eggs, one at a time, followed by the vanilla, lime juice and lime zest. Stir in the flour mixture. Pour the batter into the prepared Bundt pan. Bake until the cake springs back when touched and a tester inserted into the center comes out clean, about 60–70 minutes. Transfer to a rack and cool for 10 minutes. Loosen the edges of the cake with a knife or spatula. Invert the pan and remove the cake to a wire rack. Place waxed paper underneath.

In a small bowl stir together the confectioners' sugar with the lime juice. If mixture is too thick, add a teaspoon of water to thin. Use a skewer to poke holes into the pound cake. Pour the glaze over the top and allow it to seep into the cake. Cool to room temperature.

To serve, cut into slices and serve with fresh berries.

MAPLE CAKE DOUGHNUTS

It's so easy to eat warm doughnuts in your own kitchen. These remind me of the ones my Grandma use to make on "Fat Tuesday," the day before Ash Wednesday. It was our splurge of comfort before a season of sacrifice.

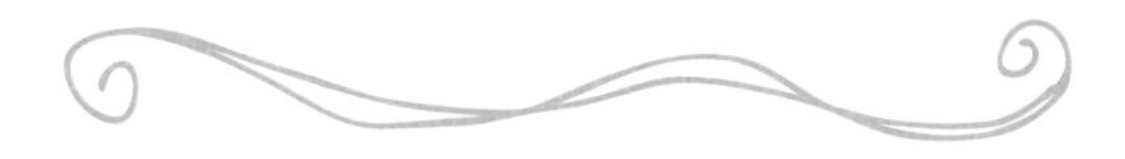

Change the flavor of these doughnuts by substituting your favorite SPICES.

In a small bowl whisk together the flour, baking powder, cinnamon, salt, and baking soda.

In a large bowl whisk together the sugar and eggs until fluffy and thick. Whisk in the orange zest, maple extract, and butter. Whisk in the sour cream. Use a rubber spatula to gently fold in the flour mixture. The dough will be sticky. Cover with plastic wrap and let rest for 1 hour.

Line 2 baking sheets with parchment paper (or use 2 Silpat liners). Dust work surface with flour. Flour a rolling pin, a 2½-inch diameter round cutter and 1-inch diameter cutter. Roll out one-third of the dough to ½-inch thickness. Cut large rounds and place onto prepared baking sheets. Use the small cutter for doughnut holes and to cut additional holes from scraps. Continue until all of the dough has been used.

Pour enough canola oil in a deep pot to come up 2 inches on the sides. Heat to 365 degrees. Line 2 baking sheets with several layers of paper towels. Use a slotted spoon to place the doughnut holes into the oil in batches. Do not crowd. Watch as they drop to the bottom of the pot. When they bob to the surface, gently turn over to evenly brown. Remove to the paper-towel-lined baking sheets. Repeat until all of the holes and doughnuts have been fried. The holes will brown in 2–3 minutes. Doughnuts will take a minute or two more.

Dust the doughnuts with confectioners' sugar while still warm.

Makes about 12 doughnuts
and a whole bunch of doughnut holes
Prep Time: 20 minutes
Cook Time: 20 minutes for all of the doughnuts

- 3½ cups unbleached all-purpose flour
- 1 tablespoon baking powder
- 1 teaspoon ground cinnamon
- ½ teaspoon salt
- ½ teaspoon baking soda
- 1 cup natural sugar
- 2 large eggs
- Zest of ½ medium orange (about 1 tablespoon)
- 1 teaspoon maple extract
- 6 tablespoons unsalted butter, melted
- 1 cup reduced-fat sour cream
- Canola oil for frying
- Confectioners' sugar for dusting

CHOCOLATE GINGERSNAPS

There is an explosion of sweet flavor in every bite of cookie. You must serve with a glass of ice-cold milk.

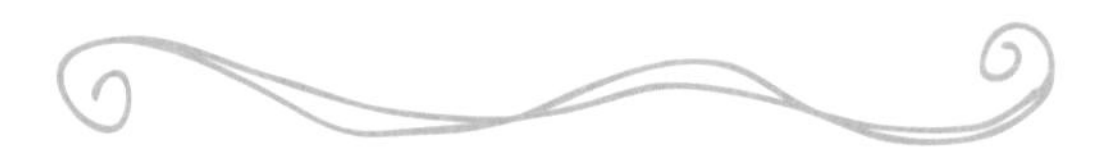

If you can find them, mini chips are an excellent choice for this cookie as they will be less visible in the end result, offering more of a surprise flavor combo. If not, don't stress—the regular ones will do just fine.

In a medium bowl whisk together the flour, ginger, cinnamon, cloves, nutmeg, cocoa powder, baking soda, and salt.

In a large bowl use an electric mixer to combine the shortening and brown sugar until fluffy. Mix in the molasses and vanilla. Stir in the flour mixture in 3 additions. Stir in the chocolate chips. Cover the dough with plastic wrap and chill for at least 1 hour.

Preheat the oven to 350 degrees. Line 2 baking sheets with parchment paper (or Silpat liners). Roll the dough into 2-inch balls and place onto baking sheets. Chill the first while you prepare the second. Remove the first batch from the refrigerator. Roll each ball in granulated sugar. Use the bottom of a glass to push the balls into disks about ½-inch thick. Bake the cookies until the bottoms just begin to turn golden, about 12–14 minutes. The cookies will not change shape after they bake. Transfer to a rack to cool completely. Repeat with remaining dough.

On Shopping Day: Make the cookie dough and divide into two disks. Cover with plastic wrap. Place 1 into a resealable plastic bag and freeze for up to 1 month. Place the second disk into the refrigerator for up to 5 days.

Makes about 4 dozen cookies, serving size 2 cookies
Prep Time: 20 minutes, plus chilling time
Cook Time: 24 minutes

- 3 cups unbleached all-purpose flour
- 2½ teaspoons ground ginger
- 1½ teaspoons ground cinnamon
- ½ teaspoon ground cloves
- ½ teaspoon ground nutmeg
- 2 tablespoons unsweetened cocoa powder
- 2 teaspoons baking soda
- ¼ teaspoon salt
- 1 cup vegetable shortening
- 1 cup dark brown sugar
- ¾ cup molasses
- 1 teaspoon pure vanilla extract
- 1 10-ounce package mini semisweet chocolate chips
- ¼ cup granulated sugar

PRETTY IN PEACH

Fresh, ripe sweet fruit is roasted with a crumbled topping, making this dessert reminiscent of Grandma's kitchen and her famous peach pie.

Makes 4 servings
Prep Time: 20 minutes
Cook Time: 25 to 35 minutes

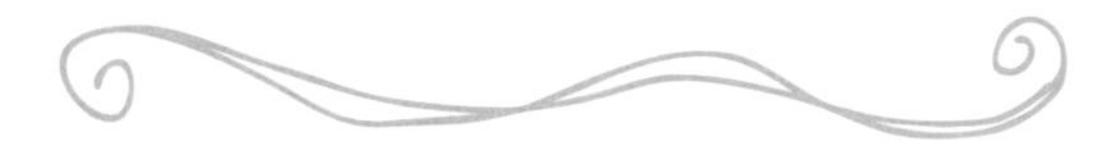

Use this recipe for any fruit CRUMBLE. Fresh, sweet cherries will work wonderfully as will a combination of apples and raspberries. You needn't stress when following a recipe—it's only a guideline for your final approval.

For the filling

- 6 medium-size ripe peaches, peeled, pitted, and sliced (about 3 cups)
- 3 tablespoons natural sugar
- 1 teaspoon cornstarch
- Juice of 1 large lemon (about 3 tablespoons)
- ½ teaspoon ground cinnamon
- ¼ teaspoon ground nutmeg

For the crumble topping

- 1 cup unbleached all-purpose flour
- ½ cup old-fashioned rolled oats
- ¼ cup natural sugar
- ¼ cup brown sugar
- ¼ teaspoon salt
- 2 teaspoons pure vanilla extract
- 6 tablespoons butter, chilled and cut into pieces
- Ice cream

Preheat the oven to 375 degrees. Place the peaches into a colander. Sprinkle with 3 tablespoons sugar and toss gently. Place the colander into a large bowl and let sit for 30 minutes. Remove the peaches and drain all but ¼ cup peach juice from the bowl. Place the peaches into a 9 x 11 x 2-inch baking dish that has been coated with vegetable oil spray. Whisk together the peach juice with the cornstarch, lemon juice, cinnamon, and nutmeg. Pour this mixture over the peaches.

In the bowl of a food processor place the flour, oats, ¼ cup sugar, brown sugar, salt, and vanilla. Pulse to combine. Add the butter and pulse to form course crumbs. Sprinkle the topping over the peaches.

Bake until the peaches are bubbly and the topping is golden, about 25–35 minutes.

To serve, spoon the peach crumble into serving bowls and top with a spoonful of ice cream.

On Shopping Day: Slice the peaches and store in an airtight container for up to 3 days.

Gorgeous Home Spa Secrets . . . for Cozy Comfort

De-stressing in the bathtub is a no-brainer—so is whipping up a home facial from organic elements. After you've enjoyed the perfect home spa experience, the party's *far* from over. When your hair comes out of its terry cloth turban, the mud mask is washed away, and your masseuse folds up her table, you can keep on relaxing with a little something called Aryuveda teas, which are thousands of years old in practice and free of irritants like caffeine. Even if you don't need it to relax, tea makes a fine after-dinner drink. There are many to choose from, so give them all a try.

Suits You to a Tea

Dating back in Indian history about 5,000 years, Ayurveda, or "the science of life," believes that mind, body, spirit, emotions, and senses should all be in perfect balance—the way nature intended. Today's holistic health care givers have interpreted Ayurveda's ancient texts and formulated three different herbal teas for those looking to get back in balance. They may be on to something. Hot, soothing beverages are just what the doctor ordered when it comes to reducing stress. When stress takes hold of a person, it can cause some discomfort in the mouth and throat. As stress escalates, fluids are diverted from nonessential locations, including the mouth. This causes dryness and difficulty in talking. (Ever get dry mouth when you're delivering a speech?) In addition, stress can cause spasms of the throat muscles, making it difficult to swallow. Ayurvedic teas promote a sense of calm and please your palate through their exceptionally fine aromas. Here's a peek at the three cups available in any natural grocery store.

Vata tea is calming and harmonizing. It's perfect for nervous nellys or a working girl with a deadline or business trip on her horizon. It contains licorice, cinnamon, cardamom, and ginger and has a full and sweet aroma *without* adding sugar.

Pitta tea soothes the savage beast. It's perfect for someone with a reputation for having fire in her belly. Its fine mixture of rose blossom petals and mild spices possesses pleasantly cooling properties. Brew up a kettle on those summer days warm enough to match hot tempers!

Kapha tea is for the lazy bones in your family, offering a revitalizing pick-me-up without the caffeine. It's quite similar to Vata in its ingredients, differing in its inclusion of saffron. Kapha is spicy and goes best with breakfast, damp and cold weather, or springtime. Cut up a lemon, add a wedge to your steaming cup, and you're good to go!

Mary Ellen Weighs In

If you're more renowned for curling up with a good book before you'd ever consider curling dumbbells, the idea of starting small on the gorgeous path to fitness is relaxing in and of itself. Just 10 minutes of exercise three times a week builds a good base for novices. Gradually build up the length of these every-other-day sessions to 30 minutes or more, allowing muscles to rest in between workouts. For fitness virgins, I recommend starting with aerobics. It's a good way to strengthen key muscle groups before taxing them with weights and Nautilus machines. Once you are in the groove, resistance training can be included 2 to 3 days a week and aerobic training can be incorporated 4 to 5 times a week.

Who Needs a Destination Spa?

If the aforementioned sounds too ambitious, your foray into the world of fitness may be the tried-and-true *brisk* walking. Destination spa resorts in the foothills of the Sierra Nevada, up in the vast canyons of the West, or the sugar sand beaches on the coast all specialize in brisk walking—they just assign it fancier names like "hiking" and happen to offer breathtaking scenery. But who says you can't make a Destination Spa out of your favorite public park or neighborhood sidewalk? Brisk walking offers the dual benefit of conditioning your body and clearing your mind of stressful thoughts.

New Age Fitness

Yoga or Tai Chi can be very effective, combining many of the benefits of breathing, muscle relaxation, and meditation while toning and stretching the muscles. The benefits of yoga are said to be considerable. Numerous studies have found it beneficial for conditions in which stress is an important factor, such as anxiety, headaches, high blood pressure, and asthma. It also elevates mood and improves concentration and ability to focus.

Class Mates

Joining an exercise class can be a great way to find encouragement during your workouts. Signing up for an aerobics class can be a great de-stressor. Be clear about which class you sign up for (beginner, intermediate, or advanced) and remember to start slow to avoid muscle soreness or injury. Find a pal in the class who has goals similar to yours. It will be harder for you to ditch your workouts if you have a friend who is expecting you.

Swim Gym

Swimming is an excellent activity. Whether you are floating on the top of the water or drifting underneath, a "pool of tranquility" offers a much-needed break from life's hectic pace. Swimming is gentle on your joints and yet is a terrific cardiovascular workout.

Pregnant women and those recouping from injury will find swimming an excellent workout choice.

Jock with a Green Thumb

Gardening is an excellent way to de-stress. Not only is working in the garden a workout, but you are also growing the vegetables that will feed the very muscles you're using. My dad would come home on a busy workday and head right to the garden to weed his vegetables, plant flowering bulbs, or just mow the lawn. This was his way of de-stressing after a busy day. Gardening activities include pushing and pulling and bending and lunging. One of the best kinds of garden for the fitness savvy is starchy vegetables, mainly the ones grown below the ground, such as carrots and potatoes. They stimulate the production of serotonin, so when you're done tending them (and simultaneously working out), you can sit down to a supper chock-full of 'em and have better luck falling asleep that night to boot.

Community Farming

If your green thumb is still in development but you are a connoisseur of fresh fruits and veggies, you might consider joining a community-supported farm (CSA). As a member, you pay a small fee that helps the farmer grow his crops throughout the season. Depending on the conditions and the research going on, you reap the benefits of a weekly or biweekly harvest. The produce box you receive will be full of everything that is grown during that season and can include heirloom tomatoes, exotic varieties of summer squash, carrots and radishes with tops intact, and every kind of fresh herb imaginable. For more information and to find a CSA near you, check out www.nal.usda.gov/afsic/csa/.

CHAPTER 15

sowing the seeds of love

"Sex appeal is fifty percent what you've got and fifty percent what people think you've got."
—Sophia Loren

If the food on your plate is aromatic, tasty, and visually appealing—as so much of gourmet cooking is—then it arouses the mind and stimulates desire. It becomes that word everyone associates with oysters and Spanish fly: aphrodisiac—a name taken from the Greek goddess of love, Aphrodite (Cupid's mom). Sensual cooking goes beyond entrées that include exotic ingredients. Sexy eating has a lot to do as well with folklore and reputation. For example, you may have heard that there is a chemical compound in chocolate that makes your brain think it's in love. Believe it or not, there is some scientific research to support this (and heck, even if it's not for real, placebos can be both delicious and powerful). Even more studies point to responsible, healthy, and vigorous sex as good for female reproductive health, your man's heart, the sense of smell, positive hormone surges, and emotional well-being. This chapter explores the benefits of erotic exercise, enticing edibles, and the history of Valentine's Day–worthy foods that ought to be served, to any and all your loved ones, 365 days a year.

Ask Dr. Moon

The doctor is in to answer your questions.

This Q&A session highlights the amazing benefits a healthy sex life brings to bear. It proves also, proverbial though it may be, that the birds and the bees aren't for the sake of reproduction alone. There are many dimensions to sexual healing, all of which will have you singing along with Marvin Gaye in no time.

Q: Which of the five senses is particularly aroused after sex?

A: That would be your sense of smell. After sex, the production of the hormone prolactin surges. This in turn causes stem cells in the brain to stimulate neurons in the brain's olfactory bulb, its smell center. Prolactin is a hormone secreted by the pituitary gland. It stimulates lactation (milk production). It also plays an essential role in maintaining the immune system.

Q: Are there any other "hormone surges" sex can help us look forward to?

A: Yes. Sex causes increased production of oxytocin. Before orgasm, oxytocin, which is released in the brain, surges up to five times the normal level, resulting in the release of endorphins—our natural pain-killing hormones. This makes sex a terrific antidote for menstrual cramping, migraines, arthritis, and other general aches and pains.

Q: Is it true that a healthy sex life reduces the risk of heart disease?

A: This particular question isn't so much for the ladies as it is for the men in their lives. Since sexual activity increases the heart rate for twenty minutes or more, it stands to reason that having sex three or more times a week can be just the type of healthy workout your partner needs. In fact, studies suggest that men who have sex several times a week reduced their risk of heart attack or stroke by half! In England, British researchers looked at 900 middle-aged men and found that the sexually active ones had a lower risk of heart attack over the course of 10 years. The study was published in 2002 in the *Journal of Epidemiology and Community Health*, leaving me to surmise that the men's cardiovascular improvement was either affected by the sex itself and/or since physically fit men (usually) have regular sex, their heart attack risk was low to begin with, a point that brings up the following well-documented fact: cases of erectile dysfunction are far more prevalent in obese men than in those who maintain a healthy weight.

Q: Does sex burn calories?

A: Sure. Sex, if nothing else, is exercise. It improves circulation quality, flexibility, and contracts the muscles in the arms, legs, and abdomen at orgasm. The pulse rate, in a person aroused, rises from about 70 beats per minute to 150, the same as that of an athlete putting forth maximum effort. Since nobody sustains that for the same length of time as, say, running up a steep incline on a treadmill, sex shouldn't replace weekly exercise, but it makes one heck of a supplement, burning up to 7,500 extra calories a year!

Q: Is sex good for battling depression?

A: The phrase "love conquers all" may as well include "especially depression." Sex benefits both parties in a loving relationship with naturally occurring mood boosters (endorphin highs). For women, a surge of oxytocin increases estrogen production, which, in addition to promoting feelings of affection, also helps maintain the health of endometrial linings and reproductive organs. In men, sex encourages the flow of testosterone, which strengthens bones and muscles. In both genders, an active, healthy sex life can moderate cholesterol levels and coat the skin in glowing perspiration that helps cleanse and exfoliate.

Q: What can sex do for the common cold?

A: In a word: MUCH. Wilkes University in Pennsylvania found that individuals who have sex once or twice a week show 30 percent higher levels of an antibody called immunoglobulin A, which is known to boost the immune system.

Q: What are Kegel exercises?

A: Experiencing orgasm strengthens the pelvic floor muscles, which improves bladder control. Ever heard of Kegel exercises? You do them, whether you know it or not, every time you stop and start the flow of urine. The same set of muscles is worked during sex. Sexperts report that performing Kegel exercises on a daily basis can improve the duration and intensity of orgasm. Here's how to do them. Contract your muscles strongly (do not strain by bearing down), hold for five to 10 seconds (keep breathing), rest, then repeat several times. Perform this a few times a day (each trip to the bathroom is as good a time as any).

Q: What is the history of aphrodisiacs and how do they work?

A: Originally, aphrodisiacs were sought out as a remedy for sexual hang-ups and a need to increase fertility. These "foods of love" were chosen on the basis of their shape and whether or not they resembled certain aspects of the male and/or female genitalia. As millennia passed, identifying vitamins and minerals in foods and how they interact with our chemistry pinpointed which foods actually increase our libidos. Some of the ancient beliefs endured and others were dispelled as myths. Popular aphrodisiacs, ones that have withstood the test of time, include garlic, mint, rosemary, sage, and thyme, which have been added to cooking, incense, massage oils, and aromatherapy.

Q: Are there foods that improve your libido?

A: Yes. Foods such as whole grains, beef, and particularly oysters are considered aphrodisiacs because they're high in zinc. Zinc is vital for the production of hormones, particularly prostaglandin, the chemical that regulates the growth and functioning of the sex organs.

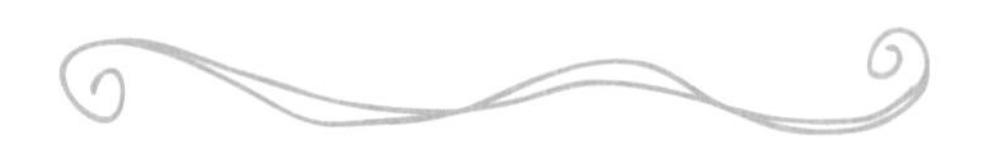

Q: What nutrients play a role in an improved sex life?

A: Vitamin E is essential for reproduction, so get plenty of leafy green veggies in your diet, making sure to include sulfur-rich ones like onions and leeks as well. These keep your sexual drive in healthy check. But don't stop with plain old salad. You'll want to decorate it with iodine-infused food, like shrimp. Iodine is needed by the thyroid gland to regulate energy and maintain the body's every function—including sex. Vitamin B_3 (niacin) increases healthy blood flow to the skin and other parts of the body. Lack of it and vitamin C have been linked to male infertility. Beta-carotene, selenium, and other antioxidants help maintain a healthy sperm count. In other words, saturated fats and simple carbohydrates are mood killers, but fresh, wholesome foods help bring back (and keep!) your mojo. Now, isn't that what we've been saying all along?!

Jorj's Seductive Glam Kitchen

If ever there was a time to roast meats in garlic, bury an entrée in arugula, stuff crabs with avocado, or sauté pine nuts until somebody's in love, it's when you're looking to stack your gorgeous meal plan with aphrodisiacal fare. The foods in this section pack a two-fold punch—both visual and fragrant. They look a certain way (you eat with your eyes first), and they smell *heavenly*. Some of the fruits, veggies, and spices used here feature an ancient past, going down in sensual history as mood enhancers that increase the likelihood of fertility—not to mention sky rocketing one's sexual appeal. Cooking the right way rewards all five senses, bewitching both palate and plate.

Exotic Aphrodisiacal Fare

There's such mythological appeal to the stories behind aphrodisiacs, particularly those of the fruit variety. The pomegranate, for instance, was what lured Persephone into the underworld and created, at least according to ancient Greek folklore, summer, spring, winter, and fall. In real life, the pomegranate hails from northern India and has been cultivated all over the Mediterranean for centuries. In the United States, this "Lebanese love fruit" is grown in California and Arizona; some may recognize its ruby red seeds from reading about it in the *Kama Sutra*.

Mucho Mojo

The Far East is no stranger to sensual fruit. The lychee tree, springing up all over China, Vietnam, and Indonesia, is rich in vitamin C and other healthy minerals one can associate with mucho mojo. Since its texture is similar to that of a grape, with a sweet and fleshy white translucent skin that's heaven to taste, it's no wonder the lychee has inspired Hawaiian growers in the continental U.S. and cultivators in California to plant its seeds, which by the way, you should be wary of: DO NOT EAT the single brown (and slightly poisonous) seed inside a lychee fruit.

The Enduring Classics . . . or What's a Heaven For?

The best way to present the enduring classics is in alphabetical order. Each "short n' sweet" definition is accompanied by a juicy anecdotal tidbit. Make sure your pantry features some (preferably all!) of the items from this abridged Dictionary of Aphrodisiacs.

A is for

Aniseed—Used as an aphrodisiac since the Greeks and the Romans, who believed aniseed had special powers. Sucking on the seeds is said to increase your desire.

Asparagus—Given its phallic shape, asparagus is frequently enjoyed as an aphrodisiac. The Vegetarian Society suggests "eating asparagus for three days for a most powerful effect."

Almond—The scent of almonds is thought to induce passion in the female.

Arugula—Popular since the first century A.D., this ingredient was added to grated orchid bulbs and parsnips and also combined with pine nuts and pistachios. Arugula greens are frequently used in salads and pasta.

Avocado—The Aztecs called the avocado tree "Ahuacuatl," which, translated, means "testicle tree."

B is for

Bananas—The banana flower has a painfully obvious phallic shape and is rich in potassium and B vitamins—necessary for the production of sex hormones.

Sweet Basil—Is said to boost fertility and lift libido. It is also said to produce a general sense of well-being for body and mind.

C is for

Cardamom—Popular in India and in Arabic cultures, cardamom used to be employed by the Chinese court to ensure nice breath.

Carrots—The phallus-shaped carrot has been associated with a male's sexual stimulation and was used by early Middle Eastern royalty to aid seduction.

Chocolate—Contains chemicals thought to affect neurotransmitters in the brain that heighten energy.

Cloves—Contains eugenol (also found in cinnamon), which is a pleasant-smelling chemical compound that is pale yellow, oily, and used in perfumeries, essential oils, flavorings, and even antiseptics. Because cloves smell so fragrant and are so aromatic, they have long been considered a stimulant of sexual feelings.

Coffee—Stimulates both the body and the mind.

Cilantro Seed—*The Arabian Nights* tells a tale of a merchant who had been childless for over 30 years but was cured by a mixture containing cilantro.

D is for

Durian—This is a thorny fruit whose sweet, custard-like flesh emits a strong and sensual odor. Not everyone is a fan, however. While some find the durian's unique scent appealing, others regard it as a stench. In fact, there are public areas in Singapore that strictly prohibit durians. The fruit can't be all bad if it has been used, over the years, in milkshakes, cakes, cappuccino, and ice cream.

F is for

Figs—An open fig is thought to resemble the female sex organs and is traditionally thought of as a sexual stimulant.

G is for

Garlic—Has been used for centuries to cure everything from the common cold to heart ailments. Make sure that you *and* your lover enjoy it at the same meal.

Ginger—Ginger root, raw, cooked, or crystallized, is a stimulant to the circulatory system. Ginger contains gingerols, zingiberene, and other characteristic agents that have made it a favored seductive flavor in Asiatic and Arabic herbal traditions.

H is for

Honey—Many medicines in Egyptian times were based on honey, including cures for sterility and impotence. Medieval seducers plied their partners with mead, a fermented drink made from honey.

M is for

Mustard—Believed to stimulate the sexual glands and increase desire.

Mangosteen—Each of these fruits can be easily divided into five perfect sections. They are said to melt in your mouth. The taste is comparable to a fat, juicy apple. Because fruit flies present a risk to U.S. growers of mangosteen, it can only be procured on your Hawaiian or Asian travels.

N is for

Nutmeg—Nutmeg was highly prized by Chinese women as an aphrodisiac. In great quantity, an overpowering aroma of nutmeg is said to produce a hallucinogenic effect because nutmeg contains myristicin and similar compounds that are related to mescalin. In smaller amounts they are traditional aphrodisiacs.

O is for

Oysters—Perhaps the most famous aphrodisiac, no higher concentration of zinc exists in a single food than in the oyster. Zinc is the most important mineral for the health of the reproductive organs.

P is for

Pepper—Piperine is found in pepper. According to ancient beliefs, this pungent agent can stimulate sexual function.

Pine Nuts—Zinc is a key mineral necessary to maintain male potency, and pine nuts are rich in it. They're predominantly thought of as an aphrodisiac in the Mediterranean.

Pineapple—Rich in vitamin C, it is used in the homeopathic treatment for impotence.

S is for

Saffron—Contains picrocrocin, which is alleged to have the ability to cause erotic sensations.

Spanish Fly—The crushed and powdered body of the emerald-green blister beetle is considered to be an aphrodisiac. When the dried and crushed body of the beetle makes contact with the skin, it causes swelling and blistering—and, some men hoped, swelling of the penis) It was believed that, if slipped into the drink of a lady, it would arouse the desire for sex. The cocktail "Spanish Fly" does not contain any crushed beetles, just a mix of tequila and cinnamon.

T is for

Truffles—The Greeks and the Romans considered the rare truffle to be an aphrodisiac. Truffles produce chemicals similar to sex hormones. These underground fungi have been proven to turn women on. Female pigs become sexually excited at the musty, chemical smell of truffles, which is why sows are used to find them (to female pigs, the smell is the same as that of a hog's breath). In laboratory tests on women, photographs of men were considered sexier when the aroma of truffles was secretly released into the room.

V is for

Vanilla—The scent and flavor of vanilla is believed to increase lust.

W is for

Walnuts—A sign of fertility in Italy.

Wine—Relaxes and helps to stimulate our senses.

Start Your Day

Main Plates

On the Side

Snacks & Sweets

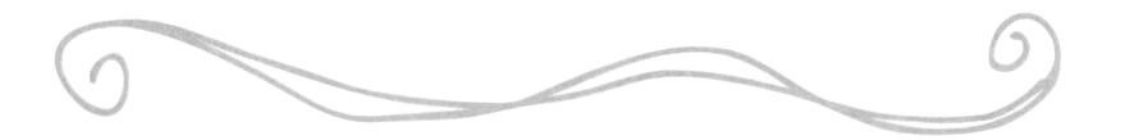

VERY SEXY SCRAMBLED EGGS

With Caviar and Peppered Strawberries

Every mouthful of this rich, creamy treat screams sexy. Eat slowly and savor every bite.

Makes 2 servings
Prep Time: 10 minutes
Cook Time: 5 minutes

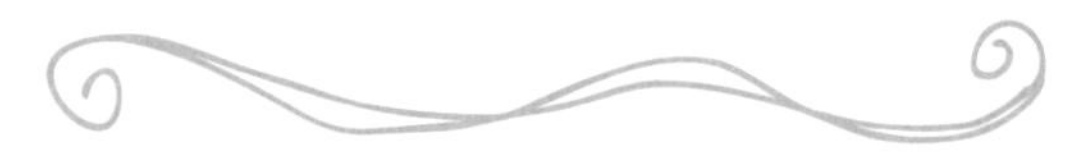

Cooking the eggs over low heat and stirring gently will produce eggs that are WET AND SOFT—the perfect consistency for this dish.

- 4 large eggs
- 4 tablespoons heavy cream
- 2 tablespoons chopped fresh chives
- 1/4 teaspoon truffle oil
- 1 tablespoon butter
- Freshly ground pepper
- 2 very thin slices pumpernickel bread, toasted
- 2 teaspoons caviar (for garnish)
- 1 tablespoon crème fraîche or sour cream (for garnish)
- 2 very large strawberries (for garnish)

Gently whisk together the eggs, cream, chives, and truffle oil. Heat the butter in a skillet over medium-low heat until melted. Pour the egg mixture into the skillet. Stir gently until the eggs are set, but still very soft, about 4–5 minutes. Season with fresh pepper.

To serve, place the toast slices onto 2 plates. Spoon the eggs over top. Garnish with a teaspoon of caviar and a dollop of crème fraîche. Dip the cut side of the strawberries into cracked black pepper and serve on the plate as an additional garnish.

CINNAMON CHOCOLATE-CHIP PANCAKES

With Whipped Cream and Warm Maple Syrup

For a late-night splurge or a morning-after indulgence, you can't beat this sweet-tasting dish.

Makes 4 servings
Prep Time: 15 minutes
Cook Time: 10 minutes

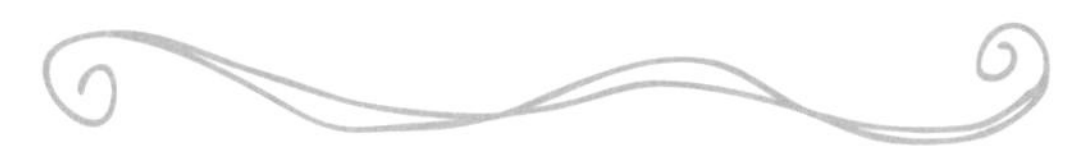

In case that can of ready-to-use WHIPPED CREAM has found another use and disappeared from your fridge, prepare your own by whipping cold, heavy cream using an electric mixer. Add in some confectioners' sugar and make sure the beaters and bowl are cold.

* * *

If you are really feeling decadent, add a drizzle of hot fudge sauce (page 395) to these pancakes.

- 2 cups unbleached all-purpose flour
- 2 tablespoons natural sugar
- 1 teaspoon baking powder
- 1 teaspoon ground cinnamon
- 1/2 teaspoon ground nutmeg
- 2 cups milk
- 2 large eggs
- 1 teaspoon vanilla
- 4 tablespoons butter, melted (1/2 stick)
- 1/2 cup semisweet chocolate chips
- Whipped cream
- Maple syrup

In a small bowl whisk together the flour, sugar, baking powder, cinnamon, and nutmeg. In a large bowl stir together the milk, eggs, vanilla, and butter. Stir the flour mixture into the wet ingredients. Fold in the chocolate chips.

Heat a griddle over medium-high heat. Coat with vegetable oil spray. Pour ¼ cup batter for each pancake onto the hot griddle. Cook until the tops bubble, about 2 minutes. Carefully turn and cook until golden on the second side, about 2 minutes more.

To serve, top each pancake with a dollop of whipped cream and a drizzle of warm maple syrup.

EGG, SAUSAGE, AND SPINACH SKILLETS

You need not run to your favorite diner for a satisfying breakfast meal. Instead, prepare these skillets in advance and bake while you sip coffee and read the paper—in bed!

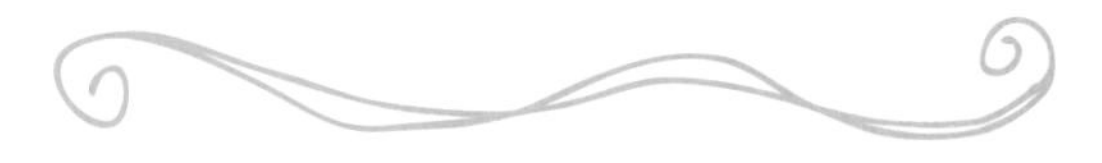

PHYLLO DOUGH makes a whimsical topping for this dish. You will find it in the frozen section of your grocery store. Thaw what you need in the refrigerator. The remaining sheets will keep in the freezer for several months.

Brown the sausage in a large skillet over medium-high heat. Use a slotted spoon to transfer the cooked sausage to a large bowl. Discard any fat remaining in the skillet. Heat the olive oil in the skillet over medium-high heat. Add the onion and the bell pepper and cook until soft, about 5 minutes. Add the garlic and cook 2 minutes more. Stir in the spinach and cook until wilted, about 5 minutes. Cool to room temperature.

Preheat the oven to 375 degrees. Pour the spinach mixture into the bowl with the sausage and toss. Whisk together the eggs. Stir the eggs and cheese into the bowl. Season with salt and pepper. Spoon the egg mixture into 4 or 6 individual skillets, casserole dishes, or ramekins.

Place the phyllo dough strips into a bowl. Toss with canola oil, paprika, and nutmeg. Mound the top of each casserole with phyllo dough pieces. Place the casseroles onto rimmed baking sheets. Bake until the eggs are cooked through and the topping is golden, about 20–30 minutes.

On Shopping Day: Prepare the casseroles, cover, and refrigerate for up to 2 days.

Makes 4 to 6 servings
Prep Time: 15 minutes
Cook Time: 20 to 30 minutes

For the filling

- 1 pound Italian sausage
- 1 tablespoon olive oil
- 1 large white onion, peeled and diced (about 1 cup)
- 1 large yellow bell pepper, seeded and diced (about 1 cup)
- 2 medium cloves garlic, minced (about 1 teaspoon)
- 3 4-ounce bags fresh spinach leaves, washed, dried and chopped (about 3 cups)
- 4 large eggs
- 4 ounces Gruyère cheese, shredded (about 1 cup)
- Salt and freshly ground pepper

For the topping

- 8 ounces frozen phyllo dough sheets, cut into thin strips
- 1/4 cup canola oil
- 1/2 teaspoon paprika
- 1/4 teaspoon nutmeg

BAKED RASPBERRY-STUFFED FRENCH TOAST

With Pecans and Maple Drizzle

Bake this dish for a leisurely weekend brunch and invite the pals to drop by and graze. The rest of the day belongs to the two of you.

Makes 8 servings
Prep Time: 10 minutes
Cook Time: 35 to 40 minutes

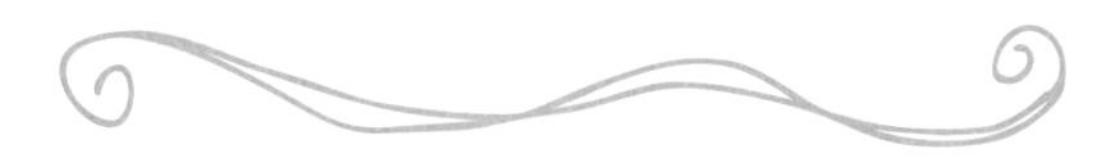

This is a sweet dish that is sure to get your sugar rush off to a BIG start. You can reduce the amount of sugar in the dish by using fresh, mashed fruit in place of the sweeter preserves.

- 1 12-ounce whole grain (French bread–style) loaf, cut into 16 (1/2-inch) slices
- 3/4 cup raspberry preserves
- 2 cups reduced-fat milk
- 5 large eggs
- 1 tablespoon vanilla extract
- 1/4 teaspoon ground cinnamon
- 1/4 teaspoon ground nutmeg
- 1/4 cup pecans, chopped
- 1/2 cup pure maple syrup
- Confectioners' sugar
- Fresh raspberries

Preheat the oven to 350 degrees. Place half of the bread slices into a large baking dish that has been coated with vegetable oil spray. Spread the raspberry preserves over the top half of the bread slices. Top with the remaining bread slices.

Whisk together the milk, eggs, vanilla, cinnamon, and nutmeg. Pour this mixture over the bread, allowing the bread to soak in the sauce. Sprinkle the pecans over the top. Cover the dish with aluminum foil. Bake for 15–20 minutes and remove the foil. Bake until the top is golden, about 15–20 minutes more. Remove from the oven. Drizzle with maple syrup. Let cool 5 minutes.

To serve, sprinkle with confectioners' sugar. Cut into 8 squares. Serve each with fresh raspberries.

GRILLED LOBSTER TAILS

With Parsley Butter Served Over Creamy Hash

The hash is a rich blend of diced potatoes and the veggies you would find in a creamy succotash. It is the perfect accompaniment for the grilled, buttery lobster.

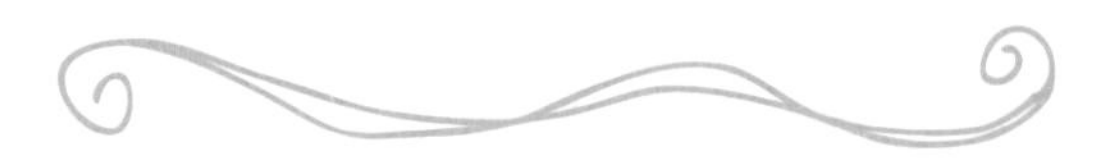

Leftover veggies would be perfect in this hash recipe. If lobster is not in your budget, substitute SHRIMP or TILAPIA. There might be enough savings for a sexy splurge.

On Shopping Day: Prepare the veggies for the hash. Store separately in an airtight container in the refrigerator for up to 3 days.

Makes 4 servings
Prep Time: 20 minutes
Cook Time: 20 minutes

For the hash

- 2 slices thick bacon, diced
- 1 small white onion, finely diced (about 1/2 cup)
- 4–6 2-inch red creamer potatoes, diced
- 1 medium red bell pepper, seeded and finely diced
- 1/4 cup chicken stock or low-sodium chicken broth
- 1/4 cup cream
- 1 cup frozen lima beans, thawed
- 1 cup frozen corn kernels, thawed
- Salt and freshly ground pepper
- 2–4 drops hot pepper sauce
- 1 tablespoon chopped fresh thyme

For the lobster

- 4 6- to 8-ounce lobster tails split in half
- Juice of 1 medium lemon (about 2 tablespoons)
- 4 tablespoons butter
- 2 tablespoons chopped fresh parsley

Cook the bacon in a skillet over medium-high heat. Add the onion, potatoes, and bell pepper. Cook until crisp, about 5 minutes. Pour in the chicken stock. Reduce the heat to medium and cook until the potatoes are soft, about 5–8 minutes. Pour in the cream and simmer until the sauce thickens. Stir in the lima beans and corn. Season with salt, pepper, and hot pepper sauce. Stir in fresh thyme. Keep the hash warm.

Heat a grill pan over medium-high heat. Season the lobster flesh with salt, pepper and lemon juice. Grill the lobster, flesh-side down, until the shells begin to turn pink, about 5 minutes. Turn and continue cooking until the lobster is cooked through, about 3 to 4 minutes more.

Melt the butter over medium-low heat. Stir in the parsley.

To serve, spoon the creamy hash onto a serving platter. Top with grilled lobster. Pour the parsley butter over the shellfish.

ORGASMIC BRAISED RIBS

With Chili and Chocolate

A hint of chocolate and a whiff of spice make this braising sauce irresistible. But then isn't everything better with chocolate?

You can prepare this dish in your slow cooker. Prepare as directed. Pour the sauce into the slow cooker. Submerge the browned ribs into the sauce and cook on medium all day. When you are ready to serve, transfer the ribs to a platter. Pour the sauce into a pot and simmer until thickened.

* * *

The secret to moist, FALL-OFF-THE-BONE ribs is to slowly simmer the dish for a long time. Don't try to rush through this; the result will not be as satisfying.

Cook the bacon in a Dutch oven with lid (or deep skillet with lid) over medium-high heat until crisp. Use a slotted spoon to remove and drain on paper towels. Season the short ribs with salt and pepper. Sear the ribs in the Dutch oven, turning to brown all sides, about 6 minutes. Transfer the ribs to a platter.

Stir in the onion, celery, carrots, and garlic. Cook until soft and just beginning to brown, about 5 minutes. Pour in the wine. Cook until most of the liquid disappears, about 6–8 minutes. Stir in the tomatoes and the beef stock. Stir in the chili powder and cocoa powder. Place the bacon and the short ribs back into the Dutch oven. Bring to a boil; reduce the heat to medium-low and slowly simmer for at least 90 minutes. (Alternatively, you can place the Dutch oven in a 325-degree oven to slowly simmer.)

Remove the lid and slowly simmer until the sauce thickens and the meat falls from the bone, about 30 minutes more. Transfer the short ribs to a platter. Bring the sauce to a boil, add the cornstarch, and simmer until very thick, about 10 minutes.

To serve, place the ribs on a serving dish. Ladle the sauce over the top. Serve with rice, pasta, or mashed potatoes.

On Shopping Day: Prepare the veggies, store in an airtight container for up to 4 days.

Makes 4 to 6 servings
Prep Time: 20 minutes
Cook Time: 3 hours

4 ounces thick bacon (about 3–4 strips)
8 meaty beef short ribs, about 4 pounds
Salt and freshly ground pepper
1 medium yellow onion, peeled and diced into ½-inch squares (about 1 cup)
2 medium celery ribs, diced (about 1 cup)
2 large carrots, diced (about 1 cup)
3 medium garlic cloves, minced (about 1½ teaspoons)
2 cups red wine (try a good Chianti)
1 28-ounce can diced tomatoes
2 cups homemade beef stock or low-sodium beef broth
1 tablespoon chili powder
1 tablespoon unsweetened cocoa powder
1 teaspoon cornstarch mixed with 1 tablespoon cold water

BUTTERNUT SQUASH RAVIOLI

With Brown Butter, Sage, and Pine Nut Sauce

When you desire a bite of something rich and delicious, this dish fills the bill. For an extra touch of decadence, add curls of shaved dark chocolate on top of the ravioli. Your lover won't know what hit him!

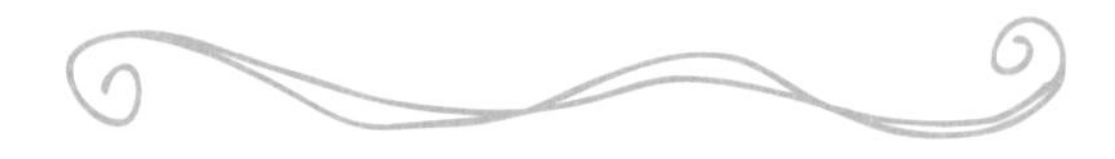

Preheat the oven to 400 degrees.

Place the squash cubes on a baking sheet that has been coated with vegetable oil spray. Generously sprinkle with chili powder, garlic powder, onion powder, dark brown sugar, ground cumin, ground cinnamon, and ground nutmeg and drizzle with olive oil. Roast until the squash just begins to turn brown and is soft, about 15–20 minutes. Remove from the oven and cool to room temperature.

Place the squash into the bowl of a food processor. Add ricotta cheese, Parmesan cheese, 2 beaten eggs and 2 tablespoons fresh sage leaves. Pulse to combine. Season with salt and pepper.

Lay 6 wonton wrappers onto your work surface. Brush the out edges of the squares with egg wash. Place a generous teaspoonful of the filling into the center of each square. Fold over the corners to form a triangle and press down to make sure that the filling is evenly placed inside. Use the tines of a fork to seal the raviolis completely. Place onto a baking sheet lined with parchment paper. Continue until all of the wonton wrappers have been used.

(Note: You can reserve extra filling by storing in an airtight container. Use to stuff shells or as a filling for manicotti.)

Bring a pot of water to boil over high heat. Add salt. Drop the ravioli (in batches) into the water and cook for 2–3 minutes. Use a slotted spoon to remove and place into a serving bowl.

Heat the butter in a skillet over high heat until just beginning to brown (watch carefully so the butter doesn't burn—adjust the heat if necessary). Stir in chopped sage and pine nuts.

To serve, pour the sauce over the ravioli. Garnish with shaved Parmesan cheese and freshly ground pepper.

Makes 6 servings
Prep Time: 30 minutes
Cook Time: 6 to 8 minutes

For the squash

- 2 large butternut squash, peeled and diced into 1-inch squares (about 6 cups)
- 2 tablespoons chili powder
- 1 tablespoon garlic powder
- 1 tablespoon onion powder
- 1 tablespoon dark brown sugar
- 2 teaspoons ground cumin
- 1 teaspoon ground cinnamon
- ½ teaspoon ground nutmeg
- 2 tablespoons olive oil

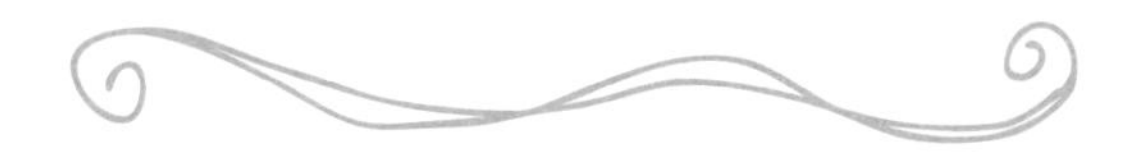

For the filling

- 1 15-ounce container reduced-fat ricotta cheese
- 4 ounces grated Parmesan cheese (about 1 cup)
- 2 large eggs, beaten
- 2 tablespoons fresh sage leaves
- Salt and freshly ground pepper

For the ravioli

- 36 wonton wrappers
- 1 large egg, beaten with 2 tablespoons cold water

For the sauce

- 1 cup unsalted butter, room temperature (2 sticks)
- 2 tablespoons chopped fresh sage leaves
- ½ cup pine nuts
- Parmesan Cheese, shaved (for garnish)

ROASTED BEEF TENDERLOIN STEAKS STUFFED WITH SPINACH AND GORGONZOLA

With Béarnaise Sauce

Okay, this is rich, and delicious and sinful and did I mention rich? Oh, what we do for love. . . .

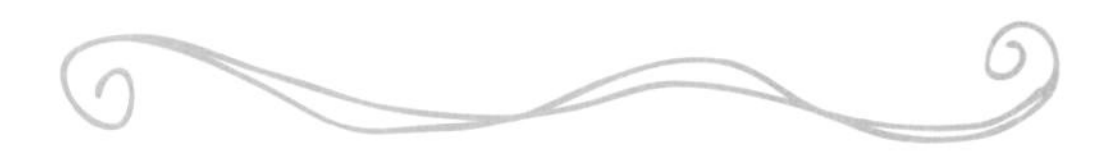

Don't let the Béarnaise sauce trip you up. If it ends up a little thick, just add water. If the eggs cook too quickly and begin to scramble, run the sauce through a blender. KEEP QUIET about it and he'll never know!

Heat the wine, shallots, tarragon, and lemon juice in a sauce pan over medium-high heat until the mixture boils. Reduce the heat to medium and simmer until the liquid is reduced to 2 tablespoons, about 5 minutes. Reduce the heat to medium low. Whisk the butter into the reduced sauce, adding a few pieces at a time. Strain this mixture through a sieve and return to the pan. Whisk in the egg yolks until the sauce is just thickened, about 2–4 minutes. Remove the pan from the heat. Whisk in the Worcestershire sauce and hot pepper sauce. Cover the pot to keep the sauce warm.

Heat 1 tablespoon olive oil in a skillet over medium-high heat. Add the shallots and cook until soft, about 2 minutes. Add the spinach and cook until wilted. Add the sherry and season with salt and pepper. Cook until the liquid disappears, about 2 minutes more. Remove the skillet from the heat. Stir in the Gorgonzola cheese and rosemary.

Preheat the oven to 400 degrees. Season the tenderloins with salt and pepper. Heat a skillet over medium-high heat. Sear the steaks until browned, about 2 minutes. Turn and sear on the second side until browned, about 2 minutes more. Transfer the steaks to a baking dish. Divide the spinach mixture among the 4 steaks and mound the filling on the top of each. Roast the steaks in the oven until medium rare, about 10 minutes (a thermometer should reach an internal temperature of 140 degrees).

To serve, place the steaks onto dinner plates. Spoon the sauce around the steak.

Makes 4 servings
Prep Time: 30 minutes
Cook Time: 10 minutes for sauce, 10 minutes for the filling, 20 minutes for tenderloins

For the Béarnaise sauce

- 1/2 cup white wine
- 2 large shallots, minced (about 2 tablespoons)
- 1 tablespoon chopped fresh tarragon
- Juice of 1/2 medium lemon (about 1 tablespoon)
- 12 tablespoons unsalted butter, cut into pieces
- 3 large egg yolks mixed with 2 tablespoons water
- 1/4 teaspoon Worcestershire sauce
- 2 drops hot pepper sauce

For the tenderloin

- 1 tablespoon olive oil
- 2 large shallots, minced (about 2 tablespoons)

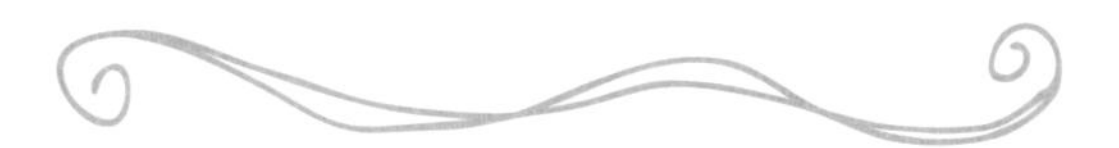

- 6 ounces fresh spinach leaves, washed, dried, and chopped (about 4 cups)
- 2 tablespoons sherry
- Salt and freshly ground pepper
- 2 ounces Gorgonzola cheese, crumbled (about $^1/_2$ cup)
- 1 tablespoon chopped fresh rosemary
- 4 6-ounce 2-inch-thick tenderloin steaks

SALTIMBOCCA

"Saltimbocca" means "jump-in-the-mouth"—in other words, irresistible! You and the dish. . . .

Makes 4 servings
Prep Time: 10 minutes
Cook Time: 10 minutes

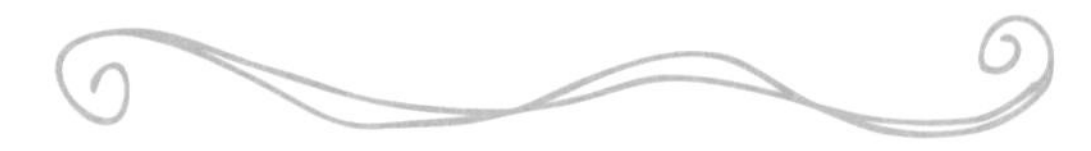

Save time by asking your butcher to POUND the veal for you (unless you need to revisit the "reduce stress" chapter).

- 1 pound veal scaloppini
- Salt and freshly ground pepper
- 4 ounces prosciutto, thinly sliced
- 2 tablespoons olive oil
- 2 tablespoons butter, plus 1 tablespoon for the sauce
- 1 cup white wine
- 2 tablespoons chopped fresh sage, plus garnish
- Lemon slices (for garnish)

Use a meat mallet to pound the veal to ¼-inch thickness. Season with salt and pepper. Top each piece with a slice of prosciutto. Heat 1 tablespoon olive oil and 1 tablespoon butter in a skillet over medium-high heat. Cook the veal, prosciutto side down, in the skillet until golden, about 2 minutes. Carefully turn, keeping the prosciutto in place and continue cooking until golden on the second side, about 2 minutes more. (Repeat using additional butter and oil as needed for all of the veal.) Transfer the veal to a platter and keep warm.

Pour the wine into the pan. Stir up any brown bits and reduce to about ½ cup. Stir in the sage. Remove from the heat and swirl in the last tablespoon of butter.

To serve, spoon the sauce over the scaloppini. Garnish with lemon slices and whole sage leaves.

CHICKEN WINGS

With Mole Sauce

This rich sauce has all of the seeds of love—and plenty of heat as well. Traditionally the dish is prepared with turkey wings. This version uses chicken wings, but anything tastes good in this sauce!

Traditional MOLE sauce is prepared using several different types of dried chilies and almonds and tortillas ground up in the sauce. This version takes some liberties—but, hey, what's fair in love and . . .

Heat the olive oil in a large skillet over medium-high heat. Add the onions and cook until soft, about 5 minutes. Place the coriander and aniseed into the bowl of a food processor or spice grinder. Pulse to crush. Stir this into the onions. Stir in the chili powder, sugar, cinnamon, and cloves and cook for 1 minute. Stir in the cocoa powder, peanut butter, chicken stock, tomatoes, raisins, and garlic and season with salt and pepper. Simmer the sauce over medium-low heat about 5–10 minutes.

Preheat the oven to broil. Cut the tips from the wings and discard (or reserve to make stock). Cut the wings into 2 pieces. Place onto a rimmed baking sheet that has been coated with vegetable oil. Season with salt and pepper. Broil until golden, about 10 minutes. Turn and broil until golden on the second side, about 10 minutes more.

Pour the sauce into the bowl of a food processor and pulse to emulsify. If the sauce is too thick, add additional chicken broth. Return the sauce to the skillet. Add the chicken wings to the sauce and simmer until cooked through, about 20 minutes.

To serve, pour the chicken wings and sauce over cooked rice. Garnish with sesame seeds and fresh cilantro.

On Shopping Day: Prepare the sauce and cool to room temperature. Store in an airtight container in the refrigerator for up to 5 days.

Makes 4 servings
Prep Time: 35 minutes
Cook Time: 30 minutes

For the mole sauce

- 3 tablespoons olive oil
- 3 medium yellow onions, peeled and diced (about 3 cups)
- 1/2 teaspoon coriander seeds
- 1/2 teaspoon aniseed
- 3 tablespoons chili powder
- 2 teaspoons natural sugar
- 3/4 teaspoon ground cinnamon
- 1/8 teaspoon ground cloves
- 2 tablespoons unsweetened cocoa powder
- 2 tablespoons peanut butter
- 2 cups homemade chicken stock or low-sodium chicken broth
- 1 16-ounce can diced tomatoes, drained
- 2 tablespoons raisins
- 3 garlic cloves, minced
- Salt and freshly ground pepper

For the chicken

- 10 chicken wings (about 2 pounds)
- Cooked rice
- Sesame seeds (for garnish)
- Chopped fresh cilantro (for garnish)

DUCK BREASTS

With Pinot Noir Red Grape Sauce

This impressive dish can be served at your next intimate dinner party. It's easy, it's fun to prepare, and it's really, really good!

Makes 4 servings
Prep Time: 5 minutes
Cook Time: 30 minutes

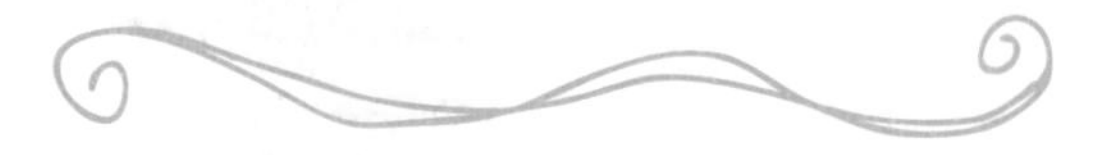

You can purchase frozen duck breasts and store in your freezer for up to 6 months. Defrost in the refrigerator at least 24 hours before cooking the dish.

- 4 6-ounce boned duck breast halves with skin
- 1 tablespoon olive oil
- Salt and freshly ground pepper
- ½ cup Pinot Noir
- 1 cup homemade chicken stock or low-sodium chicken broth
- 2 cups red seedless grapes, cut into halves
- 1 tablespoon prepared chili sauce
- 2 tablespoons butter, chilled
- 2 tablespoons chopped fresh sage, plus garnish

Score the skin of the duck breast with a sharp knife without cutting all the way through. Brush both sides with olive oil. Season with salt and pepper. Heat a skillet over medium-high heat. Place the breasts, skin-side down, into the skillet. Cook until golden, about 6–8 minutes. Turn and cook for 6–8 minutes more. Remove to a platter and keep warm.

Remove any excess fat from the skillet. Pour in the wine and cook for 5 minutes. Pour in the chicken broth and grapes. Cook for 5 minutes more. Stir in the chili sauce. Season with salt and pepper. Remove the pan from the heat and swirl in the butter and sage.

To serve, place the duck breasts onto a serving platter. Pour the sauce over the top. Garnish with additional fresh sage leaves.

GRILLED PORK CHOPS

With Cherry Ginger Chutney

Surprise your special someone with something different in the middle of the week and see what good things follow.

Makes 4 servings (with extra chutney)
Prep Time: 45 to 60 minutes for chutney
Cook Time: 8 to 10 minutes

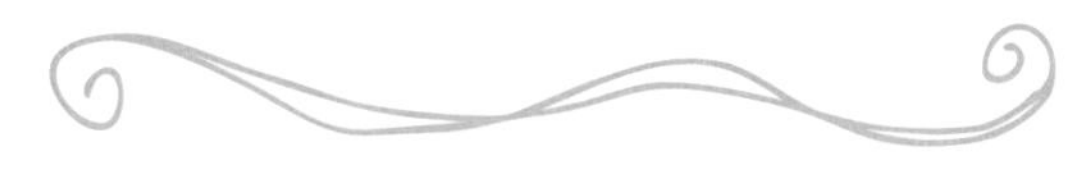

The SWEETER the cherries, the sweeter your chutney will be. Adjust your seasoning as you simmer to make sure that the final product meets your expectations.

* * *

Pitting cherries is one of my kids' favorite things to do. We use a newfangled CHERRY PITTING MACHINE. But you can use the back of a knife and a swift snap of the wrist to accomplish the same results.

For the chutney

- 1 pound cherries, stemmed, pitted, and chopped (about 3 cups)
- 1 cup brown sugar
- 1 medium apple, peeled and finely diced (about 1 cup)
- 1 small red onion, peeled and diced (about $1/2$ cup)
- $1/3$ cup apple cider vinegar
- 1 $1/2$-inch piece ginger, peeled and grated (about 2 teaspoons)
- $1/4$ teaspoon allspice
- $1/4$ teaspoon ground cinnamon
- $1/2$ teaspoon salt
- 2 tablespoons chopped fresh basil

For the pork

- 4 6- to 8-ounce $1\frac{1}{2}$-inch-thick bone-in pork loin chops, trimmed of fat
- Salt and freshly ground pepper

In a saucepan over medium heat place the cherries, brown sugar, apple, onion, cider vinegar, ginger, allspice, cinnamon, and salt. Bring to a boil. Reduce the heat and simmer until the mixture is thick and syrupy, about 45–60 minutes. Stir in the basil for the last 5 minutes.

Heat a grill pan coated with vegetable oil spray over medium-high heat. Season the pork chops with salt and pepper. Grill until the pork chops are seared on one side, about 4–5 minutes. Turn and cook until medium rare, about 5 minutes more.

To serve, spoon the cherry chutney alongside the grilled pork chops.

On Shopping Day: Prepare the chutney. Cool to room temperature. Store in an airtight container in the refrigerator for up to 1 week.

ARUGULA SALAD

With Walnut-Crusted Goat Cheese

Warm, gooey, rich goat cheese is a remarkable contrast with peppery greens and tart vinaigrette dressing in this super-sensual salad.

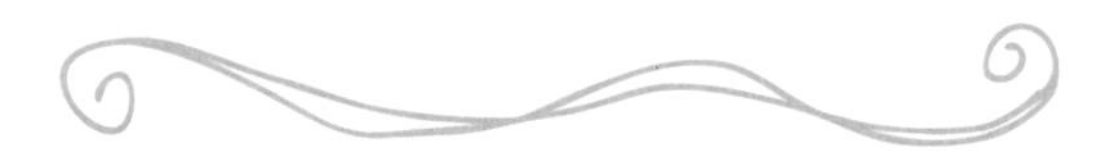

Choose a flavorful, smoky BACON like Applewood for this dish.

Cook the bacon in a skillet over medium-high heat until crisp. Use a slotted spoon to transfer to paper towels to drain.

Place the egg yolk, Dijon mustard, and lemon juice into the bowl of a food processor. Pulse to emulsify. With the machine running, slowly add the olive oil. Season with salt and pepper. Place the mesclun and arugula into a salad bowl. Chill until ready to serve.

Cut the goat cheese into 4 round slices. Place the walnuts into the bowl of a food processor. Pulse to form fine crumbs. Pour the crumbs into a shallow bowl. Place the egg white into a shallow bowl. Heat 1 tablespoon olive oil in a skillet over medium-high heat. Dip the goat cheese slices into the egg white and then into the walnut crumbs to coat. Cook in the hot oil until golden, about 20–30 seconds. Carefully turn and cook until golden on the second side, about 20 seconds more.

To serve, toss the greens with enough of the dressing to just lightly coat. Divide the greens among 4 chilled salad plates. Sprinkle bacon over the top. Place one slice of goat cheese on each plate.

On Shopping Day: Prepare the salad dressing and store in an airtight container in the refrigerator for up to 3 days. Prepare the goat cheese through coating. Store in an airtight container in the refrigerator for up to 3 days. Wash and dry the salad greens. Store in a plastic bag in the refrigerator for up to 5 days.

Makes 4 servings, plus extra vinaigrette
Prep Time: 15 minutes
Cook Time: 6 to 8 minutes

For the salad

- 8 ounces thick bacon, diced (about 6–8 strips)
- 1 large egg yolk
- 2 teaspoons Dijon mustard
- Juice of 3 medium lemons (about 1/3 cup)
- 1 cup olive oil
- Salt and freshly ground pepper
- 2 cups mesclun greens, washed and dried
- 2 cups arugula leaves, washed and dried

For the goat cheese

- 1 4-ounce goat cheese log
- 1/2 cup walnut pieces
- 1 large egg white
- 1 tablespoon olive oil

PEEL-AND-EAT JUMBO SHRIMP

With Buffalo-Style Sauce

Oh yeah, baby. This dish is certain to add some spice to your love life. It's messy and hot, hot, hot! Linger over every bite.

Makes 4 servings if you are lingering . . .
Prep Time: 10 minutes
Cook Time: 10 minutes

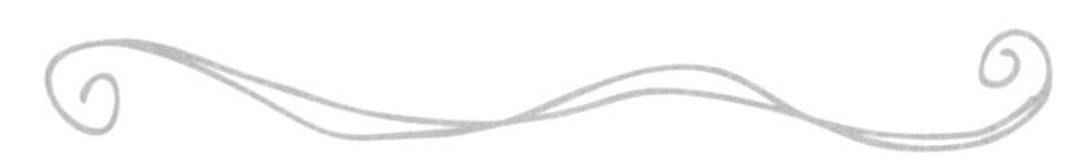

To spruce this dish up for your mother-in-law's visit, peel the shrimp before GRILLING, serve over crisp, grilled French bread slices, and hand her a fork!

For the shrimp

- 2 pounds uncooked jumbo shrimp, deveined, shells on (about 24)
- 2 tablespoons olive oil
- 1 teaspoon paprika
- 1/4 teaspoon ground cardamom
- Salt and freshly ground pepper

For the sauce

- 6 tablespoons unsalted butter, melted
- Juice of 1 medium lemons (about 2 tablespoons)
- 1 tablespoon white wine vinegar
- 2 medium garlic cloves, minced (about 1 teaspoon)
- 1–2 teaspoons hot pepper sauce (or more)
- 2 tablespoons chopped fresh cilantro (for garnish)
- Celery sticks
- Blue Cheese Dip (see page 161)

Toss the shrimp with olive oil, paprika, and cardamom. Season with salt and pepper. Heat a grill pan over medium-high heat. Grill the shrimp, turning once, until pink and opaque, about 4–5 minutes per side.

Heat the butter in a skillet over medium heat. Stir in the lemon juice, vinegar, garlic, and hot pepper sauce.

Add the shrimp to the skillet and coat with sauce.

To serve, transfer the shrimp to a serving bowl. Garnish with fresh cilantro. Use your fingers to peel the shrimp. Deposit shells into another bowl. Serve with blue cheese dip and celery sticks. One for him—one for you. . . .

BAKED OYSTERS

With Pancetta Topping

Choose very fresh, very plump oysters for this dish. Then pick a perfect setting to share with that special someone.

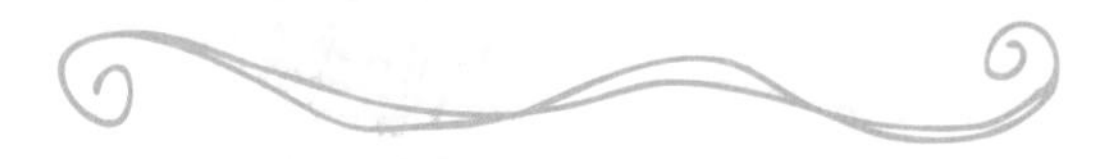

If you are not planning to shuck the oysters yourself, make sure you prepare them very soon after you purchase them from your fishmonger.

On Shopping Day: Prepare the filling. Cool to room temperature. Store in an airtight container in the refrigerator for up to 3 days.

Makes 4 servings
Prep Time: 20 minutes
Cook Time: 25 minutes

- 1 tablespoon unsalted butter
- 1 tablespoon unbleached all-purpose flour
- 1/2 cup half and half
- 2 ounces pancetta, finely diced
- 2 large shallots, minced (about 2 tablespoons)
- 2 medium celery ribs, diced (about 1/2 cup)
- 1 tablespoon sherry
- 1 ounce Gruyère cheese, shredded (about 1/4 cup)
- Salt and freshly ground pepper
- 1 dozen fresh oysters, shucked
- Juice of 1 medium lemon, about 2 tablespoons
- 1/2 cup fresh breadcrumbs
- Lemon slices (for garnish)

Melt the butter in a pot over medium heat. Whisk in the flour until smooth. Pour in the half and half. Simmer this mixture until thickened, about 5 minutes. Remove from the heat.

Heat the pancetta in a small skillet over medium-high heat. Add the shallots and celery. Cook until the pancetta is crisp and the veggies are soft, about 3–4 minutes. Add the sherry and simmer until the liquid is absorbed. Pour the cream mixture into the pancetta mixture. Simmer for 2 minutes. Add the cheese and season with salt and pepper. Bring the filling to room temperature.

Preheat the oven to 450 degrees. Place the oysters onto a rimmed baking sheet. (You can pour a layer of rock salt onto the baking dish to make sure that the oysters lay flat during cooking.) Drizzle with lemon juice. Mound the filling on top of each oyster. Top with breadcrumbs. Bake until the oysters are cooked through and the topping is golden and bubbling, about 10–15 minutes.

To serve, lay the oysters onto a serving platter and garnish with additional lemon slices.

OLIVE, ONION, AND ROASTED PEPPER BRUSCHETTA

The perfect romantic picnic includes a loaf of bread, a bottle of wine, a hunk of cheese, and a container filled with olive tapenade. Well, the latter is taking a little liberty; however, this topping is so good and the ingredients are so sexy that adding this dish makes every picnic a little bit better.

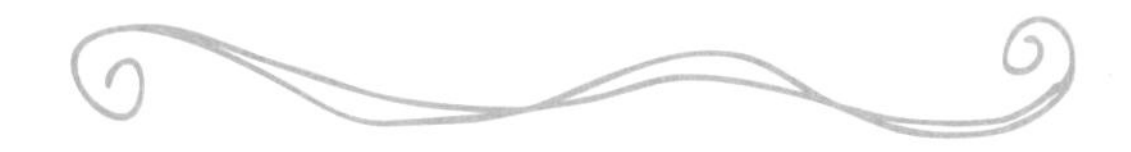

This is an excellent topping for fish or chicken as well as a perfect start for a PASTA SAUCE. There's no end to the foods that this rustic tapenade will flavor.

Makes 4 servings
Prep Time: 15 minutes

For the tapenade

- 1 cup frozen pearl onions, thawed
- 1 jarred roasted red pepper, diced
- 1 jarred roasted yellow pepper, diced
- 1 cup Kalamata olives, pitted and roughly chopped
- 2 large garlic cloves, peeled and minced (about 1 teaspoon)
- 2 tablespoons chopped fresh oregano
- 1 teaspoon crushed red pepper flakes
- ¼ cup olive oil
- ¼ cup red wine vinegar

For the bruschetta

- 1 12-ounce loaf French-style bread, cut into ½-inch slices
- 2 tablespoons olive oil
- 2 teaspoons garlic powder

Place the onions into a microwave-safe bowl with 1 inch of water. Cover and microwave on high for 4–5 minutes. Drain and cut each onion in half. Place the onions into a medium bowl. Add the roasted peppers, olives, garlic, oregano, and red pepper flakes. Pour in the ¼ cup olive oil and the vinegar. Chill in the refrigerator for at least 1 hour.

Preheat the oven to 350 degrees. Place the bread slices onto a rimmed baking sheet that has been coated with vegetable oil spray. Combine the 2 tablespoons olive oil with garlic powder. Brush each bread slice with this mixture. Bake until the bread is golden, about 5–7 minutes.

To serve, remove the tapenade from the refrigerator. Drain off excess liquid. Place into a bowl. Surround with bruschetta.

On Shopping Day: Prepare the tapenade. Store in an airtight container in the refrigerator for up to 3 days.

PEANUT BUTTER CHOCOLATE BARS

When peanut butter meets chocolate, the mouth waters and the senses come alive. These rich bars blend peanut butter shortbread with a rich, brownie-like filling. Oh yum . . .

I like GHIRARDELLI'S 60 percent cocoa BITTERSWEET chocolate bar for this recipe—but feel free to use the best chocolate you can find.

Prepare the chocolate filling by combining the chocolate and butter pieces in a bowl. Melt together by putting the bowl into a microwave on medium-high heat, checking and stirring every 30 seconds. Cool this mixture to room temperature.

In a small bowl whisk together ¾ cup flour, ½ teaspoon baking powder, and ¼ teaspoon salt. Use an electric mixer to combine 2 eggs and ½ cup sugar until this mixture is pale and thick. Stir in 1 teaspoon vanilla. Add the chocolate mixture to the egg and sugar mixture. Mix well. Pour in the flour mixture until just combined. Set aside.

Prepare the peanut butter dough by whisking together 3 cups flour, 1 teaspoon baking powder, and ¼ teaspoon salt in a small bowl. In a large bowl use an electric mixer to combine 1 cup butter, 2 cups peanut butter, and 1½ cups sugar until soft and fluffy. Mix in 2 eggs, one at a time, and 1 teaspoon vanilla. Stir the flour mixture into the peanut butter mixture to form soft dough.

For the bars, preheat the oven to 350 degrees. Coat the bottom of a 9 x 13 x 2-inch baking dish with vegetable oil spray. Line with parchment paper, allowing some paper to overhang. Spray the parchment paper. Pat half of the peanut butter dough into the bottom of the pan. Pour the chocolate mixture over top. Crumble the remaining peanut butter dough over top of the chocolate mixture.

Bake until golden, about 45 minutes. Cool in the pan.

To serve, remove the bars by lifting the parchment paper out of the baking dish. Cut into squares.

Makes 24 cookie bars
Prep Time: 20 minutes
Cook Time: 45 minutes

For the chocolate filling

- 4 ounces bittersweet chocolate, broken into pieces
- ½ cup unsalted butter, room temperature (1 stick), cut into pieces
- ¾ cup unbleached all-purpose flour
- ½ teaspoon baking powder
- ¼ teaspoon salt
- 2 large eggs
- ½ cup natural sugar
- 1 teaspoon vanilla extract

For the peanut butter dough

- 3 cups unbleached all-purpose flour
- 1 teaspoon baking powder
- ¼ teaspoon salt
- 1 cup unsalted butter, room temperature (2 sticks)
- 18 ounces creamy peanut butter, (about 2 cups)
- 1½ cups natural sugar
- 2 large eggs
- 1 teaspoon vanilla extract

INDIVIDUAL BROWNIE CAKES LOADED WITH CHOCOLATE CHUNKS AND WALNUTS

Served with Ice Cream and Hot Fudge Sauce

I know, I know—but this dessert is guaranteed to produce the desired response!

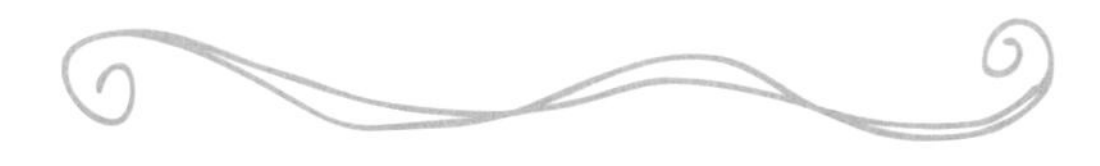

These little cakes are way too scrumptious to keep on hand. Share with your BESTEST FRIENDS and spare yourself the temptation.

Preheat the oven to 350 degrees. Melt the semisweet chocolate and butter together until smooth. (You can use the microwave oven or a double boiler. In either case, melt slowly to prevent burning.) Cool to room temperature. Place the melted chocolate into a bowl. Whisk in the eggs, sugar, vanilla, and salt. Gently stir in the flour until just incorporated. Stir in the chocolate chunks and walnuts. Spoon the batter into a muffin tin with paper liners. Bake until the cakes spring back when touched and a tester inserted into the center comes out clean, about 34–40 minutes. Cool on wire racks.

Heat the corn syrup and chocolate chips in a saucepan over medium heat until smooth. Remove from the heat and stir in the cream. Keep warm.

To serve, split 1 brownie cake in half horizontally. Place the bottom half into a shallow dessert bowl. Top with a scoop of ice cream. Ladle warm sauce over top. Place the top half of the brownie on top. Ladle with extra sauce. Use 2 spoons!

On Shopping Day: Prepare the hot fudge sauce. Cool to room temperature and store in an airtight container for up to 1 week.

Makes 12 mini cakes and about 1½ cups hot fudge sauce
Prep Time: 20 minutes
Cook Time: 40 minutes

For the mini cakes

- 1 11.5-ounce package semisweet chocolate chips (about 2 cups)
- 10 tablespoons unsalted butter
- 4 large eggs
- 3/4 cup natural sugar
- 1 teaspoon pure vanilla extract
- 1/4 teaspoon salt
- 1 cup unbleached all-purpose flour
- 1 cup milk chocolate chunks
- 1 cup chopped walnuts

For the sauce

- 1/4 cup corn syrup
- 1 cup semisweet chocolate chips
- 3/4 cup heavy cream
- Vanilla Ice cream

LEMON VANILLA PUDDING

With Mixed Berries

Refreshing and creamy, this delicious dessert is just what you need for a midnight snack. Serve one with two spoons.

Makes 4 servings
Prep Time: 10 minutes
Cook Time: 10 minutes, plus chilling

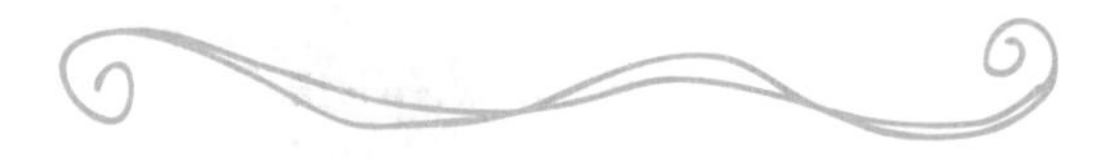

Change the FLAVOR of this dessert by substituting with peach juice, apple juice, or blueberries.

- 3 large egg yolks
- 1/2 cup natural sugar
- 2 tablespoons cornstarch
- Zest of 1 large lemon (about 1 tablespoon)
- 1 teaspoon pure vanilla extract
- 1/4 teaspoon salt
- 1 3/4 cups reduced-fat milk
- Juice of 3 large lemons (1/2 cup)
- 2 cups mixed berries

In a saucepan whisk together the egg yolks, sugar, cornstarch, lemon zest, vanilla, salt, and milk. Whisk until smooth. Place the pan over medium heat and simmer, stirring constantly until thick and pale, about 5–8 minutes. Remove the pan from the heat and whisk in the lemon juice. If the pudding has lumps, strain through a colander. Pour into 4 ramekins and place into the refrigerator for at least 2 hours. (If you are serving later on, cover the pudding with plastic wrap after it has cooled.)

To serve, mound berries on top of the pudding and dig in!

BASIL-ROASTED STRAWBERRY CHEESECAKE

With Rich Chocolate Crust

This delicious dessert is perfect for a celebration. It's sweet and creamy and chocolaty, and designed for a party. Don't worry, when the crowd goes home, there will be plenty left over for just the two of you.

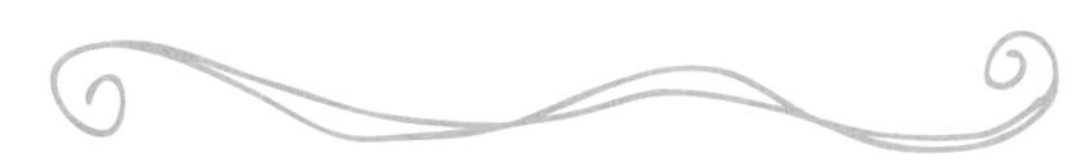

CHOCOLATE WAFER COOKIES are usually found in the ice-cream cone section in your grocery store. My grandmother use to make icebox cake with these delicious morsels.

* * *

If your celebration is a little more INTIMATE than a party for a crowd, you can easily divide this recipe in half and bake in a 9-inch springform pan. The amount of baking time may be reduced.

Preheat the oven to 300 degrees. Place the strawberries onto a rimmed baking sheet. Drizzle with corn syrup and toss with basil. Bake until the strawberries are quite soft and syrupy, about 90 minutes. Use a spatula to scrape the strawberries and syrup into a large bowl. Use a whisk to roughly mash the fruit.

Increase the oven temperature to 350 degrees. Place the wafers into the bowl of a food processor. Pulse to form crumbs. Add the sugar, melted butter, and salt. Pulse to combine. Pour this mixture into the bottom of a 12-inch springform pan. Use the back of a fork to press into the bottom and up the sides of the pan. Bake for 10 minutes. Remove to a wire rack to cool to room temperature. Wrap the bottom of the pan in aluminum foil.

Reduce the oven temperature to 325 degrees. Place the cream cheese into the bowl of an electric mixer. Beat until smooth. Stir in 1½ cups sugar. Stir in the eggs, one at a time. Stir in the vanilla and mascarpone cheese.

Spoon two-thirds of the cream cheese mixture into the bowl with the strawberries. Stir to combine. Pour this mixture into the foil-wrapped springform pan. Top with the remaining cream cheese mixture.

Place the pan into a large roasting pan. Pour hot water into the pan halfway up the sides of the springform pan. Place into the oven. Cook until the middle of the cheesecake is just slightly wiggling, about 1 hour or up to 1 hour and 20 minutes. Turn off the oven and open the oven door. Cool in the oven for 15 minutes. Remove the roasting pan from the oven. Carefully remove the springform pan to a rack. Carefully unwrap the pan. Cool to room temperature. Run a knife around the inside of the pan. Cover with plastic wrap and chill overnight.

To serve, remove the outer ring of the pan. Cut into 1-inch slices.

Makes 12 or more servings
Prep Time: 20 minutes, plus roasting and chill time
Cook Time: 60 to 80 minutes

For the strawberries

- 3 pounds fresh strawberries, stems removed
- 1/4 cup light corn syrup
- 2 tablespoons chopped fresh basil

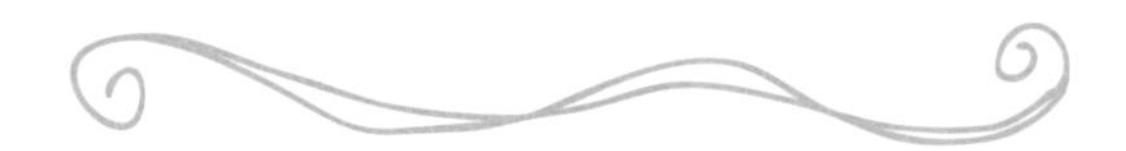

For the crust

- 1 1/2 9-ounce packages chocolate wafer cookies (3 cups cookie crumbs)
- 3 tablespoons natural sugar
- 4 tablespoons butter, melted (1/2 stick)
- 1/8 teaspoon salt

For the filling

- 3 pounds cream cheese, room temperature
- 1 1/2 cups natural sugar
- 4 large eggs
- 1 tablespoon vanilla
- 2 8-ounce containers mascarpone cheese

Gorgeous Home Spa Secrets . . . Just for the Two of You

A steamy soak in a Jacuzzi tub . . . lights dimmed . . . scented candles ablaze. . . . The scene is set, and yet the traditional ideas on sensual bathing could use some global inspiration every once in a while. Conjuring up the new and improved, we look to romantic spa rituals in lands far, far away. The sudsy concoctions introduced here can't help but appeal to your wanderlust. They smell divine, soften the skin, and better yet, to look upon these tubs of water is pure poetry.

Who Says the Honeymoon's Over?

In Javanese tradition, brides-to-be are pampered with 40 days worth of coconut oil massages and jasmine-scented baths. For a modern version, reduce the length of indulgence (whittled down to an hour or so) but include every last drop of sensual Indonesian aromatherapy. Add a few drops of each of these easily obtained essential oils: jasmine, coconut, sandalwood, and rose, with dashes of turmeric to your bath. Follow up with his-and-her massages with Plumeria moisturizer, available at many bath stores.

Green-Wise Ambience

The sweet-smelling protocol for Javanese newlyweds can work for you too. Filling your bathroom with fragrant, living things creates an atmosphere of verdant fertility and can't help but lend a more natural, organic flair when you're bathing—one that really makes you feel like you're getting in touch with your inner, sexy animal. Great indoor plant choices (ones that will thrive in your loo) are bonsai, philodendron, and spider plants, as well as Lucky Bamboo. If you're going to line your bathtub with candles, look for the kind that possess interiors or casings partially made of leaves, flowers, fruit, or bark, or come in a coconut husk. Throw red roses into the mix and you'd swear you were a Javanese girl crossing the threshold of her honeymoon suite.

A Bath & Sauna Hour Cocktail

Javenese brides sipped a traditional drink made of turmeric, ginger, egg yolk, and healing herbs, like mint and sweet basil, during their lulu baths. They also enjoyed a specific kind of hot sauna afterward. You can imitate that sauna by splashing sandalwood onto your major pulsepoints before entering the steam room.

Photogenic Baths

Our **Lavender Sea Soak** bath is visually enhanced with food coloring, allowing you to wash every last care away in a pretty bath of brilliant purple. You can impress your sweetheart further by scattering a few white and yellow rose petals (maybe even lotus flowers if you're feeling extra creative) on the colored water. To prepare this bath, mix together 1 cup Epsom salts with 1 cup sea salt. Stir in 1 cup baking soda. Add purple food coloring (4 drops blue and 6 drops red makes purple), 15 drops lavender essential oil, 8 drops ylang ylang essential oil, and 8 drops Neroli essential oil. Use a spoonful or two in your bathwater.

A Blue Blood's Bath

Made popular by Anne Marie Orsini, the seventeenth-century Italian Duchess of Neroli (a part of Rome), Neroli oil is similar to bergamot and comes from the blossom of the bitter orange tree. Duchess Orsini is responsible for its spread in popularity, using the oil to perfume her gloves and bathwater. Neroli has a refreshing and distinctive, spicy aroma with sweet and flowery notes. Because it's a nontoxic, nonirritating, nonsensitizing, nonphototoxic substance, more than 12 percent of today's quality perfumes use Neroli as their principal ingredient. It's rumored to be an ingredient in Coca-Cola as well and is said to have a soothing effect on the nervous system—hence its use in massage oils and in aromatic candles.

For your next bath, evoke the essence of Coco Chanel and tap into the blue-blooded sensibilities of an Italian duchess by mixing up what we like to call "Lost in the Rose Forest." Just mix together 2 cups Epsom salts, 1 cup sea salt, 10 drops of sandalwood essential oil, 5 drops of ylang ylang essential oil, 3 drops Neroli oil, and 10 drops of rose essential oil. In a large bowl mix salts first, then add the other ingredients slowly. Add a spoonful or two to your next bath and feel the aristocratic sensuality.

Your Honeymoon Suite

Make your bedroom a room that you look forward to entering by adding a couple of fun enhancements. Light candles and fill vases with fresh flowers. Spray rosewater onto your sheets—the aroma is sensual and invigorating. For those special moments, toss a few rose petals over your pillows. The smell and the texture will leave you breathless. To quench your thirst, keep a pitcher of herb-and-fruit-scented ice water on your bedside table. A few spoonfuls of pomegranate juice will delightfully flavor your chilled water. Scent your shower by placing a few drops of essential oil onto a washcloth. Tuck the washcloth into the corner of your shower and turn on the water. Wait a few minutes, allowing the steam to spread the scent all through the bathroom. Set your alarm and open the shutters so that you and your partner can watch the sun rise from you bedroom window. The colors are explosive and the experience is renewing. And, yes, a decadently rich, wrapped chocolate, conveniently placed on his pillow, will get a sweet result.

The Love Gym: Mary Ellen Weighs In

When we think of exercise that really makes a difference, like the cardiovascular intensity of spinning and Tae Bo, we see how the resulting conditioning and toning can improve our sex lives. The same is true for lower-impact exercises. They too can create an immediate sense of ultra-femininity. An emerging twenty-first-century trend to extrapolate, then work out to, the sexier parts of yoga, Pilates, belly dancing, and even jazzercise offers the dual results of toning up while spicing up your marriage. Check out these moves to see what I mean.

Yoga and Desire

Yoga, an ancient set of practices that originated in India and is revered worldwide today, is a path to enlightenment and physical fitness that does, at times, seem like a contradiction in terms. What it entails (mastery over the body, mind, and emotional self and the transcendence of desire) is odd when one considers how erotic some of yoga's postures (asanas) are. The breathing and stretching exercises make a person more agile, limber, open-minded, and calm—an invitation to improve your sex life. Luckily, weekly yoga classes don't ask you to "transcend your desire"—that's left up to the hardcore practitioners, like yogis and monks. These exercises, which originated in yoga and can't help but stimulate eroticism, make for great foreplay!

FOURGASMS: 4 Yoga-Inspired Exercises for the Bedroom

Downward and upward facing dog, cat, and cow poses, and the cobra (oh my!) are all yoga moves that inspire you to new heights. Perhaps there's something to learn from these (much simpler!) yoga moves.

1) *Open Your Hips*
    - Start by opening your hips. Do this by assuming the Lotus position: In this sitting position the right foot is placed on the left thigh and the left foot on the right thigh with the soles of the feet turned up; the spine is kept straight.
    - De-pretzel yourself and assume this new position: Bring the soles of your feet together, put your hands on your ankles, allow your knees to relax toward the floor, and hinge forward at the hips as far as is comfortable. Hold for 10 to 15 complete breaths (inhale and exhale). Alternate between this and the Lotus, so that you've done each posture at least twice. Daily reps of these will turn a once squeaky gate into a well-oiled machine when it comes to opening your hips.

2) *Strengthen Your Pelvic Floor*

It's the same idea behind the Kegel exercise, but there's a name for it in Sanskrit too. It's a practice in yoga called the Mula Bandha, and it's discreet enough that you can do it behind your desk at work.

- Seated or standing, contract and then release the pubococcygeus muscle, located between the pubic bone and the tailbone.
- Do this 10 times in sets of three.

3) *Intensify Your Climax*

- Tighter abs can mean better orgasms!
- Start in the push-up position, arms extended.
- Engage your abs as you lower your body slowly toward the floor.
- Stop when your torso is about 2 to 3 inches away.
- Keeping elbows in, hold there for 5 breaths, then lower to the floor.
- Repeat three times at first, and build up to five.

4) *Heighten Your Sense of Emotional Well-Being*

- Lie on your back with one hip touching a wall.
- Swing your legs up and turn your body so you face the wall, legs resting against it from heels to butt, arms at your sides.
- Bring your awareness to your breath and focus on it for 5 minutes.
- This position allows more oxygen-rich blood to flow from your lower body and back up to the heart and the brain so you'll have energy for pillow talk afterward!

Bridge to Passion

Back pain can be a serious mood killer, which brings to mind the core philosophy of Pilates, which teaches awareness of neutral alignment of the spine and strengthening the deep postural muscles that support it. Often indistinguishable from yoga, Pilates features a pelvic lift that is highly beneficial to sexually relevant areas of the body. It makes your body look like a bridge and is performed as follows:

- Lie on your back with knees bent and slightly apart.
- Feet should be flat on the floor and arms at your side.
- Inhale, clenching your abdominals and buttocks and lifting the pelvis until your back is straight and buttocks held about a foot off the floor.
- Take care not to arch your back.
- Breathe as you hold the position for at least 10 seconds. Exhale as you lower your body and repeat the exercise.

Grab Your Partner!

You'll need a little help with this one. Don't worry—I'm sure there's, ahem, *somebody* who'd be happy to spot you! It's called The Butterfly and you do it like so:

- Lie on your back on your bed with knees bent. Feet should be together and flat on the bed.
- Next, pull your feet in until they touch your buttocks. Turn your ankles so the soles of your feet are facing each other and touching. Your knees will point out to the sides of the bed.
- Lower your knees toward the bed, taking care not to force them down. You or your partner may gently press downward on your inner thighs.
- When your knees are as far apart as is comfortable, hold for 60 seconds.
- Gently bring the knees back together with your hands and relax.

Like a Pair of Bookends

The aforementioned exercise can also be done sitting up, back-to-back with your partner.

- Sit up as straight as possible with your spines pressed gently together.
- Relax your shoulders and keep your head in line with your spine.
- Bring your feet in as close to your body as possible, and turn them so your soles touch and knees point out. Clasp your feet. Breathe deeply and watch as your knees begin to lower, taking care not to force the knees down.
- Repeat 5 to 10 reps—depending on how eager you are to get down to business!

Workout Mates

Whichever exercises you choose to embrace, remember to start off slow and only do what you can. Gradually work up to more weight, more repetitions, and more difficult movements. Also remember to work out with your mate. Take walks together, go to the gym together, sign up for a class together. A satisfying sex life is more than the act—it's about intimacy. A what's more intimate than holding your lover's hand while strolling in the moonlight. . . .

PART FOUR

gorgeous lifestyle guide for fresh, healthy, balanced living

We have assembled all of the information in this book into a gorgeous lifestyle guide that includes daily activities, meal plans, spa and relaxation techniques, volunteering, and tried-and-true techniques for balancing work and parenting. With these weekly plans, you will have all of the tools necessary to achieve truth, love, and beauty.

CHAPTER 16

a day-to-day guide to living the gorgeous lifestyle

Choose from any of the 52 weekly lifestyle plans in this chapter to get started on your path to *gorgeous*. You can incorporate all of the information found in this book into your own personal guide to fulfill your personal goals. Included in the weekly guides are suggestions for daily exercise and stress relievers, healthy meal plans, personal spa time (at home and at the spa), tips on improving personal appearance, and how to find time to be charitable as well as suggestions for igniting romance, balancing work and parenting, and valuing your relationships with family, friends, and coworkers.

After you choose your plan from the ones in this section, go to: www.GorgeousLifestyleGuide.com to get specific tips for that week, like a printable grocery shopping list and shopping day tips. We'll also give you current info to make sure that your path to *gorgeous* is totally up to date, and we are available to answer any questions you might have.

Now, it's time to get *gorgeous*. . . .

gorgeous lifestyle guide week 1 — skin-savvy

Day	Breakfast	Lunch	Dinner	Revitalizing Activity
saturday	Whip up a batch of Banana Flaxseed Bread with Warm Strawberry Sauce (pg. 75). Make extras for later in the week.	While you are running your errands, take a lunch break. Stop at the market for your favorite fresh veggie salad.	Date night! Invite pals for Chicken Thighs with Sage and Caramelized Peaches (pg. 65) and Peach Gingerbread with Walnut Streusel (pg. 76).	Start the day with a 40-minute POWER WALK with a pal! Today is Shopping Day! Hit the farmer's market.
sunday	Gather the gang for a super breakfast of Breakfast Burritos with Red Pepper Salsa (pg. 60).	**Afternoon** Nibble on leftover Banana Flaxseed Bread.	Serve a light supper of Grilled Halibut with Salsa Verde (pg. 64), Rosemary Roasted Carrot Sticks (pg. 72), and Oven-Roasted Fruit with Vanilla Yogurt Sorbet (pg. 77). Save extras for later in the week.	Me time! Luxuriate with an MINT FACIAL STEAM (pg. 78).
monday	Blend up Fruit and Yogurt Breakfast Parfaits with Granola Crunch (pg. 59).	Brown bag it! Fill your lunch tote with brightly colored foods containing antioxidants.	Prepare Mediterranean Tuna Melts (pg. 62) while the kids do their homework.	Give your dull skin a creamy shine with a MILKY CLEANSER (pg. 78). Take a 30-minute POWER WALK.
tuesday	Pecan Bananadana Muffins (pg. 90). Make extras for snacks later in the week.	Sip on a steamy bowl of Butternut Squash Soup Flavored with Orange and Tarragon (pg. 70).	Supper comes together easily. Serve Sushi-Style Salmon Wraps (pg. 61) and Sweet Potato Apple Salad with Honey, Ginger, and Mustard Dressing (pg. 63). Make extra salad for tomorrow's lunch.	Me time! Luxuriate with an OATMEAL PEEL (pg. 79). Visit the cosmetic counter and treat yourself to a makeover.
wednesday	Blend your favorite Juiced-Up Fruit-and-Herb Breakfast Drinks (Cantaloupe-Tarragon, pg. 57).	Nibble on leftover Sweet Potato Apple Salad.	The gang will love Open-Faced Chicken Tacos (pg. 68), Stewed Tomatoes with Garlic and Black Beans (pg. 71), and Roasted Figs with Sweetened Orange Sauce (pg. 74).	Stretch out your arms and legs. Check out the latest audio book during your rush-hour drive.
thursday	Make Fresh Fruit Salad with Citrus Basil Dressing (pg. 58) the night before.	Brown bag it! Remember that cornucopia of colors. A salad or veggie sandwich will work here.	Serve a rainbow dinner of Spinach Salad with Warm Chipotle Chili Vinaigrette Topped with Chicken Strips and Crisp Sweet Potato (pg. 66) and Peach Gingerbread with Walnut Streusel (pg. 76).	Me time! Apply a HONEY MASK (pg. 79). Don't forget that 30-minute POWER WALK.
friday	More fruit for you. Blend up your favorite Juiced-Up Fruit-and-Herb Breakfast Drinks (Apple-Mint, pg. 57).	A great way to add veggies to your diet. Bake up several Stuffed Sweet Potatoes with Spinach and Corn (pg. 73) and share with the carpool moms.	A perfect Friday's fish supper. Prepare Roasted Tomato Basil Soup with Sea Bass Center (pg. 69) and finish with leftover Peach Gingerbread.	Start the day with a 40-minute POWER WALK with a pal! Discuss the latest novels.

For Week 1 Grocery Shopping List and Shopping Day Prep Tips visit www.GorgeousLifestyleGuide.com

gorgeous lifestyle guide week 2 — good hair

	Breakfast	Lunch	Dinner	Revitalizing Activity
saturday	Make a batch of Pecan Bananadana Muffins (pg. 90). Use extras for weekday grab-and-go breakfasts.	This is Shopping Day, so while you are running errands stop and treat yourself to your favorite deli sandwich. Remember to choose whole grain bread, fresh veggies, and lean meats.	Date night! Invite friends for an over-the-top supper of Lobster in an Orange Curry Butter Sauce (pg. 93) and Baked Pears in Brandy Sauce (pg. 104).	Start the day with a 40-minute POWER WALK with a pal! Today is Shopping Day! Hit the farmer's market and smell the . . . oranges.
sunday	Gather the gang for a brunch of Creamy French-Style Eggs Garnished with Chopped Tomatoes and Chives (pg. 87).	**Afternoon:** Nibble on a salad of fresh veggies topped with a bit of olive oil and balsamic vinegar.	A Sunday comfort supper includes Roasted Pork Tenderloin with Swiss Chard (pg. 96) and Toasted Corn with Sautéed Spinach and Cherry Tomatoes (pg. 103).	Me time! Luxuriate with an OLIVE OIL HAIR MASK (pg. 110).
monday	Blend up a batch of Juiced-Up Fruit-and-Herb Breakfast Drinks (Apple-Mint, pg. 57).	Brown bag it! Pack up a fresh veggie salad that's filled with all of the colors of the rainbow.	Not your mama's Monday night supper of Grilled Skirt Steak and Veggie Open-Faced Sandwich (pg. 95) and Rhubarb and Strawberry Frozen Yogurt with Fresh Mint (pg. 105).	Give your dull hair a COLOR LIFT (pg. 109). Don't forget to squeeze in your 30-minute POWER WALK.
tuesday	Reheat a Pecan Bananadana Muffin to go with a hot cup of morning java.	Sip on a steaming cup of Creamy Cauliflower Soup with Arugula and Crispy Bacon Garnish (pg. 101). Save extras for lunch later in the week.	Serve a simple supper of Rosemary Roasted Chicken Breasts with Smoky Almond Sauce (pg. 91) and Oatmeal Snack Cake (pg. 106). Make extras for later in the week.	Me Time! Luxuriate with an OLIVE OIL HAIR MASK (pg. 110). Buy a magazine and try out a *new* hairdo.
wednesday	Blend up a batch of Juiced-Up Fruit-and-Herb Breakfast Drinks (Cantaloupe-Tarragon, pg. 57).	Invite your GORGEOUS gal pals for a special luncheon of Mussels with Brussels in a White Wine Butter Sauce (pg. 94).	Serve the family a super supper of Lamb Chops with Skillet Coconut Sauce (pg. 92) and Louisiana-Style Red Beans (pg. 102).	Stretch out your neck and shoulders to reduce stress. Let your fingers do the walking to make an appointment with a hip hairstylist.
thursday	Bake a batch of Raspberry Oatmeal Muffins with Macadamia Nut Butter (pg. 89). Save extras for later in the week.	Brown bag it! Build a super sandwich on whole grain bread using Tuesday's leftover chicken topped with fresh veggies.	Good-for-you Calf's Liver with Golden Onions (pg. 97) makes for a fun meal. Finish with Oatmeal Snack Cake baked earlier in the week.	Me time! Start your day with a 30-minute POWER WALK. Later that night treat yourself to a fruit HAIR MASK (pg. 109).
friday	Spend an extra 5 minutes to prepare Egg White Omelets with Bell Peppers and Turkey Sausage (pg. 88). You'll be satisfied all day!	Heat up a cup of leftover Creamy Cauliflower Soup.	TGIF. Celebrate with Paella with Chorizo, Asparagus, and Shellfish (pg. 98), Fried Plantains (pg. 100), and Sautéed Bananas with Sweet Mascarpone and Walnut Crunch (pg. 107).	Grab a pal and start the day with a 40-minute POWER WALK. Let the gossip flow!

For Week 2 Grocery Shopping List and Shopping Day Prep Tips visit www.GorgeousLifestyleGuide.com

gorgeous lifestyle guide week 3 — eye-catching

Day	Breakfast	Lunch	Dinner	Revitalizing Activity
saturday	**Breakfast** Start your busy day with a super breakfast of Poached Eggs in Spicy Tomato Sauce (pg. 119).	**Lunch** This is Shopping Day, so while you are running errands, stop and treat yourself to your favorite fresh veggie salad.	**Dinner** Date night! Invite pals for an excellent supper of Grilled New York Strip Steaks with Garlic Herb Oil (pg. 125), Sweet Balsamic Onions (pg. 129), and Pear and Strawberry Crisp (pg. 133).	**Revitalizing Activity** Start the day with a 40-minute POWER WALK with a pal! Today is Shopping Day! Hit the farmer's market.
sunday	**Breakfast** Enjoy a fruity breakfast of Melon Bowls with Strawberry Ginger Sauce (pg. 120).	**Afternoon** Build your favorite deli sandwich. Choose whole grain breads, lots of veggies, and lean meat.	**Dinner** Sunday's comfort supper includes Chicken Paprikash Served over Egg Noodles (pg. 122), Buttermilk Rolls with Sweet Onion Filling (pg. 130), and Orange-Glazed Yogurt Cake (pg. 134).	**Revitalizing Activity** Lighten dark circles and smooth puffiness with raw ingredients like potatoes and egg whites.
monday	**Breakfast** Blend up a batch of Juiced-Up Fruit-and-Herb Breakfast Drinks (Apple-Mint, pg. 57).	**Lunch** Brown bag it! Take along a fresh veggie salad topped with leftover Sirloin Steak from Saturday's meal.	**Dinner** Have breakfast for dinner. Serve an Italian-Style Strata (pg. 126).	**Revitalizing Activity** Make FROZEN EYE PADS (pg. 138). Relax with eyes closed for 15 minutes. Did you remember your 30-minute POWER WALK?
tuesday	**Breakfast** Take five to prepare Scrambled Eggs with Red Grape and Avocado Salsa (pg. 118).	**Lunch** You will love a lunch of Roasted Veggie Stuffed Tomatoes (pg 131). Make extras to share with coworkers.	**Dinner** Gather the gang for a quick and flavorful dinner of Stir-Fry Chicken and Broccoli with Chopped Peanuts (pg. 123).	**Revitalizing Activity** See clearly. Identify something beautiful in your environment and appreciate the sight. Pull out the digital camera and create a picture to frame for your desk.
wednesday	**Breakfast** Add more fruit to your daily diet with a power breakfast of Broiled Grapefruit with Honey Mascarpone Cream (pg. 117).	**Lunch** Invite your GORGEOUS gal pals to share Mushroom and Spinach-Filled Frittata (pg. 128) for lunch.	**Dinner** You and the kids will love Roasted Veggie Burritos with Chipotle Chili Tomato Sauce (pg. 121), Unfried Fried Onions (pg. 132), and Orange-Glazed Yogurt cake left over from Sunday's supper.	**Revitalizing Activity** Stretch out your neck and shoulders to reduce stress. Make an appointment with your favorite department store's cosmetic counter expert. Test the new seasonal eye makeup colors.
thursday	**Breakfast** Blend up your favorite Juiced-Up Fruit-and-Herb Breakfast Drinks (Apple-Mint, pg. 57).	**Lunch** Make a smart choice when you eat out for lunch. Look for fresh veggies, whole grain breads, and just a dash of salad dressing or mayonnaise.	**Dinner** Prepare a quick and easy meal of Grilled Skirt Steak and Veggie Open Faced Sandwich (pg. 95) with Cranberry Wedding Cookies (pg. 135).	**Revitalizing Activity** Start the day with a 30-minute POWER WALK. Don't forget your shades. Add a few crunches to "see" how you feel.
friday	**Breakfast** Spoon up Fruit and Yogurt Breakfast Parfaits with Granola Crunch (pg. 59).	**Lunch** Sip on a savory Butternut Squash Soup Flavored with Orange and Tarragon (leftovers from your freezer).	**Dinner** Make Friday fresh with Spaghetti Squash Carbonara (pg. 124) served with Chocolate Ricotta-Filled Crepes (pg. 136) for dessert.	**Revitalizing Activity** Start the day with a 40-minute POWER WALK with a pal! Enjoy spending time with a good friend.

For Week 3 Grocery Shopping List and Shopping Day Prep Tips visit www.GorgeousLifestyleGuide.com

gorgeous lifestyle guide week 4 — smile pretty

Day	Breakfast	Lunch	Dinner	Revitalizing Activity
saturday	Prepare warm Oatmeal with Caramelized Fruit Topping (pg. 149) for a filling breakfast on your busy day.	This is Shopping Day, so while you are running errands, stop and treat yourself to your favorite deli sandwich made with whole grain bread, fresh veggies, and lean meats.	Date night! Invite pals for Blue Cheese Dip with All Kinds of Dippers (pg. 161), Swiss Cheese Wafers (pg. 160), Lemon Veal with Sautéed Spinach, Pine Nuts, & Goat Cheese (pg. 158), and Mango-Walnut Crumble (pg. 165).	Start the day with a 40-minute POWER WALK that includes 10 minutes of jogging! Today is Shopping Day! Hit the farmer's market.
sunday	Gather the gang for Spicy Roasted Veggie and Shrimp Salsa with Fried Egg and Warm Cheese Sauce (pg. 146).	**Afternoon** Nibble on a favorite snack of Artichoke and Asiago Crostini (pg. 162).	Sunday's comfort supper includes Crispy Roasted Chicken with Penne Pasta (pg. 154) and New York-Style Cheesecake (pg. 164). Make extras for lunchboxes later in the week.	Prepare your own homemade mouthwash (pg. 167) for the freshest smile possible.
monday	Blend up a smoothie of Juiced-Up Fruit-and-Herb Breakfast Drinks (Blueberry-Basil, pg. 57).	Brown bag it! Take along a fresh veggie salad topped with chicken left over from Sunday's supper.	Perk up your everyday weeknight meal by serving Seared Jumbo Scallops with Herb Butter Sauce (pg. 152) and Orange and Tarragon-Infused Crème Brûlées with Slice Bananas (pg. 163).	After your 30-minute POWER WALK, curl up with a good book and a cup of non-teeth-staining herbal tea.
tuesday	Another fast fruity treat for breakfast is a batch of Coconut Tropical Smoothies (pg. 148).	Prepare refreshing Shrimp Salad with Mango and Cucumber (pg. 159), share extras with coworkers, and save the rest for Thursday's lunch.	Turn your kitchen into a super sandwich shop by serving Turkey with Caramelized Onion and Smoked Gouda Panini (pg. 151) and Emergency Key Lime Pie (pg. 166) for dessert.	Grab your someone special and take an after-dinner walk to work off that pie.
wednesday	How about an encore of Oatmeal with Caramelized Fruit Topping (pg. 149) for a mid-week breakfast that keeps you going strong.	Invite your GORGEOUS gal pals to share a fun lunch of Buffalo Chicken Cobb Salad with Buttermilk Dressing (pg. 150).	Create your favorite quesadilla using leftover chicken from Sunday night. Add roasted pepper, Jack cheese, and sauteed mushrooms. Serve leftover cheesecake for dessert.	Stretch out your lower back and legs. Take a 30-minute power walk to start your day. Make an appointment with the cosmetic counter to test out the new seasonal lipstick colors.
thursday	Jazz up your fruity breakfast fare with Fresh Papaya and Grapefruit with Yogurt and Mint (pg. 147).	Brown bag it! Take along a sandwich stuffed with leftover Shrimp Salad. Choose whole grain bread; add dark green lettuce and slices of tomato to boost the veggie impact.	Serve a simple supper of Grilled Swordfish Steaks with Hot Papaya Relish and Herbed Compound Butter (pg. 157).	Smile at everyone you meet today and see how many smile back at you. Smile while cars pass you on your 30-minute POWER WALK.
friday	Spoon up a bowl of Fruit and Yogurt Breakfast Parfaits with Granola Crunch (pg. 59).	Teacher's workday. Prepare Double-Cheese and Sausage Calzones with Marinara Dipping Sauce (pg. 153) and share with the other classroom moms.	Serve the family an elegant entrée of Chicken with Bel Paese, Proscuitto, and Capers with White Wine Pan Sauce (pg. 156).	Start the day with a 40-minute POWER WALK with a pal that includes 10 minutes of jogging!

For Week 4 Grocery Shopping List and Shopping Day Prep Tips visit www.GorgeousLifestyleGuide.com

gorgeous lifestyle guide week 5 — good to the bones

Day	Breakfast	Lunch	Dinner	Revitalizing Activity
saturday	Bake up a batch of Whole Grain Apple Muffins with Walnut Streusel (pg. 177). Save extras for later in the week.	This is Shopping Day, so while you are running errands, stop and treat yourself to your favorite fresh veggie salad.	Date Night! Invite Pals for Watercress Salad with Raspberry Vinaigrette and Blood Orange (pg. 191), Grilled Lamb Chops with White Bean Salad (pg. 182), and Almond-Topped Ricotta Cheesecake (pg. 195).	Start the day with a 40-minute POWER WALK that includes 10 minutes of jogging! Today is Shopping Day! Hit the farmer's market.
sunday	Gather the group for a brunch of Eggs Benedict with Swiss Chard and Whole Grain English Muffins (pg. 175).	**Afternoon** Prepare Green Gazpacho Soup with Navy Bean Garnish (pg. 188)—have a small cup for lunch and reserve the rest for later in the week.	Our comfort supper includes Mustard-Garlic Roasted Chicken Served with Arugula and Artichoke Salad (pg. 179), Lentils with Wild Rice & Mushrooms (pg. 190), and Peanut Butter Sandwich Cookies (pg. 194).	After supper, while the kids and Dad do the dishes, soak in a hot tub filled with Epsom salts and lavender oil.
monday	Warm up a Whole Grain Apple Muffin for a grab-and-go Monday breakfast.	Brown bag it! Choose whole grain breads to build a sandwich stuffed with leftover sliced chicken from Sunday's supper. Add a peanut butter cookie for dessert.	Simple supper for a Monday night includes Baked Tilapia with Fresh Herbs (pg. 183) and leftover Almond-Topped Ricotta Cheesecake from the weekend.	Go to an introductory yoga class or try out some basic moves at home.
tuesday	Take an extra 5 minutes to build the best Breakfast Panini with Chicken Sausage (pg. 178).	Enjoy a bowl of Green Gazpacho Soup with Navy Bean Relish (prepared earlier in the week).	A midweek veggie meal is re-invented with Rosemary Polenta with Spinach, Red Beans, and Goat Cheese (pg. 184) and Cocktail Nut Cookie Bars (pg. 196) for dessert.	Grab the entire family for an after-dinner walk around the neighborhood. Don't forget the dog!
wednesday	Grab a bowl of warm Oatmeal with Caramelized Fruit Topping (pg. 149) for a tummy-warming breakfast.	Invite your GORGEOUS gal pals to share Sweet Potato and Country Ham Frittata (pg. 176).	Whole Wheat Spaghetti with Grilled Turkey, Broccoli Rabe, Red Peppers and Peas (pg. 180)—a perfect midweek meal.	Stretch out from head to toe. Take a 30-minute POWER WALK to start your day. Add 10 minutes of weight lifting. Remember to start light.
thursday	Warm up a Whole Grain Apple Muffin.	Brown bag it! Take a container filled with Peppery White Bean Salsa with Whole Wheat Pita Chips (pg. 189) to work to share with everyone.	A dinner of Peppered Pork Pinwheels Stuffed with Swiss Chard, Sun-Dried Tomatoes and Mozzarella (pg. 186) will leave 'em smiling.	It's POWER WALK day. Spend 30 minutes walking. Add a few lunges to stretch out those legs.
friday	Sip Coconut Tropical Smoothies (pg. 148) for breakfast.	Stay home for lunch and build a super dish packed full of veggies. Summer Squash Salad with Baby Spinach, Roasted Tomatoes, and Parmesan Cheese (pg. 192) fits the bill.	Treat the family to Parmesan Chicken Fingers with Green Cashew and Curry Dipping Sauce (pg. 181). Prepare Macadamia Nut Biscotti (pg. 193) with the kids for dessert tonight and snacks next week.	Start the day with a 40-minute POWER WALK with a PPal that includes 10 minutes of jogging and 10 minutes of stretching!

For Week 5 Grocery Shopping List and Shopping Day Prep Tips visit www.GorgeousLifestyleGuide.com

gorgeous lifestyle guide week 6 — you could be dancin'

Day	Breakfast	Lunch	Dinner	Revitalizing Activity
saturday	Bake up a batch of Whole Wheat Bran Muffins with Golden Raisins and Walnuts (pg. 207). Save extras for later in the week.	This is Shopping Day. While you are running errands, stop and treat yourself to your favorite deli sandwich made with whole grain bread, fresh veggies, and lean meat.	Date night! Invite pals for Charred Sirloin Steak with Mushroom and Red Wine Sauce (pg. 213) and Tropical Strawberry Tiramisu (pg. 224).	Start the day with a 40-minute POWER WALK that includes 10 minutes of jogging! Today is Shopping Day! Hit the farmer's market.
sunday	Gather the group for Brunch Frittata with Red Potatoes and Kale (pg. 208).	**Afternoon** Prepare Sweet Pea Panzanella Salad (pg. 221). Have a small dish for lunch and reserve the rest for later in the week.	Sunday night supper fun includes Mojo Marinated Chicken Served over Black Beans (pg. 216), Slowly Stewed Collard Greens (pg. 222) and Chilled Berry Sauce with Lime Sherbet and Coconut Garnish (pg. 225).	Stretch out those toes and soak in warm water after a long weekend.
monday	Grab a Whole Wheat Bran Muffin for the commute to work.	Brown bag it! Choose whole grain breads to build a sandwich stuffed with veggies and leftover sliced steak from the weekend.	Prepare Better Veggie Chili (pg. 218) for an easy workday supper.	Take a couple of minutes to visit the sporting goods store and update your athletic shoes. Remember to purchase a pair with just the support you need to protect your tootsie toes.
tuesday	Prepare Double-Berry Whole Wheat Pancakes (pg. 209) for the family and start the day off just fine.	Sweet Pea Panzanella Salad (made earlier in the week).	Wild Ivory King Salmon Fillets with Macadamia Nut Crust (pg. 211) and Blueberry Shortbread Bars (pg. 223). Make extra salmon for Thursday's lunch.	Get your kids together for a quick game of one-on-one.
wednesday	Blend up a batch of Juiced-Up Fruit-and-Herb Breakfast Drinks (Blueberry-Basil, pg. 57).	Invite your GORGEOUS gal pals to share a lunch of Overstuffed Beef Steak Tomatoes with Tortellini Salad (pg. 214) with leftover Blueberry Shortbread Bars.	Hoisin Beef and Veggies (pg. 212) make for a super supper.	Take a 30-minute POWER WALK to start your day. Add 15 minutes of weight lifting. Do a few more reps. Reward yourself with a pedicure appointment.
thursday	Warm up a leftover Whole Wheat Bran Muffins.	Brown bag it! Take along a container of salmon salad made from the leftover salmon from earlier in the week.	Feast on a menu of Sea Scallops with Blood Orange, Avocado, and Red Onion Salsa (pg. 215) and Pecan Graham Squares (pg. 226).	Remember your 30-minute POWER WALK. Add a few lunges to stretch out those legs and feet.
friday	Get a jumpstart on the weekend with a great breakfast of Poached Eggs with Spinach and White Beans (pg. 210).	Home for lunch? Enjoy Asparagus Cheese Toasts (pg. 219) and an extra Pecan Graham Square from last night.	Treat the whole family to veggie night with Baked Potatoes Stuffed with Swiss Chard and Black Beans (pg. 217) and Roasted Veggie Stacks with Mozzarella (pg. 220).	Start the day with a 40-minute POWER WALK with a pal that includes 10 minutes of jogging and 10 minutes of stretching!

For Week 6 Grocery Shopping List and Shopping Day Prep Tips visit www.GorgeousLifestyleGuide.com

gorgeous lifestyle guide week 7 — hands-on glam

Day	Breakfast	Lunch	Dinner	Revitalizing Activity
saturday	Bake up a stunning Blueberry Buttermilk Coffee Cake Topped with Granola (pg. 236). Save extras for later in the week.	This is Shopping Day. While you are running errands, stop and treat yourself to a fresh veggie salad with your favorite (but light) dressing.	Date night! Invite pals for Roasted Asparagus Salad with Arugula, Radishes, and Lemon Vinaigrette (pg. 248), Snapper Veronique (pg. 244), and Strike-It-Rich Chocolate Pudding with Chocolate Cookie Crumbles (pg. 252).	Start the day with a 40-minute POWER WALK that includes 10 minutes of jogging! Today is Shopping Day! Hit the farmer's market.
sunday	Breakfast: Gather the group for Walnut-Stuffed Baked Apples with Maple Syrup (pg. 238).	Afternoon: Have a snacky lunch of Black Bean and Roasted Pepper Empanadas (pg. 250). Share extras with coworkers.	Prepare Jambalaya (pg. 245) for Sunday's supper and serve with Simple Zucchini Cake with Vanilla Glaze (pg. 254), reserving leftovers for later in the week.	Give yourself a home spa manicure while you listen to your favorite new jazz cd.
monday	Blend up your favorite Juiced-Up Fruit-and-Herb Breakfast Drinks (Apple-Mint, pg. 57).	Brown bag it! Build a better tuna sandwich by adding green pepper, celery and onion to the salad. Choose whole grain breads and plenty of dark green lettuce with slices of tomato.	Surprise! Serve Sliced Chicken Breast with Red Grape Sauce (pg. 247) and Sauteed Red Cabbage with Drunken Raisins (pg. 251). (Don't tell the kids!)	Take a couple of minutes to visit the cosmetic counter and purchase a rich hand cream filled with collagen. Oh, and check out that bracelet in the glass counter!
tuesday	Dash off to work with a slice of Blueberry Buttermilk Coffee Cake made earlier in the week.	Make a fresh veggie salad topped with slices of leftover chicken and your favorite citrus vinaigrette.	The kids (big and small) will dig into Chicken and Rice Meatball Hoagies (pg. 242).	Hold hands with your special someone while you stroll through the neighborhood after supper.
wednesday	Prepare Banana Bread Snack Cake (pg. 237), reserving extras for later in the week.	Invite your GORGEOUS gal pals to share Chilled Shrimp Salad with Red Grapes (pg. 241) for a light lunch.	Enjoy a decadent supper of Poached Salmon in Infused Olive Oil with Horseradish Sauce (pg. 240) with leftover Simple Zucchini Cake slices.	Take a 30-minute POWER WALK to start your day. Add 15 minutes of weight lifting. Do a few more reps than last week. Reward yourself with a manicure appointment.
thursday	Whip up a batch of Granola Power Bars (pg. 239) for a real grab-and-go breakfast.	Brown bag it! Take along a container of veggie salad topped with slices of salmon leftovers from last evening.	Sauteed Yellowtail Snapper with Braised Cabbage and Cheesy Mashed Potatoes (pg. 246) make for a cozy hand-holding supper.	Walk this way—for 30 minutes. Add a few lunges to stretch out those legs and feet. Remember the sunscreen, especially on your hands.
friday	Grab a wedge of Banana Snack Cake on your way out the door.	After your light midday restaurant meal, splurge on a cup of Chocoholic's Crutch (pg. 255).	Treat the whole family to Turkey Meatloaf Burgers with Sweet Potato Sticks (pg. 243) and Roasted Red Grape Parfaits with Orange and Maple-Flavored Ricotta Cheese (pg. 253).	Start the day with a 40-minute POWER WALK with a pal that includes 10 minutes of jogging and 10 minutes of stretching!

For Week 7 Grocery Shopping List and Shopping Day Prep Tips visit www.GorgeousLifestyleGuide.com

gorgeous lifestyle guide week 8 — tummy-pleasing

Day	Breakfast	Lunch	Dinner	Revitalizing Activity
saturday	Blend up a batch of Juiced-Up Fruit-and-Herb Breakfast Drinks (Cantaloupe-Tarragon, pg. 57).	This is Shopping Day. While you are running errands, stop and treat yourself to your favorite deli sandwich made with whole grain breads, plenty of veggies, reduced-fat cheese, and lean meat.	Date night! Invite pals for Snapper Fillets Smothered with Caramelized Onions (pg. 272), Grilled Veggie Skewers (pg. 283), and Poached Cherry Sundaes (pg. 288).	Start the day with a 40-minute POWER WALK that includes 15 minutes of jogging! Today is Shopping Day! Hit the farmer's market.
sunday	Gather the group for Say "Ricotta Cheese" Pancakes with Very Berry Sauce (pg. 269).	**Afternoon** Have a simple lunch of roasted veggie soup made by blending leftover veggie skewers with homemade chicken broth.	Prepare Pancetta-Wrapped Turkey Medallions with Broccoli Rabe, Peppers, and Onions (pg. 278) and Fresh Lime Cake with Warm Blueberry Sauce (pg. 289), saving extra cake for later in the week.	Turn on your Pilates DVD and get down with your inner core. Stretch out those muscles and improve your squats—work your way up to a perfect teaser.
monday	Prepare Eggs in a Frame with Basil Tomatoes (pg. 270) for the gang to start off the week on the right foot.	Brown bag it! Take along a salad made with tons of fresh veggies and your favorite vinaigrette.	Roasted Chipotle Salmon with Minted Couscous (pg. 279) and Sautéed Peas with Mint (pg. 282) makes an easy weekday meal.	Sign up for an aerobics class with your best pal so that neither of you will skip out on the other.
tuesday	Dash off to work with a homemade Granola Bar saved from the batch made last week.	Enjoy Avocado and Grapefruit Salad (pg. 281) while reading the newest issue of your favorite magazine.	The kids will love Eggplant Boats Stuffed with Spicy Beef and Peas (pg. 271) with leftover slices of Fresh Lime Cake.	Rest your muscles and spend 20 minutes stretching out your tired parts, followed by a luxurious, scented bath.
wednesday	Apple Pie for Breakfast (pg. 267). Just kidding, of course!	Invite your GORGEOUS gal pals to share Southwestern Chopped Salad with Toasted Peppers and Corn (pg. 284).	Spicy Tuna Dinner Salad with Balsamic Dressing (pg. 273) and Orange Cappuccino Parfaits (pg. 285) are yummy and simple to prepare.	Take a 30-minute POWER WALK to start your day. Add 15 minutes of weight lifting. Do a few more reps than last week. Find a pal who wants to run a marathon and start training.
thursday	Blend up your favorite Juiced-Up Fruit-and-Herb Breakfast Drinks (Blueberry-Basil, pg. 57).	Brown bag it! Prepare fresh tuna salad with leftovers from last night's supper.	Prepare Baked Chicken Breasts with Artichoke and Sun-Dried Tomato Sauce (pg. 275) for an easy midweek supper.	Walk this way—for 30 minutes. Add a few lunges to stretch out those legs and butt. Add a few squats after your walk. Hold in your tummy during your workout to build muscles.
friday	Breakfast Tacos (pg. 268) are a fun Friday breakfast.	Prepare Grilled Veggie Panini with Basil Pesto Sauce (pg. 274). Make one to share with your walking buddy.	Treat the whole family to Chicken Portobello with Linguini in Butter Sauce (pg. 276; you've been so good!). Add a bite of Tropical Buttermilk Panna Cotta with Strawberry Sauce (pg. 287) for dessert.	Start the day with a 40-minute POWER WALK with a pal that includes 10 minutes of jogging and 10 minutes of stretching!

For Week 8 Grocery Shopping List and Shopping Day Prep Tips visit www.GorgeousLifestyleGuide.com

gorgeous lifestyle guide week 9 — sleepy time

Day	Breakfast	Lunch	Dinner	Revitalizing Activity
saturday	Bake up a batch of Orange Breakfast Muffins (pg. 305). Save extras for later in the week.	This is Shopping Day. While you are running errands, stop and treat yourself to your favorite fresh garden salad with whole grain bread on the side.	Date night! Invite pals for Rack of Lamb with Spinach and Breadcrumb Topping (pg. 311), Broccoli Mash (pg. 321) and Simmering Blueberries with Cinnamon Dumplings (pg. 324).	Start the day with a 40-minute POWER WALK that includes 15 minutes of jogging! Today is Shopping Day! Hit the farmer's market.
sunday	Gather the group for Sweet Potato Pancakes with Warm Raspberry Syrup (pg. 306).	**Afternoon** Have a simple lunch of Grilled Ratatouille Salad with Tomato Basil Vinaigrette (pg. 323). Save extra veggies for later in the week. They will make a great soup!	Serve a comfort meal of Roast Turkey Breast with Cornbread-Cranberry Dressing and Madeira Mushroom Gravy (pg. 310) and Stuffed Zucchini, Yellow Squash, and Eggplant (pg. 322).	After dinner relax with a warm and soothing cup of decaffeinated tea and a hot, lavender-scented bath.
monday	Enjoy rich Fruit 'N Soy Milk Drinks (pg. 307) as a start to your workweek.	Brown bag it! Choose whole grain bread to build your turkey sandwich made with leftover roasted turkey. Add dark green lettuce and sliced tomato.	Grilled Coconut Curry Shrimp with Soba Noodles (pg. 312) makes for a light and easy supper. Add leftover grilled veggies from earlier in the week.	Get to bed early with a lavender sachet tucked under your pillow.
tuesday	Dash off to work with a warmed Orange Breakfast Muffin.	Prepare Open-Faced Eggplant, Tomato, and Cheddar Grilled Cheese (pg. 309). Make extras for your workout buddy.	Gather the family for a supper of Stuffed Chicken Breasts with Mushrooms, Thyme, and Fontina Cheese (pg. 313) and Sautéed Cauliflower and Spinach Fettuccini Casserole (pg. 320).	Rest your muscles and spend 20 minutes stretching out your tired parts, followed by a luxurious, scented bath.
wednesday	Enjoy a treat of Breakfast Tomatoes with Smoke Salmon (pg. 308).	Invite your GORGEOUS gal pals to share Crab Cake Po' Boys (pg. 316) for lunch.	Simply prepared Broiled Tilapia Fillets with Arugula Aioli Sauce (pg. 315) comes together so quickly that you'll have time to bake a batch of Butterscotch Blondies (pg. 325) for dessert.	Take a 30-minute POWER WALK to start your day. Add 15 minutes of weight lifting. Schedule a Swedish massage.
thursday	Blend up your favorite Juiced-Up Fruit-and-Herb Breakfast Drinks (Apple-Mint, pg. 57).	Brown bag it! Take along a fresh garden salad topped with chicken slices from earlier in the week. Add a Butterscotch Blondie to the bag and another one for a pal.	Whip up Linguini with Mussels and Snow Peas (pg. 318) for a light meal on Thursday night. Prepare a batch of Almond Cookies Two Ways (pg. 327) and freeze half for next week.	Walk this way—for 30 minutes. Place a blank piece of paper on your bedside table and quote your sleepy time mantra as you dose off.
friday	Sip on Fruit 'N Soy Milk Drinks (pg. 307) for breakfast.	Prepare Grilled Veggie Panini with Basil Pesto Sauce (pg. 274). Make one to share with your walking buddy.	Treat the whole family to Pecan-Crusted Chicken Fingers with Apricot Mustard Dipping Sauce (pg. 319) and Simple Chocolate Mousse with Graham Cracker Crumbles (pg. 326).	Start the day with a 40-minute POWER WALK with a pal that includes 10 minutes of jogging and 10 minutes of stretching!

For Week 9 Grocery Shopping List and Shopping Day Prep Tips visit www.GorgeousLifestyleGuide.com

gorgeous lifestyle guide week 10 — stress-free

Day	Breakfast	Lunch	Dinner	Revitalizing Activity
saturday	Just for *fun*, make the gang Grilled Peanut Butter and Banana Sandwiches with Just a Touch of Honey (pg. 344) for breakfast.	This is Shopping Day. While you run your errands, stop and treat yourself to your favorite garden fresh salad and whole grain roll.	Date night. Invite pals for an easy menu of Creamy Wild Mushroom Soup with Sherry and Fresh Thyme (pg. 357), Shrimp Scampi with Angel Hair Pasta (pg. 346), and Key Lime Pound Cake (pg. 360).	Start the day with a 40-minute POWER WALK that includes 15 minutes of jogging! Today is Shopping Day! Hit the farmer's market.
sunday	Gather the group for Bacon and Asparagus Quiche (pg. 342) for brunch.	**Afternoon** Have a simple lunch of leftover Creamy Wild Mushroom Soup with Sherry and Fresh Thyme from last night's supper.	Serve Hearty Beef Stew (pg. 348) and Pretty in Peach (pg. 363) dessert to start the week off just fine.	After dinner relax with a warm and soothing cup of tea and a hot, lavender-scented bath.
monday	Fruit 'N Soy Milk Drinks (pg. 307) make an easy and nourishing breakfast.	Brown bag it! Choose whole grain bread and fresh veggies to build your favorite deli sandwich and take it on the road alongside a slice of leftover Key Lime Pound Cake.	Ginger-Marinated Tuna with Lime Butter (pg. 347) makes for a simple midweek super.	Work off that frustration by spending 20 to 30 minutes in your garden.
tuesday	Dash off to work with an Open-Faced BLT Sandwich (pg. 340).	Prepare a huge pot of Fresh Veggie Minestrone Soup with Chickpeas (pg. 356). Have a bowl for lunch and reserve leftovers for later in the week.	Old-Fashioned Turkeyloaf with Hidden Mushrooms (pg. 345) is totally comforting for a midweek supper.	Rest your muscles. Spend 20 minutes stretching. De-stress by preparing a batch of Maple Cake Doughnuts (pg. 361) to take to the office tomorrow morning. Eat one and share the rest!
wednesday	Blend up your favorite Juiced-Up Fruit-and-Herb Breakfast Drinks (Cantaloupe-Tarragon, pg. 57).	Invite your GORGEOUS gal pals for Pan Sautéed Gnocchi with Sun-Dried Tomato and Sage (pg. 355). It's to die for. . . .	Butternut Squash and Swiss Chard Roll-Ups with Sun-Dried Tomato Basil Sauce (pg. 353) are easily prepared and soothing to eat.	Take a 30-minute POWER WALK to start your day. Add 15 minutes of weight lifting. Schedule a Swedish massage. Buy an audiobook and put it in your car for rush-hour listening.
thursday	You will just love Ham and Cheese Scramble (pg. 341) for breakfast.	Brown bag it! Take along a childhood favorite—leftover meatloaf on whole grain bread. Don't forget the ketchup.	Hunter's-Style Chicken Stew with Yellow Rice (pg. 352) can be prepared in your slow cooker and served to a hungry crowd.	Remember to hold in your stomach on your 30-minute POWER WALK. Afterward, enjoy a cup of soothing tea.
friday	There's always time for Fruit 'N Soy Milk Drinks (pg. 307).	Enjoy Spicy Flank Steak Sandwich with Roasted Pepper Blue Cheese Sauce (pg. 350) shared with the other moms at the park.	Treat the whole family to Really Good Turkey Burgers with Cheddar Cheese and Horseradish Sauce (pg. 354) and The Real Deal Fries with Ketchup of Course (pg. 358).	Start the day with a 40-minute POWER WALK with a P\pal that includes 10 minutes of jogging and 10 minutes of stretching!

For Week 10 Grocery Shopping List and Shopping Day Prep Tips visit www.GorgeousLifestyleGuide.com

gorgeous lifestyle guide week 11 — sexy glam

Day	Meal	Meal	Meal	Revitalizing Activity
saturday	**Breakfast** Start off your sexy weekend with Cinnamon Chocolate-Chip Pancakes with Whipped Cream and Warm Maple Syrup (pg. 377).	**Lunch** This is Shopping Day. While you are running your errands, stop and enjoy your favorite deli sandwich filled with fresh veggies, lean meat, and reduced-fat cheese.	**Dinner** Couples' supper club menu: Baked Oysters with Pancetta Topping (pg. 392), Duck Breasts with Pinot Noir Red Grape Sauce (pg. 388), and Basil-Roasted Strawberry Cheesecake with Rich Chocolate Crust (pg. 397).	Start the day with a 40-minute POWER WALK that includes 15 minutes of jogging! Today is Shopping Day! Hit the farmer's market and the specialty wine shop.
sunday	**Breakfast** Enjoy a luxurious brunch of Very Sexy Scrambled Eggs with Caviar and Peppered Strawberries (pg. 376). Yum!	**Afternoon** Plan a workout for two—prepare a batch of Orgasmic Braised Ribs with Chili and Chocolate (pg. 381).	**Dinner** Serve Orgasmic Braised Ribs with Chili and Chocolate (pg. 381), Arugula Salad with Walnut Crusted Goat Cheese (pg. 390), and a small sliver of last night's cheesecake.	After dinner relax with a warm and soothing cup of tea and a hot, revitalizing bath.
monday	**Breakfast** For a quick pick-me-up, choose Fruit 'N Soy Milk Drinks (pg. 307) for breakfast.	**Lunch** Brown bag it! Build a take-along salad full of fresh veggies.	**Dinner** Monday . . . Monday's dinner is purrrfect when it stars Grilled Pork Chops with Cherry Ginger Chutney (pg. 389).	Grab your partner and enter the "Love Gym." Work on your Pilates moves.
tuesday	**Breakfast** Whip up Juiced-Up Fruit-and-Herb Breakfast Drinks (Blueberry-Basil, pg. 57).	**Lunch** Lighten up with Avocado and Grapefruit Salad (pg. 281) for a quick lunch.	**Dinner** Saltimbocca is a dish that comes together quickly when you want to "spice up" that weeknight meal.	Rest your muscles and spend 20 minutes stretching. De-stress further by preparing a batch of Peanut Butter Chocolate Bars (pg. 394) to take to the office tomorrow morning.
wednesday	**Breakfast** Grab a Granola Bar from that stash in your freezer.	**Lunch** Invite your GORGEOUS gal pals for a luscious lunch of Butternut Squash Ravioli with Brown Butter, Sage, and Pine Nut Sauce (pg. 382).	**Dinner** Reconnect as you graze over Peel-and-Eat Jumbo Shrimp with Buffalo-Style Sauce (pg. 391).	Take a 30-minute POWER WALK to start your day. Add 15 minutes of weight lifting. After supper, grab his hand for an evening stroll around the neighborhood.
thursday	**Breakfast** Start the day off with a hearty breakfast of Egg, Sausage, and Spinach Skillets (pg. 378). You might have to call in late for work!.	**Lunch** Brown bag it! Take along spicy shrimp salad, using up the shrimp you couldn't finish last evening.	**Dinner** Take advantage of your slow cooker when you prepare Chicken Wings with Mole Sauce (pg. 387) and eat at your leisure.	Walk this way—for 30 minutes, followed by a cup of soothing tea and a neck and shoulder massage from your honey.
friday	**Breakfast** Baked Raspberry-Stuffed French Toast with Pecans and Maple Drizzle (pg. 379) is an excellent way to start the weekend.	**Lunch** Enjoy a light lunch of Olive, Onion, and Roasted Pepper Bruschetta (pg. 393).	**Dinner** Dinner for two stars Grilled Lobster Tails with Parsley Butter Served over Creamy Hash (pg. 380). Does it get any better than this?	Start the day with a 40-minute POWER WALK with a your significant other that includes 10 minutes of jogging and 10 minutes of stretching!

For Week 11 Grocery Shopping List and Shopping Day Prep Tips visit www.GorgeousLifestyleGuide.com

gorgeous lifestyle guide week 12 — eye-catching, skin-savvy

Day	Breakfast	Lunch	Dinner	Revitalizing Activity
saturday	Fruit and Yogurt Breakfast Parfaits with Granola Crunch (pg. 59) make for a stellar Saturday splurge.	This is Shopping Day. While you are running your errands treat yourself to a Fresh Fruit Salad with Citrus Basil Dressing (pg. 58).	Date night! Invite pals for a menu of Butternut Squash Soup Flavored with Orange and Tarragon (pg. 70), Grilled New York Strip Steaks with Garlic Herb Oil (pg. 125), and Chocolate Ricotta-Filled Crepes (pg. 136).	Start the day with a 40-minute POWER WALK with a pal! Today is Shopping Day! Hit the farmer's market.
sunday	Enjoy a luxurious brunch of Breakfast Burritos with Red Pepper Salsa (pg. 60) with the gang.	**Afternoon**: Mediterranean Tuna Melts (pg. 62) make an easy lunch sandwich—especially during "football Sunday."	Bring the family to the table for a supper of Chicken Thighs with Sage and Caramelized Peaches (pg. 65) with Rosemary Roasted Carrot Sticks (pg. 72).	Luxuriate with an OATMEAL PEEL (pg. 79). Visit the cosmetic counter for a new makeover.
monday	Broiled Grapefruit with Honey Mascarpone Cream (pg. 117) is an easy and yummy breakfast.	Brown bag it! Build a take-along salad full of fresh veggies. Add a thermos of leftover Butternut Squash Soup from the weekend.	Try a meal of Grilled Halibut with Salsa Verde (pg. 64) to beat the Monday blues.	Lighten dark circles and smooth puffiness with raw ingredients like potatoes and egg whites.
tuesday	Juiced-up Fruit-and-Herb Breakfast Drink (Apple-Mint, pg. 57).	Enjoy Sweet Potato Apple Salad with Honey, Ginger and Mustard Dressing (pg. 63). Make extras to take to coworkers.	Spice up your Tuesday night with Roasted Veggie Burritos with Chipotle Chili Tomato Sauce (pg. 121) and Orange-Glazed Yogurt Cake (pg. 134) for dessert.	Apply a HONEY MASK (pg. 79) and relax for 20 minutes. Don't forget to squeeze in your 30-minute POWER WALK.
wednesday	Perk up the midweek with a breakfast of Scrambled Eggs with Red Grape and Avocado Salsa (pg 118).	Invite your GORGEOUS gal pals for Spinach Salad with Warm Chipotle Chili Vinaigrette, Chicken Strips, & Crisp Sweet Potato (pg. 66) and Cranberry Wedding Cookies (pg. 135) for dessert.	Please the kids with Open-Faced Chicken Tacos (pg. 68) and leftover cookies.	Take a 30-minute POWER WALK to start your day. See clearly. Identify something beautiful in your environment and appreciate the sight.
thursday	Melon Bowls with Strawberry Ginger Sauce (pg. 120) are a great way to start your day.	Brown bag it! Take along Sushi-Style Salmon Wraps (pg. 61) and surprise someone special with a desk-top picnic.	Dinner comes together quickly when you prepare Stir-Fry Chicken and Broccoli with Chopped Peanuts (pg. 123). You'll find extra time to make Oven-Roasted Fruit with Vanilla Yogurt Sorbet (pg. 77).	Work in a 30-minute POWER WALK followed by a cup of soothing tea and a neck and shoulder massage.
friday	Poached Eggs in Spicy Tomato Sauce (pg. 119) start off the weekend.	Enjoy a make-ahead lunch of Stuffed Sweet Potatoes with Spinach and Corn (pg. 73). Very veggie!	Dinner for two stars Spaghetti Squash Carbonara (pg. 124) and Roasted Figs with Sweetened Orange Sauce (pg. 74) for dessert.	Stretch out your neck and shoulders. Make an appointment with the cosmetic counter expert at the department store to test out the new seasonal eye makeup colors.

For Week 12 Grocery Shopping List and Shopping Day Prep Tips visit www.GorgeousLifestyleGuide.com

gorgeous lifestyle guide week 13 — skin-savvy, good to the bones

	Breakfast	Lunch	Dinner	Revitalizing Activity
saturday	Bake up a batch of Whole Grain Apple Muffins with Walnut Streusel (pg. 177). Make extras for later in the week.	It's Shopping Day. While you are running errands, stop at the market for your favorite deli sandwich stuffed with fresh veggies and piled onto whole grain bread.	Date night! Invite pals for Grilled Lamb Chops with White Bean Salad (pg. 182) and Almond-Topped Ricotta Cheesecake (pg. 195).	Start the day with a 40-minute POWER WALK with a Pal! Today is Shopping Day! Hit the farmer's market.
sunday	Enjoy a good-for-you brunch that includes Eggs Benedict with Swiss Chard and Whole Grain English Muffins (pg. 175).	**Afternoon** Nibble on Peppery White Bean Salsa with Whole Wheat Pita Chips (pg. 189).	Sunday supper includes Baked Tilapia with Fresh Herbs (pg. 183), Lentils with Wild Rice and Mushrooms (pg. 190), and Peanut Butter Sandwich Cookies (pg. 194). Save extra cookies for treats later in the week.	Soak in a hot tub filled with Epsom salts and lavender oil.
monday	Fruit and Yogurt Breakfast Parfaits with Granola Crunch (pg. 59) are a great Monday morning breakfast.	Brown bag it! Take along a container of Green Gazpacho Soup with Navy Bean Garnish (pg. 188).	Parmesan Chicken Fingers with Green Cashew and Curry Dipping Sauce (pg. 181) will become a family favorite supper.	Give your dull skin a creamy shine with a MILKY CLEANSER (pg. 78). Remember that POWER WALK!
tuesday	A grab-and-go Whole Grain Apple Muffin warmed in the microwave is terrific.	Summer Squash Salad with Baby Spinach, Roasted Tomatoes, and Parmesan Cheese (pg. 192) is a perfect veggie salad for midday.	Prepare a fast and fabulous meal of Whole Wheat Spaghetti with Grilled Turkey, Broccoli Rabe, Red Peppers, and Peas (pg. 180). Remember those extra cookies?	Luxuriate with an OATMEAL PEEL (pg. 79). Visit the cosmetic counter for a new makeover.
wednesday	Take five and prepare Breakfast Panini with Chicken Sausage (pg. 178).	Sushi-Style Salmon Wraps (pg. 61) are simple and suave for a desk-side picnic.	Roasted Tomato Basil Soup with Sea Bass Center (pg. 69) and Cocktail Nut Cookie Bars (pg. 196).	Stretch out from head to toe. Take a 30-minute POWER WALK to start your day. Add 10 minutes of weight lifting. Remember to start light.
thursday	Fresh Fruit Salad with Citrus Basil Dressing (pg. 58) is yummy and full of fabulous fruit power.	Invite your GORGEOUS gal pals for a lunch of Watercress Salad with Raspberry Vinaigrette and Blood Orange (pg. 191) with Rosemary Polenta with Spinach, Red Beans, and Goat Cheese (pg. 184).	Prepare a light supper of Spinach Salad with Warm Chipotle Chili Vinaigrette Topped with Chicken Strips and Crisp Sweet Potato (pg. 66).	Apply a HONEY MASK (pg. 79). Remember that POWER WALK? Add a few lunges to stretch out those legs.
friday	Blend up your favorite Juiced-Up Fruit-and-Herb Breakfast Drinks (Apple-Mint, pg. 57).	Prepare a couple of Mediterranean Tuna Melts (pg. 62) and share with the moms at the PTA meeting.	Gather the family for Mustard Garlic Roasted Chicken Served with Arugula and Artichoke Salad (pg. 179) and Macadamia Nut Biscotti Dipped in Chocolate and Coconut (pg. 193).	Start the day with a 40-minute POWER WALK with a pal! Discuss the latest novel.

For Week 13 Grocery Shopping List and Shopping Day Prep Tips visit www.GorgeousLifestyleGuide.com

gorgeous lifestyle guide week 14 — skin-savvy, hands-on glam

Day	Breakfast	Lunch	Dinner	Revitalizing Activity
saturday	Make a batch of Granola Power Bars (pg. 239). Save extras for later in the week.	Enjoy a fast, light lunch of Chilled Shrimp Salad with Red Grapes (pg. 241).	Date night! Invite pals for Sautéed Yellowtail Snapper with Braised Cabbage and Cheesy Mashed Potatoes (pg. 246) served with Chocoholic's Crutch (p. 255).	Start the day with a 40-minute POWER WALK with a pal! Today is Shopping Day! Hit the farmer's market.
sunday	Gather the gang for a brunch of Breakfast Burritos with Red Pepper Salsa (pg. 60).	**Afternoon:** Sip on a bowl of warm Butternut Squash Soup Flavored with Orange and Tarragon (pg. 70).	Gather the family for a festive evening meal featuring Jambalaya (pg. 245), Sweet Potato Soufflé (pg. 249), and Roasted Red Grape Parfaits with Orange and Maple-Flavored Ricotta Cheese (pg. 253).	Luxuriate with a MINT FACIAL STEAM (pg. 78).
monday	Start the workweek with Blueberry Buttermilk Coffee Cake Topped with Granola (pg. 236).	Brown bag it! Make up a few Chicken and Rice Meatball Hoagies (pg. 242) and share with coworkers.	Keep it light with Roasted Asparagus Salad with Arugula, Radishes, and Lemon Vinaigrette (pg. 248) and Poached Salmon in Infused Olive Oil with Horseradish Sauce (pg. 240).	Give yourself a home spa manicure while you listen to your favorite new jazz cd.
tuesday	Bake up a batch of Pecan Bananadana Muffins (pg. 90). Save some for next week.	Dig into Black Bean and Roasted Pepper Empanadas (pg. 250).	Serve the workweek crowd Turkey Meatloaf Burgers with Spicy Sweet Potato Sticks (pg. 243) and Strike-It-Rich Chocolate Pudding with Chocolate Cookie Crumbles (pg. 252).	Luxuriate with an OATMEAL PEEL (pg. 79). Visit the cosmetic counter for a new makeover.
wednesday	Choose your favorite Juiced-Up Fruit-and-Herb Breakfast Drinks (Cantaloupe-Tarragon, pg. 57).	Sweet Potato Apple Salad with Honey, Ginger, and Mustard Dressing (pg. 63) is purrfect for lunch.	Serve a family favorite of Open-Faced Chicken Tacos (pg. 68), Stewed Tomatoes with Garlic and Black Beans (pg. 71), and Roasted Figs with Sweetened Orange Sauce (pg. 74).	Hold hands with your special someone while you stroll through the neighborhood after supper.
thursday	Grab a Granola Power Bar for the drive to work.	Invite your GORGEOUS gal pals for Roasted Tomato Basil Soup with Sea Bass Center (pg. 69) and Simple Zucchini Cake with Vanilla Glaze (pg. 254).	Serve a colorful meal of Sliced Chicken Breast with Red Grape Sauce (pg. 247) and Sautéed Red Cabbage with Drunken Raisins (pg. 251).	Apply a HONEY MASK (pg. 79) and relax for 20 minutes. Did you remember your POWER WALK today?
friday	Prepare Walnut-Stuffed Baked Apples with Maple Syrup (pg. 238) the night before and bake in the morning while you get ready for your day.	Sushi-Style Salmon Wraps (pg. 61) are perfect for lunch at home or on the run.	Friday fish night—updated. Serve Snapper Veronique (pg. 244) with Rosemary Roasted Carrot Sticks (pg. 72) and leftover Zucchini Cake.	Take a 30-minute POWER WALK to start your day. Add 15 minutes of weight lifting. Do a few more reps than last week. Reward yourself with a manicure appointment.

For Week 14 Grocery Shopping List and Shopping Day Prep Tips visit www.GorgeousLifestyleGuide.com

gorgeous lifestyle guide week 15 — skin-savvy, sleepy time

Day	Breakfast	Lunch	Dinner	Revitalizing Activity
saturday	Fruit 'N Soy Milk Drinks (pg. 307) make a fast and nutritious start to a busy day.	Open-Faced Eggplant, Tomato, and Cheddar Grilled Cheese (pg. 309) are perfect to keep your energy level up.	Date night! Invite pals for Rack of Lamb with Spinach and Breadcrumb Topping (pg. 311), Stuffed Zucchini, Squash, and Eggplant (pg. 322), and Key Lime Pound Cake (pg. 360).	Start the day with a 40-minute POWER WALK with a pal! Today is Shopping Day! Hit the farmer's market
sunday	Gather the clan for a brunch of Sweet Potato Pancakes with Warm Raspberry Syrup (pg. 306).	**Afternoon:** Serve a yummy dish to the gathering clan. Sweet Potato Apple Salad with Honey, Ginger, and Mustard Dressing (pg. 63) fits the bill.	Keep it light this Sunday with Broiled Tilapia Fillets with Arugula Aioli Sauce (pg. 315) and Broccoli Mash (pg. 321).	Rest your muscles and spend 20 minutes stretching out your tired parts, followed by a luxurious, scented bath.
monday	Fruit and Yogurt Breakfast Parfaits with Granola Crunch (pg. 59) spoon up easily.	Brown bag it! Take along Mediterranean Tuna Melts (pg. 62) and share with coworkers.	Surprise the Monday night crowd with Roast Turkey Breast with Cornbread-Cranberry Dressing with Madeira Mushroom Gravy (pg. 310).	Give your dull skin a creamy shine with a MILKY CLEANSER (pg. 78). Don't forget your 30-minute POWER WALK.
tuesday	Open-Faced BLT Breakfast Sandwiches (pg. 340) are so good for a Tuesday start.	Use leftover turkey to build a super sandwich that includes whole grain bread, leafy lettuce, thick slices of tomato, and a dab of reduced-fat mayo.	Keep it simple with Linguini with Mussels and Snow Peas (pg. 318) and Almond Cookies Two Ways (pg. 327—save extras for snacks).	Start the day with a 30-minute POWER WALK. Place a blank piece of paper on your bedside table and quote your sleepy time mantra as you dose off this evening.
wednesday	Every day is a good day for your favorite Juiced-Up Fruit-and-Herb Breakfast Drinks (Blueberry-Basil, pg. 57).	There's probably still some turkey in the fridge! Make turkey salad with red grapes and celery.	It's comfort food on Wednesday! Serve Stuffed Chicken Breast with Mushrooms, Thyme, and Fontina Cheese (pg. 313) with Sautéed Cauliflower and Spinach Fettuccini Casserole (pg. 320).	Stretch out your arms and legs. Try out some Pilates moves. Check out the latest audiobooks.
thursday	Fresh Fruit Salad with Citrus Basil Dressing (pg. 58) is a great way to add fruit to your diet.	Invite your GORGEOUS gal pals for a lunch of Grilled Coconut Curry Shrimp with Soba Noodles (pg. 312) and Simple Chocolate Mousse with Graham Cracker Crumbles (pg. 326).	Prepare Grilled Halibut with Salsa Verde (pg. 64) with leftover Cauliflower Casserole and serve at least one Almond Cookie.	Apply a HONEY MASK (pg. 79) and relax for 20 minutes. Remember to squeeze in a 30-minute POWER WALK.
friday	Breakfast Tomatoes with Smoked Salmon (pg. 308) are a perfect breakfast treat.	Sip a savory bowl of Butternut Squash Soup Flavored with Orange and Tarragon (pg. 70).	Gather the kids for Pecan-Crusted Chicken Fingers with Apricot Mustard Dipping Sauce (pg. 319) and Butterscotch Blondies (pg. 325).	Take a 30-minute POWER WALK to start your day. Add 15 minutes of weight lifting. Schedule a Swedish massage.

For Week 15 Grocery Shopping List and Shopping Day Prep Tips visit www.GorgeousLifestyleGuide.com

gorgeous lifestyle guide week 16 — skin-savvy, sexy glam

Day	Breakfast	Lunch	Dinner	Revitalizing Activity
saturday	Enjoy your favorite Juiced-Up Fruit-and-Herb Drinks (Apple-Mint, pg. 57).	It's Shopping Day. While you are running errands, stop at your favorite deli and enjoy a sandwich made on whole grain bread with leafy lettuce, thick tomato, and lean meat.	Date night dinner for two offers Arugula Salad with Walnut-Crusted Goat Cheese (pg. 390), Grilled Lobster Tails with Parsley Butter Served over Creamy Hash (pg. 380), and Pretty in Peach (pg. 363).	Start the day with a 40-minute POWER WALK with a pal! Today is Shopping Day! Hit the farmer's market.
sunday	Enjoy the Morning After with Very Sexy Scrambled Eggs with Caviar and Peppered Strawberries (pg. 376).	**Afternoon:** Nibble on Olive, Onion, and Roasted Pepper Bruschetta (pg. 393).	Grilled Pork Chops with Cherry Ginger Chutney (pg. 389) make a wonderful Sunday supper.	Luxuriate with a MINT FACIAL STEAM (pg. 78) in a warm bath.
monday	Fruit and Yogurt Breakfast Parfaits with Granola Crunch (pg. 59) are simply spoonable!	Brown bag it! Surprise him with a desk-side picnic for two that includes Mediterranean Tuna Melts (pg. 62).	Use your crock pot to help prepare Chicken Wings with Mole Sauce (pg. 387) so you can spend your time together.	Give your dull skin a creamy shine with a MILKY CLEANSER (pg. 78). Ask him to join you for a 30-minute POWER WALK. If he declines, you still go!
tuesday	Egg, Sausage, and Spinach Skillets (pg. 378) are a yummy start.	Bring him home from work for Peel-and-Eat Jumbo Shrimp with Buffalo-Style Sauce (pg. 391).	Saltimbocca (pg. 386), Stewed Tomatoes with Garlic and Black Beans (pg. 71), and Peanut Butter Chocolate Bars (pg. 394) make a wonderful midweek supper.	Luxuriate with an OATMEAL PEEL (pg. 79) for 20 minutes. Visit the cosmetic counter for a makeover.
wednesday	Fresh Fruit Salad with Citrus Basil Dressing (pg. 58) is easy and yummy.	Open-Faced Chicken Tacos (pg. 68) are perfect for teacher's workday when the kids are home from school.	Everyone will gather for Really Good Turkey Burgers with Cheddar Cheese and Horseradish Sauce (pg. 354).	Stretch out your arms, back, and legs. Check out the latest audiobooks for your rush-hour drive.
thursday	Cinnamon Chocolate-Chip Pancakes with Whipped Cream and Warm Maple Syrup (pg. 377) are faster to make than they are to say.	Invite your GORGEOUS gal pals for a lunch of Butternut Squash Ravioli with Brown Butter, Sage, and Pine Nut Sauce (pg. 382). They will love you!	Tonight's dinner is Spinach Salad with Warm Chipotle Chili Vinaigrette Topped with Chicken Strips and Crisp Sweet Potato (pg. 66).	Apply a HONEY MASK (pg. 79) after your 30-minute POWER WALK.
friday	Baked Raspberry-Stuffed French Toast with Pecans and Maple Drizzle (pg. 379) is decadent, dastardly, and definitely purrfect for a Friday breakfast.	Have a very veggie lunch of Stuffed Sweet Potatoes with Spinach and Corn (pg. 73).	Tonight offers a simple Friday supper of Roasted Tomato Basil Soup with Sea Bass Center (pg. 69).	Start the day with a 40-minute POWER WALK with a pal! Discuss the latest novels or magazine articles.

For Week 16 Grocery Shopping List and Shopping Day Prep Tips visit www.GorgeousLifestyleGuide.com

gorgeous lifestyle guide week 17 — good hair, smile pretty

Day	Breakfast	Lunch	Dinner	Revitalizing Activity
saturday	Bake up a batch of Pecan Bananadana Muffins (pg. 90). Use extras for weekday grab-and-go breakfasts.	This is Shopping Day, so treat yourself to your favorite deli sandwich. Choose whole grain bread and lean meats.	Date night! Invite pals for Paella with Chorizo, Asparagus, and Shellfish (pg. 98), Fried Plantains (pg. 100), and Baked Pears in Brandy Sauce (pg. 104).	Start the day with a 40-minute POWER WALK with a pal! Today is Shopping Day! Hit the farmer's market!
	Breakfast	**Afternoon**	**Dinner**	**Revitalizing Activity**
sunday	Invite the gang for Spicy Roasted Veggie and Shrimp Salsa with Fried Egg and Warm Cheese Sauce (pg. 146).	Splurge on Artichoke and Asiago Crostini (pg. 162).	Gather the family for a Sunday supper of Crispy Roasted Chicken with Penne Pasta (pg. 154) and Emergency Key Lime Pie (pg. 166).	Luxuriate with an OLIVE OIL HAIR MASK (pg. 110). Smile at everyone you meet today and see how many smile back!
	Breakfast	**Lunch**	**Dinner**	**Revitalizing Activity**
monday	Fresh Papaya and Grapefruit with Yogurt and Mint (pg. 147) has tons of flavor.	Brown bag it! Take along a grab-and-go container of Shrimp Salad with Mango and Cucumber (pg. 159).	Perk up your everyday weeknight meal by serving Seared Jumbo Scallops with Herb Butter Sauce (pg. 152) and Orange and Tarragon-Infused Crème Brûlées with Slice Bananas (pg. 163).	Stretch out your lower back and legs. Take a 30-minute POWER WALK to start your day. Make an appointment with the cosmetic counter to test out the new seasonal lipstick colors.
tuesday	Warm up Pecan Bananadana Muffins!	Treat yourself to Swiss Cheese Wafers (pg. 160) and Blue Cheese Dip with All Kinds of Dippers (pg. 161). Make extras for coworkers or neighbors. Remember, you CAN eat just one!	Prepare a simple supper of Roasted Pork Tenderloin with Swiss Chard (pg. 96), Toasted Corn with Sauteed Spinach and Cherry Tomatoes (pg. 103), and Mango-Walnut Crumble (pg. 165) for dessert.	Luxuriate with an OLIVE OIL HAIR MASK (pg. 110) for 20 minutes and try out a new hairdo.
wednesday	Warm Oatmeal with Caramelized Fruit Topping (pg. 149) is a satisfying starter.	Invite your GORGEOUS gal pals for a lunch of Creamy Cauliflower Soup with Arugula and Crispy Bacon Garnish (pg. 101) and Turkey with Caramelized Onion and Smoked Gouda Panini (pg. 151).	WACKY Wednesday Party: Lamb Chops with Skillet Coconut Sauce, Louisiana-Style Red Beans (pg. 102), and Sautéed Bananas with Sweet Mascarpone and Walnut Crunch (pg. 107).	Stretch out your neck and shoulders. Make an appointment with a hip-happening hairstylist!
thursday	Prepare a batch of Raspberry Oatmeal Muffins with Macadamia Nut Butter (pg. 89). Save extras for next week.	Brown bag it! Prepare Grilled Skirt Steak and Veggie Open-Faced Sandwiches (pg. 95) for a desk-side picnic.	Have a light meal of Mussles with Brussels in a White Wine Butter Sauce (pg. 94).	Apply a FRUIT HAIR MASK (pg. 109). Walk this way—for 30 minutes.
friday	Creamy French-Style Eggs Garnished with Chopped Tomatoes and Chives (pg. 87) are really, really good.	Prepare Buffalo Chicken Cobb Salad with Buttermilk Dressing (pg. 150). Save extras for Shopping Day!	Serve a special supper of Lemon Veal with Sauteed Spinach, Pine Nuts, and Goat Cheese (pg. 158) and Oatmeal Snack Cake (pg. 106). Yum!	Start the day with a 40-minute POWER WALK with a pal! Today is Shopping Day! Hit the farmer's market!

For Week 17 Grocery Shopping List and Shopping Day Prep Tips visit www.GorgeousLifestyleGuide.com

gorgeous lifestyle guide week 18 — good hair, you could be dancin'

Day	Breakfast	Lunch	Dinner	Revitalizing Activity
saturday	Bake up a batch of Whole Wheat Bran Muffins with Golden Raisins and Walnuts (pg. 207). Make extras for later in the week.	This is Shopping Day, so treat yourself to your favorite deli sandwich. Choose whole grain bread, lean meats, and lots of fresh veggies.	Date night! Invite pals for Wild Ivory Salmon Fillets with Macadamia Nut Crust (pg. 211), Toasted Corn with Sautéed Spinach and Cherry Tomatoes (pg. 103), and Tropical Strawberry Tiramisu (pg. 224).	Start the day with a 40-minute POWER WALK with a pal! Today is Shopping Day! Hit the farmer's market.
sunday	Breakfast: Invite the gang for a brunch of Poached Eggs with Spinach and White Beans (pg. 210).	Afternoon: Splurge on Overstuffed Beefsteak Tomatoes with Tortellini Salad (pg. 214).	Gather the family for Sunday supper that includes Charred Sirloin Steak with Mushrooms and Red Wine Sauce (pg. 213), Roasted Veggie Stacks with Mozzarella (pg. 220), and Blueberry Shortbread Bars (pg. 223).	Luxuriate with an OLIVE OIL HAIR MASK (pg. 110). Stretch out those toes and soak in warm water after a long weekend.
monday	Grab a warm Whole Wheat Bran Muffin for the ride to work.	Prepare a batch of Better Veggie Chili (pg. 218) and take along a thermosful to work.	Serve Grilled Skirt Steak and Veggie Open-Faced Sandwiches (pg. 95) with Rhubarb and Strawberry Frozen Yogurt with Fresh Mint (pg. 105).	Give your dull hair a COLOR LIFT (pg. 108). Remember to squeeze in your 30-minute POWER WALK.
tuesday	Enjoy a fast breakfast of Egg White Omelets with Bell Peppers and Turkey Sausage (pg. 88).	Sip on a cup of Creamy Cauliflower Soup with Arugula and Crispy Bacon Garnish (pg. 101).	Lighten up with Baked Potatoes Stuffed with Swiss Chard and Black Beans (pg. 217) for extra veggie goodness.	Take a couple of minutes to visit the sporting goods store and update your athletic shoes. Remember to purchase a pair with just the support that you need to protect your tootsie toes.
wednesday	Double-Berry Whole Wheat Pancakes (pg. 209) make a great midweek breakfast.	Invite your GORGEOUS gal pals for Asparagus Cheese Toasts (pg. 219), Sea Scallops with Blood Orange, Avocado, and Red Onion Salsa (pg. 215), and Chilled Berry Sauce with Lime Sherbet and Coconut Garnish (pg. 225).	Sneak in some Calf's Liver with Golden Onions (pg. 97) and reward everyone at home with Pecan Graham Squares (pg. 226).	Stretch out your neck and shoulders. Make an appointment with the hippest hairstylist you know.
thursday	Bake up a batch of Pecan Bananadana Muffins (pg. 90). Keep extras for shopping day!	Brown bag it! Take along Sweet Pea Panzanella Salad (pg. 221) for your desk-side picnic with coworkers.	Thursday night is FUN night with Mojo Marinated Chicken Served over Black Beans (pg. 216) and Fried Plantains (pg. 100).	Apply a FRUIT HAIR MASK (pg. 109) for 20 minutes. Keep walking! Add a few lunges to stretch out those legs and feet.
friday	Creamy French-Style Eggs Garnished with Chopped Tomatoes and Chives (pg. 87) are so good for breakfast.	Make a huge veggie salad and top it with extra slices of Mojo Marinated Chicken Served over Black Beans (pg. 216).	Gather the kids for Hoisen Beef and Veggies (pg. 212) and Pear and Strawberry Crisp (pg. 133).	Start the day with a 40-minute POWER WALK with a pal!

For Week 18 Grocery Shopping List and Shopping Day Prep Tips visit www.GorgeousLifestyleGuide.com

gorgeous lifestyle guide week 19 — good hair, tummy-pleasing

Day	Breakfast	Lunch	Dinner	Revitalizing Activity
saturday	Bake a batch of Raspberry Oatmeal Muffins with Macadamia Nut Butter (pg. 89). Save some for later in the week.	This is Shopping Day, so treat yourself to your favorite deli sandwich. Choose whole grain bread, leafy veggies, and lean meats.	Date night! Invite pals for Roasted Chipotle Salmon with Minted Couscous (pg. 279), Sautéed Peas with Mint (pg. 282), and Fresh Lime Cake with Warm Blueberry Sauce (pg. 286).	Start the day with a 40-minute POWER WALK that includes 15 minutes of jogging! Today is Shopping Day! Hit the farmer's market.
sunday	Start the day with a power breakfast. Say "Ricotta Cheese" Pancakes with Very Berry Sauce (pg. 269) is just what's needed.	**Afternoon** Splurge on Avocado and Grapefruit Salad (pg. 281).	Bring the family together for a Sunday supper that includes Chicken Portobello with Linguini in Butter Sauce (pg. 276) and Poached Cherry Sundaes (pg. 288).	Turn on your Pilates DVD and get down with your inner core. Stretch out those muscles and improve your squats—work your way up to a perfect teaser.
monday	Egg in A Frame with Basil Tomatoes (pg. 270) is a wonderful way to start your day.	Brown bag it! Prepare Grilled Veggie Panini with Basil Pesto Sauce (pg. 274) and take to work for a desk-side picnic with coworkers.	Bring the kids together for an etiquette lesson at the table and dine on Roasted Pork Tenderloin with Swiss Chard (pg. 96) and Orange Cappuccino Parfaits (pg. 285).	Give your dull hair a COLOR LIFT (pg. 108). Sign up for an aerobics class with your best pal so that neither of you will skip out on the other.
tuesday	Raspberry Oatmeal Muffins (reheated of course!) are perfect for a grab-and-go breakfast.	Prepare Southwestern Chopped Salad with Toasted Peppers and Corn (pg. 284) and dig in!	For supper tonight prepare Pancetta-Wrapped Turkey Medallions with Broccoli Rabe, Peppers, and Onions and Oatmeal Snack Cake (pg. 106).	Luxuriate with an OLIVE OIL HAIR MASK (pg. 110). Rest your muscles and spend 20 minutes stretching out your tired parts, followed by a luxurious, scented bath.
wednesday	Prepare a nourishing breakfast of Egg White Omelets with Bell Peppers and Turkey Sausage (pg. 88).	Invite your GORGEOUS gal pals for a lunch of Lobster in an Orange Curry Butter Sauce (pg. 93) and Sautéed Bananas with Sweet Mascarpone and Walnut Crunch (pg. 107).	A light weekday supper of Spicy Tuna Dinner Salad with Balsamic Dressing (pg. 273) is just perfect for a midweek meal.	Stretch out your neck and shoulders. Don't forget your POWER WALK!
thursday	Breakfast Tacos (pg. 268) are perfect on Thursday!	Brown bag it! Create your own fresh tuna salad with last evening's leftovers.	For dinner tonight serve Rosemary Roasted Chicken Breasts with Smoky Almond Sauce (pg. 91).	Apply a fruit HAIR MASK (pg. 109). Take a 30-minute POWER WALK to start your day. Add 15 minutes of weight lifting. Do a few more reps than last week. Find a pal who wants to run a marathon.
friday	Today it's Apple Pie for Breakfast (pg. 267)! Just kidding . . .	Have a yummy lunch of Grilled Skirt Steak and Veggie Open-Faced Sandwich (pg. 95).	Friday fish night is reinvented with Snapper Fillets Smothered with Caramelized Onions (pg. 272).	Start your day with a 30-minute POWER WALK. Add a few lunges to stretch out those legs and butt. Add a few squats after your walk. Hold in your tummy during your workout.

For Week 19 Grocery Shopping List and Shopping Day Prep Tips visit www.GorgeousLifestyleGuide.com

gorgeous lifestyle guide week 20 — good hair, stress-free

	Breakfast	Lunch	Dinner	Revitalizing Activity
saturday	Start the day with a batch of Maple Cake Doughnuts (pg. 361). Save extras to share with friends.	This is Shopping Day, so treat yourself to your favorite deli salad filled with the freshest veggies and topped with reduced-fat cheese.	Date night! Invite the pals for Butternut Squash and Swiss Chard Roll-Ups with Sun-Dried Tomato Basil Sauce (pg. 350) and Pretty in Peach (pg. 363).	Start the day with a 40-minute POWER WALK with a pal! Today is Shopping Day! Hit the farmer's market.
sunday	Gather for a brunch of Egg White Omelets with Bell Peppers and Turkey Sausage (pg. 88).	**Afternoon** Enjoy a light lunch of Fresh Veggie Minestrone Soup with Chickpeas (pg. 356). Save extras for later in the week.	Gather the family for a Sunday comfort supper of Old-Fashioned Turkeyloaf with Hidden Mushrooms (pg. 345), Louisiana-Style Red Beans (pg. 102), and Chocolate Gingersnaps (pg. 362).	After dinner relax with a warm and soothing cup of tea and a hot, lavender-scented bath. Luxuriate with an OLIVE OIL HAIR MASK (pg. 110) for 20 minutes.
monday	Prepare a batch of Raspberry Oatmeal Muffins with Macadamia Nut Butter (pg. 89). Save extras for later in the week.	Brown bag it! Prepare a cold Turkey Loaf sandwich with whole grain bread.	Spruce up Monday with Shrimp Scampi with Angel Hair Pasta (pg. 346) and extra Chocolate Gingersnaps.	Give your dull hair a COLOR LIFT (pg. 108). Squeeze in that 30-minute POWER WALK.
tuesday	Grab Grilled Peanut Butter and Banana Sandwiches with Just a Touch of Honey (pg. 344) as you make a dash for carpool.	Prepare Spicy Flank Steak Sandwiches with Roasted Pepper Blue Cheese Sauce (pg. 353) and share with coworkers.	Light-night supper has Mussels with Brussels in a White Wine Butter Sauce (pg. 94) on the menu.	Work off that frustration by spending 20 to 30 minutes in your garden. Luxuriate with an OLIVE OIL HAIR MASK (pg. 110). Try out a *new* hairdo!
wednesday	Heat up a Raspberry Oatmeal Muffin to take along on the morning drive.	Invite your GORGEOUS gal pals for a lunch of Ginger Marinated Tuna with Dill Lime Butter (pg. 347) and Baked Pears in Brandy Sauce (pg. 104).	Use your crock pot to ease the preparation of Hearty Beef Stew (pg. 348).	Stretch out your neck, back, and shoulders. Make an appointment with the hippest hairstylist. Are you walking?
thursday	Creamy French-Style Eggs Garnished with Chopped Tomatoes and Chives (pg. 87) start your Thursday.	Brown bag it! Use extras from yesterday's lunch to create a fresh garden salad topped with tuna.	Lamb Chops with Coconut Skillet Sauce (pg. 92) make a great midweek meal.	Take a 30-minute POWER WALK to start your day. Add 15 minutes of weight lifting. Schedule a Swedish massage. Buy an unabridged audiobook to listen to during rush hour.
friday	Grab a fruit smoothie on your way to work—remember to choose "fruit only" with none of the sugary extras.	Sip from a warm bowl of Creamy Wild Mushroom Soup with Sherry and Fresh Thyme (pg. 357).	Kids' favorites re-invented. Serve Really Good Turkey Burgers with Cheddar Cheese and Horseradish Sauce (pg. 354) and The Real Deal Fries with Ketchup of Course! (pg. 358).	Start the day with a 40-minute POWER WALK with a Pal! Talk over the weightiest current affairs.

For Week 20 Grocery Shopping List and Shopping Day Prep Tips visit www.GorgeousLifestyleGuide.com

gorgeous lifestyle guide week 21 — eye-catching, good hair

	Breakfast	Lunch	Dinner	Revitalizing Activity
saturday	Bake a batch of Pecan Bananadana Muffins (pg. 90). Have one this morning and save the rest for later in the week.	This is Shopping Day, so treat yourself to your favorite fresh veggie salad.	Invite pals for game night. Serve Grilled Skirt Steak and Veggie Open-Faced Sandwiches (pg. 95), Roasted Veggie-Stuffed Tomatoes (pg. 131), and Pear and Strawberry Crisp (pg. 133).	Start the day with a 40-minute POWER WALK with a pal! Today is Shopping Day! Hit the farmer's market.
sunday	Invite the group for Scrambled Eggs with Red Grape and Avocado Salsa (pg. 118).	**Afternoon:** Create a fresh garden salad made with leftover veggies and top it with leftover Steak.	Bring the family together for a Sunday supper of Chicken Paprikash Served over Egg Noodles (pg. 122), Buttermilk Rolls with Sweet Onion Filling (pg. 130), and Oatmeal Snack Cake (pg. 106).	Lighten dark circles and smooth puffiness with raw ingredients like potatoes and egg whites. Luxuriate with an OLIVE OIL HAIR MASK (pg. 110). Try out a new hairdo.
monday	Broiled Grapefruit with Honey Mascarpone Cream (pg. 117) comes together quickly in the morning.	Brown bag it! Choose a sandwich prepared with whole grain bread and piled high with fresh veggies, reduced-fat cheese and lean meat.	Enjoy a healthful dinner of Pork Medallions with Asparagus and Sweet Potatoes (pg. 127).	Make FROZEN EYE PADS (pg. 138) Relax with eyes closed for 15 minutes. Stretch out your neck and shoulders. Make an appointment with the hippest hairstylist you can find.
tuesday	Grab a warmed Pecan Bananadana Muffin on your way out the door.	Have breakfast for lunch! Serve an Italian-Style Strata (pg. 126) to coworkers.	Stir-Fry Chicken and Broccoli with Chopped Peanuts (pg. 123) comes together in minutes. Serve with Chocolate Ricotta-Filled Crepes (pg. 136) for dessert.	See clearly. Identify something beautiful in your environment and appreciate the sight. Don't forget that POWER WALK.
wednesday	Melon Bowls with Strawberry Ginger Sauce (pg. 120) are simple to make and oh-so-good to eat.	Invite your GORGEOUS gal pals to share a spicy lunch of Roasted Veggie Burritos with Chipotle Chili Tomato Sauce (pg. 121).	Cook out (or in). Serve Grilled New York Strip Steaks (make extras) with Garlic Herb Oil (pg. 125), Sweet Balsamic Onions (pg. 129), and Baked Pears in Brandy Sauce (pg. 104).	Stretch out your neck, back, and shoulders. Make an appointment at the mall to test out the new seasonal eye makeup colors.
thursday	Coconut Tropical Smoothies (pg. 148) are fast and fabulous.	Brown bag it! Choose your favorite veggie salad dressed with olive oil and vinegar and topped with leftover Sirloin Steak.	Serve a totally veggie supper of Spaghetti Squash Carbonara (pg. 124), Buttermilk Rolls with Sweet Onion Filling (pg. 130), and Cranberry Wedding Cookies (pg. 135).	Wear sunglasses during your 30-minute POWER WALK.
friday	Enjoy a warm bowl of Oatmeal with Caramelized Fruit Topping (pg. 149).	Whip up a batch of Mussels with Brussels in a White Wine Butter Sauce (pg. 94) and invite your sister to lunch. She'll be surprised!	Gather the gang for a festive supper of Paella with Chorizo, Asparagus and Shellfish (pg. 98), Fried Plantains (pg. 100), and Orange-Glazed Yogurt Cake (pg. 134) for dessert.	Start the day with a 40-minute POWER WALK with a pal! Catch up on the neighborhood gossip. . . .

For Week 21 Grocery Shopping List and Shopping Day Prep Tips visit www.GorgeousLifestyleGuide.com

gorgeous lifestyle guide week 22 — eye-catching, smile pretty

Day	Breakfast	Lunch	Dinner	Revitalizing Activity
saturday	Start your busy day with a Coconut Tropical Smoothie (pg. 148).	This is Shopping Day, so while you are running errands, stop and treat yourself to your favorite fresh veggie salad with citrus vinaigrette.	Date night! Invite pals for a excellent dinner of Seared Jumbo Scallops with Herbed Butter Sauce (pg. 152), Buttermilk Rolls with Sweet Onion Filling (pg. 130), and New York-Style Cheesecake (pg. 164) for dessert.	Start the day with a 40-minute POWER WALK with a Pal! Today is Shopping Day! Hit the Farmer's market.
sunday	Invite the gang for a brunch that makes everyone smile. Serve Spicy Roasted Veggie and Shrimp Salsa with Fried Eggs and Warm Cheese Sauce (pg. 146).	**Afternoon** Build a fun sandwich. Serve Turkey with Caramelized Onion and Smoked Gouda Panini (pg. 151) for lunch.	Sunday's comfort supper includes Grilled Swordfish Steaks with Hot Papaya Relish and Herbed Compound Butter (pg. 157) with Pear and Strawberry Crisp (pg. 133) for dessert.	Lighten dark circles and smooth puffiness with raw ingredients like potatoes and egg whites. Smile at everyone you meet today and see how many smile back at you.
monday	Enjoy Melon Bowls with Strawberry Ginger Sauce (pg. 120) for good start to a busy week.	Brown bag it! Take along Shrimp Salad with Mango and Cucumber (pg. 159). Tuck in a buttermilk roll left over from the weekend.	Invite the family next door to share a meal of Chicken Paprikash Served over Egg Noodles (pg. 166) and dessert of Emergency Key Lime Pie (pg. 122).	Make FROZEN EYE PADS (pg. 138). Relax with eyes closed for 15 minutes. Did you remember your 30-minute POWER WALK?
tuesday	Take five to prepare Scrambled Eggs with Red Grape and Avocado Salsa (pg. 118).	You will love a lunch of Roasted Veggie-Stuffed Tomatoes (pg. 151). Make extras to share with coworkers.	Gather the gang for a quick and flavorful dinner of Stir-Fry Chicken and Broccoli with Chopped Peanuts (pg. 123).	See clearly. Identify something beautiful in your environment and appreciate the sight. Pull out the digital camera and create a picture to frame for your desk.
wednesday	Add more fruit to your daily diet with a power breakfast of Broiled Grapefruit with Honey Mascarpone Cream (pg. 117).	Invite your GORGEOUS gal pals to share Buffalo Chicken Cobb Salad with Buttermilk Dressing (pg. 150).	You and the kids will love Double-Cheese and Sausage Calzone with Marinara Dipping Sauce (pg. 153) and Orange Glazed Yogurt Cake (pg. 134) for dessert.	Stretch out your neck and shoulders to reduce stress. Make an appointment with your department store's cosmetic counter expert. Check out the new seasonal eye makeup colors.
thursday	Oatmeal with Caramelized Fruit Topping (pg. 149) is a tummy-filling start to a full day.	Make a smart choice when you eat out for lunch. Look for fresh veggies, whole grain bread and just a dash of salad dressing or mayonnaise.	Prepare a quick and easy meal of Chicken with Bel Paese, Proscuitto, and Capers with White Wine Pan Sauce (pg. 156) with Cranberry Wedding Cookies (pg. 135).	Start the day with a 30-minute POWER WALK. Don't forget your shades. Add a few crunches to "see" how you feel.
friday	Enjoy a dish of Scrambled Eggs with Red Grape and Avocado Salsa (pg. 118).	Prepare a batch of Swiss Cheese Wafers with a side of Blue Cheese Dip to Nibble on with Coworkers.	Surprise the gang with a super supper that includes Grilled New York Strip Steaks with Garlic Herb Oil (pg. 125) and Unfried Fried Onions (pg. 132). Leftover cookies are perfect for dessert.	Start the day with a 40-minute POWER WALK with a pal! Enjoy spending time with a good friend.

For Week 22 Grocery Shopping List and Shopping Day Prep Tips visit www.GorgeousLifestyleGuide.com

gorgeous lifestyle guide week 23 — eye-catching, you could be dancin'

Day	Breakfast	Lunch	Dinner	Revitalizing Activity
saturday	Bake up a batch of Whole Wheat Bran Muffins with Golden Raisins and Walnuts (pg. 207) and save extras for later in the week.	This is Shopping Day, so while you are running errands, stop and treat yourself to a fresh deli sandwich built with whole grain bread, lean meats, and fresh veggies.	Date night! Invite pals for an excellent supper of Charred Sirloin Steak with Mushroom and Red Wine Sauce (pg. 213), Roasted Veggie Stacks with Mozzarella (pg. 220), and Tropical Tiramisu (pg. 224).	Start the day with a 40-minute POWER WALK with a pal! Today is Shopping Day!! Hit the farmer's market.
sunday	Grab the gang for Brunch Frittata with Red Potatoes and Kale (pg. 208).	**Afternoon:** Nibble on Asparagus Cheese Toasts (pg. 219) for a light and simple luncheon treat.	Sunday's comfort supper includes Wild Ivory King Salmon Fillets with Macadamia Nut Crust (pg. 211), Slowly Stewed Collared Greens (pg. 222), and Blueberry Shortbread Bars (pg. 223).	Lighten dark circles and soothe puffiness with raw ingredients like potatoes and egg whites.
monday	It's Monday—so grab a muffin on your way to carpool.	Brown bag it! Take along a fresh veggie salad topped with leftover Sirloin Steak from Saturday's meal.	Have breakfast for dinner. Serve Mushroom and Spinach-Filled Frittata (pg. 128).	Make FROZEN EYE PADS (pg. 138). Relax with eyes closed for 15 minutes. Did you remember your 30-minute POWER WALK?
tuesday	Take five to prepare Scrambled Eggs with Red Grape and Avocado Salsa (pg. 118).	You will love a lunch of Overstuffed Beefsteak Tomatoes with Tortellini Salad (pg. 214). Serve extras to share with coworkers.	Gather the gang for a quick and flavorful dinner of Hoisin Beef and Veggies (pg. 212). Serve leftover shortbread bars for dessert.	See clearly. Identify something beautiful in your environment and appreciate the sight. Pull out the digital camera and create a picture to frame for your desk.
wednesday	Add more fruit to your daily diet with a power breakfast of Broiled Grapefruit with Honey Mascarpone Cream (pg. 117).	Invite your GORGEOUS gal pals to share Italian-Style Strata (pg. 126) with Sweet Pea Panzanella Salad (pg. 221), and Pecan Graham Squares (pg. 226).	You and the kids will love Better Veggie Chili (pg. 218). Save extras for later in the week.	Stretch out your neck and shoulders to reduce stress. Make an appointment with your department store's cosmetic counter expert. Test the new seasonal eye makeup colors.
thursday	Melon Bowls with Strawberry Ginger Sauce (pg. 120) are a wonderful way to start your day with extra fruit!	A simple lunch of Baked Potatoes Stuffed with Swiss Chard and Black Beans (pg. 217) is filled with good-for-you stuff to keep you going all day long!	Prepare a quick and easy meal of Mojo Marinated Chicken Served over Black Beans (pg. 217) with Sweet Balsamic Onions (pg. 129).	Start the day with a 30-minute POWER WALK. Wear sunglasses. Add a few crunches to "see" how you feel.
friday	Surprise the gang by whipping up a batch of Double-Berry Whole Wheat Pancakes (pg. 209).	Heat up a bowl of Better Veggie Chili for a quick and satisfying lunch.	Make Friday fresh with Sea Scallops with Blood Orange, Avocado, and Red Onion Salsa (pg. 215).	Start the day with a 40-minute POWER WALK with a pal! Enjoy spending time with a good friend.

For Week 23 Grocery Shopping List and Shopping Day Prep Tips visit www.GorgeousLifestyleGuide.com

gorgeous lifestyle guide week 24 — eye-catching, tummy-pleasing

	Breakfast	Lunch	Dinner	Revitalizing Activity
saturday	Start your busy shopping day with a super breakfast of Egg in a Frame with Basil Tomatoes (pg. 270).	This is Shopping Day, so while you are running errands, stop and treat yourself to your favorite fresh veggie salad.	Date night! Invite Pals for an excellent supper of Roasted Chipotle Salmon with Minted Couscous (pg. 279), Sauteed Peas with Mint (pg. 282), and Poached Cherry Sundaes (pg. 288).	Start the day with a 40-minute POWER WALK with a pal! Today is Shopping Day! Hit the farmer's market.
sunday	Gather the gang for a Sunday brunch that includes Say "Ricotta Cheese" Pancakes with Very Berry Sauce (pg. 269).	**Afternoon** Enjoy a light lunch of Avocado and Grapefruit Salad (pg. 281).	Sunday's comfort supper includes Baked Chicken Breasts with Artichoke and Sun-Dried Tomato Sauce (pg. 275), Grilled Vegetable Skewers (pg. 283), and Fresh Lime Cake with Blueberry Sauce (pg. 286).	Take a 30-minute POWER WALK to start your day. Add 15 minutes of weight lifting. Do a few more reps than last week. Find a pal who wants to run a marathon and start training.
monday	Prepare Breakfast Tacos (pg. 268) for an on-the-run breakfast.	Brown bag it! Take along a fresh veggie salad topped with leftover Chicken Breasts from last night's supper.	Monday's special stars Eggplant Boats Stuffed with Spicy Beef and Peas (pg. 271).	Walk this way—for 30 minutes. Add a few lunges to stretch out those legs and butt. Add a few squats after your walk. Hold in your tummy during your workout to build muscles.
tuesday	Melon Bowls with Strawberry Ginger Sauce (pg. 120) is perfect for Tuesday's quick breakfast.	You will love a lunch of Southwestern Chopped Salad with Toasted Peppers and Corn (pg. 284). Share extras with coworkers.	Gather the gang for a quick and flavorful dinner of Five-Spice Beef Wraps with Orange Ginger Dipping Sauce (pg. 280) and Tropical Buttermilk Panna Cotta with Strawberry Sauce (pg. 287).	See clearly. Identify something beautiful in your environment and appreciate the sight. Pull out the digital camera and create a picture to frame for your desk.
wednesday	Add more fruit to your daily diet with a power breakfast of Broiled Grapefruit with Honey Mascarpone Cream (pg. 117).	Invite your GORGEOUS gal pals to share Spicy Tuna Dinner Salad with Balsamic Dressing (pg. 273) and Chocolate Ricotta-Filled Crepes (pg. 136).	You and the kids will love Chicken Portobello with Linguini in Butter Sauce (pg. 276).	Stretch out your neck and shoulders to reduce stress. Make an appointment with your favorite department store's cosmetic counter expert. Take a look at the new seasonal eye makeup colors.
thursday	Add veggies to your morning meal. Serve Poached Eggs in Spicy Tomato Sauce (pg. 119).	Make a smart choice when you eat our for lunch. Look for fresh veggies, whole grain bread, and just a dash of salad dressing or mayonnaise.	Prepare a quick and easy meal of Stir-Fry Chicken and Broccoli with Chopped Peanuts (pg. 123) and Cranberry Wedding Cookies (pg. 135) for dessert.	Start the day with a 30-minute POWER WALK. Don't forget your sunglasses. Add a few crunches to "see" how you feel.
friday	Calling all Kiddos. It's time for Apple Pie for Breakfast (pg. 267). Just kidding, of course!	Enjoy a special lunch of Grilled Veggie Panini with Basil Pesto Sauce (pg. 274) and share with your carpool moms.	Perk up Friday's fish night with Snapper Fillets Smothered with Caramelized Onions (pg. 272), Sautéed Peas with Mint (pg. 282) and leftover Cranberry Wedding Cookies for dessert.	Start the day with a 40-minute POWER WALK with a pal! Enjoy spending time with a good friend.

For Week 24 Grocery Shopping List and Shopping Day Prep Tips visit www.GorgeousLifestyleGuide.com

gorgeous lifestyle guide week 25 — eye-catching, stress-free

Day	Breakfast	Lunch	Dinner	Revitalizing Activity
saturday	Start your busy shopping day with an Open Faced BLT Breakfast Sandwich (pg. 340).	This is Shopping Day, so while you are running errands, stop and treat yourself to your favorite fresh deli sandwich with tons of veggies, whole grain bread, and lean meats.	Date night! Invite pals for an excellent supper of Ginger-Marinated Tuna with Dill Lime Butter (pg. 347), Roasted Veggie Stuffed Tomatoes (pg. 131), and Key Lime Pound Cake (pg. 360).	Start the day with a 40-minute POWER WALK with a pal! Today is Shopping Day! Hit the farmer's market.
sunday	Gather the gang for a Sunday brunch that includes Scrambled Eggs with Red Grape and Avocado Salsa (pg. 118).	**Afternoon** Make a batch of Fresh Veggie Minestrone Soup with Chickpeas (pg. 356). Save extras for later in the week.	Sunday's comfort supper includes Hunter's-Style Chicken Stew with Yellow Rice (pg. 352) and Chocolate Gingersnaps (pg. 362).	Lighten dark circles and smooth puffiness with raw ingredients like potatoes and egg whites.
monday	Broiled Grapefruit with Honey Mascarpone Cream (pg. 117) is a great way to start the workweek.	Brown bag it! Take along a thermos filled with leftover Fresh Veggie Minestrone Soup with Chickpeas.	Make monday night special. Serve Shrimp Scampi with Angel Hair Pasta (pg. 346). Pass around extra cookies for dessert.	Make FROZEN EYE PADS (pg. 138). Relax with eyes closed for 15 minutes. Did you remember your 30-minute POWER WALK?
tuesday	Melon Bowls with Strawberry Ginger Sauce (pg. 120) add extra fruit to start your busy day.	You will love Spicy Flank Steak Sandwich with Roasted Pepper Blue Cheese Sauce (pg. 353) so much that you can't help but share some with your special someone at his desk-side picnic.	Gather the gang for a quick and flavorful dinner of Italian-Style Strata (pg. 126). t's Breakfast for dinner!	Take a 30-minute POWER WALK to start your day. Add 15 minutes of weight lifting. Schedule a Swedish massage. Buy an audiobook and put it in your car for rush-hour listening.
wednesday	Calling all Kiddos! It's time for a breakfast treat of Grilled Peanut Butter and Banana Sandwiches with Just a Touch of Honey (pg. 344).	Whip up a creamy batch of Creamy Wild Mushroom Soup with Sherry and Fresh Thyme (pg. 357). Sip a bowl now, save the rest for later.	You and the kids will love Old-Fashioned Turkeyloaf with Hidden Mushrooms (pg. 345) with Unfried Fried Onions (pg. 132).	Stretch out your neck and shoulders to reduce stress. Make an appointment with your department store's cosmetic counter expert. Try the new seasonal eye makeup colors.
thursday	How about a little Ham and Cheese Scramble (pg. 341) to wake up the minions?	Invite your GORGEOUS gal pals to share Pan Sautéed Gnocchi with Sun-Dried Tomato and Sage (pg. 355) with Pretty in Peach (pg. 363) for dessert. You are their hero!	Prepare a quick and easy meal of Spaghetti Squash Carbonara (pg. 124) and Roasted Veggie-Stuffed Tomatoes (pg. 131) for a mega, very veggie fix!	Remember to hold in your stomach on your 30-minute POWER WALK. Afterward, enjoy a cup of soothing tea.
friday	A quick breakfast of Poached Eggs in Spicy Tomato Sauce (pg. 119) will start off a great weekend.	Sip on a bowl of leftover, savory Creamy Wild Mushroom Soup.	It's F-R-I-D-A-Y! Celebrate with Really Good Turkey Burgers with Cheddar Cheese and Horseradish Sauce (pg. 354) and The Real Deal Fries with Ketchup of Course (pg. 358)!	Start the day with a 40-minute POWER WALK with a pal! Enjoy spending time with a good friend.

For Week 25 Grocery Shopping List and Shopping Day Prep Tips visit www.GorgeousLifestyleGuide.com

gorgeous lifestyle guide week 26 — smile pretty, skin-savvy

Day	Breakfast	Lunch	Dinner	Revitalizing Activity
saturday	Bake up Banana Flaxseed Bread with Warm Strawberry Sauce (pg. 75). Save extras for snacks later in the week.	This is Shopping Day, so while you are running errands, stop and treat yourself to your favorite deli salad made with plenty of fresh veggies and whole grain roll on the side.	Date night! Invite pals for Grilled Halibut with Salsa Verde (pg. 64), Stewed Tomatoes with Garlic and Black Beans (pg. 71), and Peach Gingerbread with Walnut Streusel (pg. 76).	Start the day with a 40-minute POWER WALK that includes 10 minutes of jogging! Today is Shopping Day! Hit the farmer's market.
	Breakfast	Afternoon	Dinner	Revitalizing Activity
sunday	Gather the gang for Spicy Roasted Veggie and Shrimp Salsa with Fried Egg and Warm Cheese Sauce (pg. 146).	Nibble on a favorite snack of Artichoke and Asiago Crostini (pg. 162).	Sunday's comfort supper includes Chicken Thighs with Sage and Caramelized Peaches (pg. 65), Rosemary Roasted Carrot Sticks (pg. 72), and New York-Style Cheesecake (pg. 164).	Prepare your own homemade mouthwash for the freshest smile possible. Me time! Luxuriate with an OATMEAL PEEL (pg. 79). Visit the cosmetic counter and update your look.
	Breakfast	Lunch	Dinner	Revitalizing Activity
monday	Blend up a smoothie of Juiced-Up Fruit-and-Herb Breakfast Drinks (Blueberry-Basil, pg. 57).	Brown bag it! Take along a container of Shrimp Salad with Mango and Cucumber (pg. 159). Tuck in a piece of Banana Flaxseed Bread made earlier in the week.	Perk up your everyday weeknight meal by serving Lemon Veal with Sautéed Spinach, Pine Nuts, and Goat Cheese (pg. 158).	After your 30-minute POWER WALK, curl up with a good book and a cup of non-teeth-staining herbal tea.
	Breakfast	Lunch	Dinner	Revitalizing Activity
tuesday	Enjoy a simple yet spicy breakfast of Breakfast Burritos with Red Pepper Salsa (pg. 60).	Enjoy a fun lunch of Mediterranean Tuna Melt (pg. 62). Serve half to your walking buddy.	Make your kitchen a super sandwich shop with Turkey with Caramelized Onion and Smoked Gouda Panini (pg. 151) and Emergency Key Lime Pie (pg. 166) for dessert.	Grab your someone special and take an after-dinner walk to work off that pie. Me time! Apply a HONEY MASK (pg. 79). Don't forget that 30-minute POWER WALK.
	Breakfast	Lunch	Dinner	Revitalizing Activity
wednesday	Fruit and Yogurt Parfaits with Granola Crunch (pg. 59) will keep your tummy smilin' until lunchtime!	Invite your GORGEOUS gal pals to share a fun lunch of Spinach Salad with Warm Chipotle Chili Vinaigrette Topped with Chicken Strips and Crisp Sweet Potato (pg. 66).	Create your favorite taco by using the recipe for Open-Faced Chicken Tacos (pg. 68) as your guideline. Add Mango-Walnut Crumble (pg. 165) and watch 'em smile!	Stretch out your lower back and legs. Take a 30-minute POWER WALK to start your day. Make an appointment with the cosmetic counter to test out the new seasonal lipstick colors.
	Breakfast	Lunch	Dinner	Revitalizing Activity
thursday	Jazz up your fruity breakfast fare with Fresh Fruit Salad with Citrus Basil Dressing (pg. 58).	Invite the carpool moms for a fun lunch of Turkey with Caramelized Onion and Smoked Gouda Panini (pg. 151).	Serve a simple supper of Grilled Swordfish Steaks with Hot Papaya Relish and Herbed Compound Butter (pg. 157).	Smile at everyone you meet today and see how many smile back at you. Smile while cars pass you on your 30-minute POWER WALK.
	Breakfast	Lunch	Dinner	Revitalizing Activity
friday	Start the weekend with a tropical flair. Serve Coconut Tropical Smoothies (pg. 148) to the gang as you go out the door.	Sushi-Style Salmon Wraps (pg. 61) make a fun lunchbox treat.	The kids will love Double-Cheese and Sausage Calzone with Marinara Dipping Sauce (pg. 153). Add dessert of Oven-Roasted Fruit with Vanilla Yogurt Sorbet (pg. 77).	Start the day with a 40-minute POWER WALK with a pal that includes 10 minutes of jogging!

For Week 26 Grocery Shopping List and Shopping Day Prep Tips visit www.GorgeousLifestyleGuide.com

gorgeous lifestyle guide week 27 — smile pretty, eye-catching

	Breakfast	Lunch	Dinner	Revitalizing Activity
saturday	Start your busy day with a refreshing Coconut Tropical Smoothie (pg. 148).	This is Shopping Day, so while you are running errands, stop and treat yourself to your favorite deli sandwich made with whole grain bread, fresh veggies, and lean meats.	Date night! Invite pals for Blue Cheese Dip with All Kinds of Dippers (pg. 161), Swiss Cheese Wafers (pg. 160), Lemon Veal with Sautéed Spinach, Pine Nuts & Goat Cheese (pg. 158), and Mango-Walnut Crumble (pg. 165).	Start the day with a 40-minute POWER WALK that includes 10 minutes of jogging! Today is Shopping Day! Hit the farmer's market.
	Breakfast	Afternoon	Dinner	Revitalizing Activity
sunday	Gather the family for a fun brunch of Spicy Roasted Veggie and Shrimp Salsa with Fried Egg and Warm Cheese Sauce (pg. 146).	Nibble on a favorite snack of leftover Blue Cheese Dip with All Kinds of Dippers from last night's partee.	Sunday's comfort supper includes Chicken Paprikash Served over Egg Noodles (pg. 122) with Chocolate Ricotta-Filled Crepes (pg. 136).	Prepare your own homemade mouthwash (pg. 167) for the freshest smile possible.
	Breakfast	Lunch	Dinner	Revitalizing Activity
monday	Fresh Papaya and Grapefruit with Yogurt and Mint (pg. 147) makes a fabulous Monday starter.	Brown bag ilt! Take along a fresh veggie salad topped with chicken leftover from Sunday's supper.	Perk up your everyday weeknight meal by serving Stir-Fry Chicken and Broccoli with Chopped Peanuts (pg. 123).	After your 30-minute POWER WALK, curl up with a good book and a cup of non-teeth-staining herbal tea.
	Breakfast	Lunch	Dinner	Revitalizing Activity
tuesday	A bowl of warm Oatmeal with Caramelized Fruit Topping (pg. 149) is yummy on Tuesday.	Prepare refreshing Shrimp Salad with Mango and Cucumber (pg. 159) and share extras with coworkers.	Make your kitchen a super sandwich shop with Turkey with Caramelized Onion and Smoked Gouda Panini (pg. 151) and Emergency Key Lime Pie (pg. 166) for dessert.	Stretch out your neck and shoulders to reduce stress. Make an appointment with your department store's cosmetic counter expert. Check out the seasonal eye makeup colors.
	Breakfast	Lunch	Dinner	Revitalizing Activity
wednesday	It's a great day for eggs! How about Scrambled Eggs with Red Grape and Avocado Salsa (pg. 118) for breakfast?	Invite your GORGEOUS gal pals to share a fun lunch of Grilled Swordfish Steaks with Hot Papaya Relish and Herbed Compound Butter (pg. 157) with Cranberry Wedding Cookies (pg. 135).	Serve the gang a super supper of Grilled New York Strip Steaks with Garlic Herb Oil (pg. 125) with Unfried Fried Onions (pg. 132).	Stretch out your lower back and legs. Take a 30-minute POWER WALK to start your day. Make an appointment with the cosmetic counter to check out the seasonal lipstick colors.
	Breakfast	Lunch	Dinner	Revitalizing Activity
thursday	Jazz up your fruity breakfast fare with Melon Bowls with Strawberry Ginger Sauce (pg. 120).	Brown bag it! Take along a sandwich stuffed with extra New York Strip Steak. Choose whole grain bread and add dark green lettuce and slices of tomato to boost the veggie impact.	Light fare for Thursday includes Mushroom and Spinach-Filled Frittata (pg. 128), Roasted Veggie Stuffed Tomatoes (pg. 131), and leftover Cranberry Wedding cookies for dessert.	Smile at everyone you meet today and see how many smile back at you. Smile while cars pass you on your 30-minute POWER WALK.
	Breakfast	Lunch	Dinner	Revitalizing Activity
friday	A light breakfast of Broiled Grapefruit with Honey Mascarpone Cream (pg. 117) will start your TGIF just fine.	Teacher's workday. Prepare Double-Cheese and Sausage Calzones with Marinara Dipping Sauce (pg. 153) and share with the other classroom moms.	Bring the Friday night gang together for Crispy Roasted Chicken with Penne Pasta (pg. 154) and Orange-Glazed Yogurt Cake (pg. 134) for dessert. Yum!	Start the day with a 40-minute POWER WALK with a pal that includes 10 minutes of jogging!

For Week 27 Grocery Shopping List and Shopping Day Prep Tips visit www.GorgeousLifestyleGuide.com

gorgeous lifestyle guide week 28 — smile pretty, good to the bones

Day	Breakfast	Lunch	Dinner	Revitalizing Activity
saturday	Whip up a batch of Whole Wheat Bran Muffins with Golden Raisins and Walnuts (pg. 207). Save extras for later in the week.	This is Shopping Day, so while you are running errands, stop and treat yourself to your favorite deli sandwich made with whole grain bread, fresh veggies, and lean meats.	Date night! Invite pals for Peppered Pork Pinwheels Stuffed with Swiss Chard, Sun-Dried Tomatoes, and Mozzarella (pg. 186) and Almond-Topped Ricotta Cheesecake (pg. 195).	Start the day with a 40-minute POWER WALK that includes 10 minutes of jogging! Today is Shopping Day! Hit the farmer's market.
	Breakfast	Afternoon	Dinner	Revitalizing Activity
sunday	Gather the gang for a brunch of Eggs Benedict with Swiss Chard and Whole Grain English Muffin (pg. 175).	Green Gazpacho Soup with Navy Bean Garnish (pg. 188) is a light and yummy lunch.	Sunday supper for friends and family includes Crispy Roasted Chicken with Penne Pasta (pg. 154). Make extras for salads and sandwiches later in the week.	Prepare your own homemade mouthwash (pg. 167) for the freshest smile possible.
	Breakfast	Lunch	Dinner	Revitalizing Activity
monday	Start the week off with a refreshing Coconut Tropical Smoothie (pg. 148).	Brown bag it! Take along a fresh veggie salad topped with chicken leftover from Sunday's supper.	Perk up your weeknight by serving Whole Wheat Spaghetti with Grilled Turkey, Broccoli Rabe, Red Peppers, and Peas (pg. 180) and Orange and Tarragon-Infused Crème Brûlées with Sliced Bananas (pg. 163).	After your 30-minute POWER WALK, curl up with a good book and a cup of non-teeth-staining herbal tea.
tuesday	Grab a Whole Wheat Bran Muffin as you drive into carpool.	Prepare refreshing Shrimp Salad with Mango and Cucumber (pg. 159) and share extras with coworkers.	Make your kitchen a super sandwich shop with Turkey with Caramelized Onion and Smoked Gouda Panini (pg. 151) and Emergency Key Lime Pie (pg. 166) for dessert.	Stretch out from head to toe. Take a 30-minute POWER WALK to start your day. Add 10 minutes of weight lifting. Remember to start light.
wednesday	Split a Breakfast Panini with Chicken Sausage (pg. 178) with your Sweetie!	Invite your GORGEOUS gal pals to share Sweet Potato and Country Ham Frittata (pg. 176) and Summer Squash Salad with Baby Spinach, Roasted Tomatoes, and Parmesan Cheese (pg. 192).	Enjoy a simple supper of Parmesan Chicken Fingers with Green Cashew and Curry Dipping Sauce (pg. 181) with Mango Walnut Crumble (pg. 165).	Stretch out your lower back and legs. Take a 30-minute POWER WALK to start your day. Make an appointment with the cosmetic counter to check out the new seasonal lipstick colors.
thursday	Fresh Papaya and Grapefruit with Yogurt and Mint (pg. 147) will start off your day with gusto!	Brown bag it! Take along a sandwich stuffed with extra Shrimp Salad. Choose whole grain bread and add dark green lettuce and slices of tomato to boost the veggie impact.	Serve a yummy supper of Grilled Swordfish Steaks with Hot Papaya Relish and Herbed Compound Butter (pg. 157).	Smile at everyone you meet today and see how many smile back at you. Smile while cars pass you on your 30-minute POWER WALK.
friday	Start the weekend with a healthful bowl of Oatmeal with Caramelized Fruit Topping (pg. 149).	Teacher's workday. Prepare Double-Cheese and Sausage Calzones with Marinara Dipping Sauce (pg. 152) and share with the other classroom moms.	Serve the family an elegant entrée of Grilled Lamb Chops with White Bean Salad (pg. 182).	Start the day with a 40-minute POWER WALK with a pal that includes 10 minutes of jogging!

For Week 28 Grocery Shopping List and Shopping Day Prep Tips visit www.GorgeousLifestyleGuide.com

gorgeous lifestyle guide week 29 — smile pretty, hands-on glam

	Breakfast	Lunch	Dinner	Revitalizing Activity
saturday	Whip up a batch of Banana Bread Snack Cake (pg. 237). Save extras for later in the week.	This is Shopping Day, so while you are running errands, stop and treat yourself to your favorite deli sandwich made with whole grain bread, fresh veggies, and lean meats.	Date night! Invite pals for Roasted Asparagus Salad with Arugula, Radishes and Lemon Vinaigrette (pg. 248) and Crispy Roast Chicken with Penne (pg. 154).	Start the day with a 40-minute POWER WALK that includes 10 minutes of jogging! Today is Shopping Day! Hit the farmer's market.
sunday	Gather the gang for a brunch of Eggs Benedict with Swiss Chard and Whole Grain English Muffins (pg. 175).	**Afternoon** Artichoke and Asiago Crostini (pg. 162) is a light and yummy lunch.	Sunday's comfort supper includes Turkey Meatloaf Burgers with Spicy Sweet Potato Sticks (pg. 243) and Strike-It-Rich Chocolate Pudding with Chocolate Cookie Crumbles (pg. 252).	Prepare your own homemade mouthwash (pg. 167) for the freshest smile possible. Hold hands with your special someone while you stroll through the neighborhood after supper.
monday	Start the week off with a refreshing Coconut Tropical Smoothie (pg. 148).	Brown bag it! Take along a fresh veggie salad topped with chicken leftover from Saturday's supper.	Perk up your week night by serving Jambalaya (pg. 245) with Roasted Red Grape Parfaits with Orange and Maple Flavored Ricotta Cheese (pg. 253).	After your 30-minute POWER WALK, curl up with a good book and a cup of non-teeth-staining herbal tea.
tuesday	Grab a slice of Banana Bread Snack Cake as you drive into carpool.	Prepare refreshing Shrimp Salad with Mango and Cucumber (pg. 159) and share extras with coworkers.	Turn your kitchen into a super sandwich shop with Turkey with Caramelized Onion and Smoked Gouda Panini (pg. 151) and Emergency Key Lime Pie (pg. 166) for dessert.	Stretch out from head to toe. Take a 30-minute POWER WALK to start your day. Add 10 minutes of weight lifting. Remember to start light.
wednesday	Bake up a batch of Walnut-Stuffed Baked Apples with Maple Syrup (pg. 238). It's like eating dessert for breakfast!	Invite your GORGEOUS gal pals to share Chicken and Rice Meatball Hoagies (pg. 242) and Mango-Walnut Crumble (pg. 165). Yum!	Enjoy a simple supper of Seared Jumbo Scallops with Herbed Butter Sauce (pg. 152).	Stretch out your lower back and legs. Take a 30-minute POWER WALK to start your day. Make an appointment with the cosmetic counter to test out the new seasonal lipstick colors.
thursday	Fresh Papaya and Grapefruit with Yogurt and Mint (pg. 147) will start off your day with gusto!	Brown bag it! Take along Buffalo Chicken Cobb Salad with Buttermilk Dressing (pg. 150) and share extras with coworkers.	Serve a yummy supper of Grilled Swordfish Steaks with Hot Papaya Relish and Herbed Compound Butter (pg. 157) and Simple Zucchini Cake with Vanilla Glaze (pg. 254).	Smile at everyone you meet today and see how many smile back at you. Smile while cars pass you on your 30-minute POWER WALK.
friday	Start the weekend with a healthful batch of Granola Power Bars (pg. 239) and save extras for weekend grab-and-go snacks.	Teacher's workday. Prepare Black Bean and Roasted Pepper Empanadas (pg. 250) and share with the other classroom moms.	Serve the family an elegant entrée of Sautéed Yellowtail Snapper with Braised Cabbage and Cheesy Mashed Potatoes (pg. 246).	Start the day with a 40-minute POWER WALK with a pal that includes 10 minutes of jogging!

For Week 29 Grocery Shopping List and Shopping Day Prep Tips visit www.GorgeousLifestyleGuide.com

gorgeous lifestyle guide week 30 — smile pretty, sleepy time

Day	Breakfast	Lunch	Dinner	Revitalizing Activity
saturday	Bake up a batch of Orange Breakfast Muffins (pg. 305). Save extras for later in the week.	This is Shopping Day, so while you are running errands, stop and treat yourself to your favorite veggie salad and simple vinaigrette with a whole grain roll on the side.	Date night! Rack of Lamb with Spinach and Breadcrumb Topping (pg. 311), Broccoli Mash (pg. 321), and Simmering Blueberries with Cinnamon Dumplings (pg. 324).	Start the day with a 40-minute POWER WALK that includes 10 minutes of jogging! Today is Shopping Day! Hit the farmer's market.
sunday	Gather the gang for Sweet Potato Pancakes with Warm Raspberry Syrup (pg. 306).	Afternoon: Nibble on a favorite salad of Grilled Ratatouille with Tomato Basil Vinaigrette. (pg. 323). Turn extras into a fresh veggie soup for later in the week.	Sunday's comfort supper includes Crispy Roasted Chicken with Penne Pasta (pg. 154) and New York-Style Cheesecake (pg. 164) (make extras for lunchboxes later in the week).	Prepare your own homemade mouthwash (pg. 167) for the freshest smile possible.
monday	Blend up a batch of Fruit 'N Soy Milk Drinks (pg. 307) for breakfast.	Brown bag it! Take along fresh veggie soup made with leftover grilled veggies.	Perk up your everyday weeknight meal by serving Grilled Coconut Curry Shrimp with Soba Noodles (pg. 312) and Butterscotch Blondies (pg. 325).	After your 30-minute POWER WALK, curl up with a good book and a cup of non-teeth-staining herbal tea.
tuesday	Another fast fruity treat for breakfast is a batch of Coconut Tropical Smoothies (pg. 148).	Prepare refreshing Shrimp Salad with Mango and Cucumber (pg. 159) and share extras with coworkers.	Make your kitchen a super sandwich shop with Crab Cake Po' Boys (pg. 316) and Emergency Key Lime Pie (pg. 166) for dessert.	Grab your someone special and take an after-dinner walk to work off that pie. Rest your muscles and spend 20 minutes stretching out your tired parts, followed by a scented bath.
wednesday	How about Oatmeal with Caramelized Fruit Topping (pg. 149) for a mid-week breakfast that keeps you going strong.	Invite your GORGEOUS gal pals to share a fun lunch of Linguini with Mussels and Snow Peas (pg. 318) with extra Butterscotch Blondies for dessert.	Serve a kid friendly meal of Pecan-Crusted Chicken Fingers with Apricot Mustard Dipping Sauce (pg. 319).	Stretch out your lower back and legs. Take a 30-minute POWER WALK to start your day. Make an appointment at the cosmetic's counter to check out the new seasonal lipstick colors.
thursday	Jazz up your fruity breakfast fare with Breakfast Tomatoes with Smoked Salmon (pg. 308).	Brown bag it! Take along a sandwich stuffed with extra Shrimp Salad. Choose whole grain bread and add dark green lettuce and slices of tomato to boost the veggie impact.	Serve a comfort supper of Roast Turkey Breast with Cornbread-Cranberry Dressing and Madeira Mushroom Gravy (pg. 310).	Smile at everyone you meet today and see how many smile back at you. Smile while cars pass you on your 30-minute POWER WALK.
friday	Spoon up a bowl of Fruit and Yogurt Breakfast Parfaits with Granola Crunch (pg. 59).	Prepare your favorite panini sandwich by using the recipe for Turkey with Caramelized Onion and Smoked Gouda Panini (pg. 151) as a guideline.	Serve the family a fun supper of Lemon Veal with Sautéed Spinach, Pine Nuts, and Goat Cheese (pg. 158) with Almond Cookies (one of) Two Ways (pg. 327)!	Start the day with a 40-minute POWER WALK. Place a blank piece of paper on your bedside table and quote your sleepy time mantra as you dose off.

For Week 30 Grocery Shopping List and Shopping Day Prep Tips visit www.GorgeousLifestyleGuide.com

gorgeous lifestyle guide week 31 — good to the bones, good hair

	Breakfast	Lunch	Dinner	Revitalizing Activity
saturday	Bake up a batch of Whole Grain Apple Muffins with Walnut Streusel (pg. 177). Save extras for later in the week.	This is Shopping Day, so while you are running errands, stop and treat yourself to your favorite fresh veggie salad.	Date night! Invite pals for Watercress Salad with Raspberry Vinaigrette (pg. 191), Lobster in Orange Curry Butter Sauce (pg. 93), and Almond-Topped Ricotta Cheesecake (pg. 195).	Start the day with a 40-minute POWER WALK that includes 10 minutes of jogging! Today is Shopping Day! Hit the farmer's market.
sunday	Gather the Group for a brunch of Eggs Benedict with Swiss Chard and Whole Grain English Muffins (pg. 175).	**Afternoon** Prepare Green Gazpacho Soup with Navy Bean Garnish (pg. 188)—have a small cup for lunch and reserve the rest for later in the week.	Our comfort supper includes Mustard-Garlic Roasted Chicken Served with Arugula and Artichoke Salad (pg. 179), Lentils with Wild Rice & Mushrooms (pg. 190), and Oatmeal Snack Cake (pg. 106).	After supper, while the kids and Dad do the dishes, soak in a hot tub filled with Epsom salts and lavender oil.
monday	Warm up a Whole Grain Apple Muffin for a grab-and-go Monday breakfast.	Brown bag it! Choose whole grain breads to build a sandwich stuffed with leftover sliced chicken from Sunday's supper. Add an oatmeal snack cake for dessert.	Simple supper for a Monday night includes Grilled Skirt Steak and Veggie Open-Faced Sandwich (pg. 95) and leftover Almond-Topped Ricotta from the weekend.	Go to an introductory Yoga class or try out some basic moves at home. *Me time!* Luxuriate with an OLIVE OIL HAIR MASK (pg. 110).
tuesday	Take an extra five minutes to prepare Egg White Omelets with Bell Peppers and Turkey Sausage (pg. 88) for a terrific mid-week starter.	Enjoy a bowl of Green Gazpacho Soup with Navy Bean Relish (prepared earlier in the week).	A midweek veggie meal is re-invented with Rosemary Polenta with Spinach, Red Beans, and Goat Cheese (pg. 184) and Sautéed Bananas with Sweet Mascarpone and Walnut Crunch (pg. 107) for dessert.	Grab the entire family for an after-dinner walk around the neighborhood. Don't forget the dog!
wednesday	Grab a bowl of warm Oatmeal with Caramelized Fruit Topping (pg. 149) for a tummy warming breakfast.	Invite your GORGEOUS gal pals to lunch and serve Rosemary Roasted Chicken Breasts with Smoky Almond Sauce (pg. 91).	Whole Wheat Spaghetti with Grilled Turkey, Broccoli Rabe, Red Peppers, and Peas (pg. 180)—a perfect midweek meal.	Stretch out from head to toe. Take a 30-minute POWER WALK to start your day. Add 10 minutes of weight lifting. Remember to start light.
thursday	Bake up a batch of Pecan Bananadana Muffins (pg. 90) and save extras for the weekend.	Brown bag it! Take along a container of Peppery White Bean Salsa with Whole Wheat Pita Chips (pg. 189) to work to share with friends.	A dinner of Roasted Pork Tenderloin with Swiss Chard (pg. 96) will leave 'em smiling.	It's POWER WALK day. Spend 30 minutes walking. Add a few lunges to stretch out those legs. Let your fingers do the walking and make an appointment with a hip hairstylist.
friday	Creamy French-Style Eggs Garnished with Chopped Tomatoes and Chives (pg. 87) will start your weekend with a bang!	Stay home for lunch. Build a super dish packed full of veggies. Summer Squash Salad with Baby Spinach, Roasted Tomatoes, and Parmesan Cheese (pg. 192) fits the bill.	Treat the family to Paella with Chorizo, Asparagus, and Shellfish (pg. 98). Prepare Macadamia Nut Biscotti (pg. 193) with the kids for dessert tonight and snacks next week.	Start the day with a 40-minute POWER WALK with a pal that includes 10 minutes of jogging and 10 minutes of stretching!

For Week 31 Grocery Shopping List and Shopping Day Prep Tips visit www.GorgeousLifestyleGuide.com

gorgeous lifestyle guide week 32 — good to the bones, you could be dancin'

	Breakfast	Lunch	Dinner	Revitalizing Activity
saturday	Bake up a batch of Whole Grain Apple Muffins and Walnut Streusel (pg. 177). Save extras for later in the week.	This is Shopping Day, so while you are running errands, stop and treat yourself to your favorite fresh veggie salad with citrus-filled vinaigrette.	Date night! Invite pals for Watercress Salad with Raspberry Vinaigrette (pg. 191), Mojo Marinated Chicken Served Over Black Beans (pg. 217), and Almond-Topped Ricotta Cheesecake (pg. 195).	Start the day with a 40-minute POWER WALK that includes 10 minutes of jogging! Today is Shopping Day! Hit the farmer's market.
sunday	Gather the group for Brunch Frittata with Red Potatoes and Kale (pg. 208).	**Afternoon:** Prepare Green Gazpacho Soup with Navy Bean Garnish (pg. 188)—have a small cup for lunch and reserve the rest for later in the week.	Our comfort supper includes Charred Sirloin Steak with Mushroom and Red Wine Sauce (pg. 213), Lentils with Wild Rice & Mushrooms (pg. 190,) and Peanut Butter Sandwich Cookies (pg. 194).	After supper, while the kids and Dad do the dishes, soak in a hot tub filled with Epsom salts and lavender oil.
monday	Warm up a Whole Grain Apple Muffin for a grab-and-go Monday breakfast.	Brown bag it! Choose whole grain breads to build a sandwich stuffed with leftover sliced chicken from Saturday's supper. Add a peanut butter cookie for dessert.	Simple supper for a Monday night includes Better Veggie Chili (pg. 218) and leftover cheesecake from the weekend.	Go to an introductory yoga class or try out some basic moves at home. Stretch out those toes and soak in warm water after a long weekend.
tuesday	Take an extra 5 minutes to whip up a batch of Double-Berry Whole Wheat Pancakes (pg. 209).	Enjoy a bowl of Green Gazpacho Soup with Navy Bean Relish (prepared earlier in the week).	A midweek veggie meal is re-invented with Rosemary Polenta with Spinach, Red Beans, and Goat Cheese (pg. 184) and Pecan Graham Squares for dessert (pg. 226).	Grab the entire family for an after-dinner walk around the neighborhood. Don't forget the dog!
wednesday	Grab a bowl of warm Oatmeal with Caramelized Fruit Topping (pg. 149) for a tummy-warming breakfast.	Invite your GORGEOUS gal pals to lunch. Serve Sweet Pea Panzanella Salad (pg. 221) with Sea Scallops with Blood Orange, Avocado, and Red Onion Salsa (pg. 215). Yum!	Whole Wheat Spaghetti with Grilled Turkey, Broccoli Rabe, Red Peppers, and Peas (pg. 180)—a perfect midweek meal.	Stretch out from head to toe. Take a 30-minute power walk to start your day. Add 10 minutes of weight lifting. Remember to start light.
thursday	Poached Eggs with Spinach and White Beans (pg. 210) makes a powerful starter.	Brown bag it! Take along a container of Peppery White Bean Salsa with Whole Wheat Pita Chips (pg. 189) to work to share with friends.	A dinner of Baked Potatoes Stuffed with Swiss Chard and Black Beans (pg. 217) will leave 'em smiling.	It's power walk day. Spend 30 minutes walking. Add a few lunges to stretch out those legs. Get your kids together for a quick game of one-on-one.
friday	Sip Coconut Tropical Smoothies (pg. 148) for breakfast.	Stay home for lunch. Build a super dish packed full of veggies. Summer Squash Salad with Baby Spinach, Roasted Tomatoes, and Parmesan Cheese (pg. 192) fits the bill.	Treat the family to Parmesan Chicken Fingers with Green Cashew and Curry Dipping Sauce (pg. 181). Prepare Macadamia Nut Biscotti (pg. 193) with the kids for dessert tonight and snacks next week.	Start the day with a 40-minute POWER WALK with a pal that includes 10 minutes of jogging and 10 minutes of stretching!

For Week 32 Grocery Shopping List and Shopping Day Prep Tips visit www.GorgeousLifestyleGuide.com

gorgeous lifestyle guide week 33 — good to the bones, tummy-pleasing

Day	Breakfast	Lunch	Dinner	Revitalizing Activity
saturday	Bake up a batch of Whole Grain Apple Muffins with Walnut Streusel (pg. 177). Save extras for later in the week.	This is Shopping Day, so while you are running errands, stop and treat yourself to your favorite fresh veggie salad.	Date night! Invite pals for Snapper Fillets Smothered with Caramelized Onions (pg. 272) and Orange Cappuccino Parfaits (pg. 285).	Start the day with a 40-minute POWER WALK that includes 10 minutes of jogging! Today is Shopping Day! Hit the farmer's market.
sunday	Gather the group for a brunch of Say "Ricotta Cheese" Pancakes with Very Berry Sauce (pg. 269).	**Afternoon** Prepare Green Gazpacho Soup with Navy Bean Garnish (pg. 188)—have a small cup for lunch and reserve the rest for later in the week.	Our comfort supper includes Baked Chicken Breasts with Artichoke and Sun-Dried Tomato Sauce (pg. 275) and Poached Cherry Sundaes (pg. 288).	Turn on your Pilates DVD and get down with your inner core. Stretch out those muscles and improve your squats—work your way up to a perfect teaser.
monday	Warm up a Whole Grain Apple Muffin for a grab-and-go Monday breakfast.	Brown bag it! Choose whole grain bread to build a sandwich stuffed with leftover sliced chicken from Sunday's supper. Add a peanut butter cookie for dessert.	Simple supper for a Monday night includes Grilled Veggie Panini with Basil Pesto Sauce (pg. 274).	POWER WALKING for 30 minutes starts your day. Add a few lunges to stretch out those legs and butt. Add a few squats. Hold in your tummy during your workout to build muscles.
tuesday	Take an extra 5 minutes to build Egg in a Frame with Basil Tomatoes (pg. 270) for breakfast.	Enjoy a bowl of Green Gazpacho Soup with Navy Bean Relish (prepared earlier in the week).	A midweek veggie meal is re-invented with Rosemary Polenta with Spinach, Red Beans, and Goat Cheese (pg. 184) and Cocktail Nut Cookie Bars (pg. 196) for dessert.	Grab the entire family for an after-dinner walk around the neighborhood. Don't forget the dog!
wednesday	Grab a bowl of warm Oatmeal with Caramelized Fruit Topping (pg. 149) for a tummy-warming breakfast.	Invite your GORGEOUS gal pals to lunch. Serve Roasted Chipotle Salmon with Minted Couscous (pg. 279).	Whole Wheat Spaghetti with Grilled Turkey, Broccoli Rabe, Red Peppers, and Peas (pg. 180)—a perfect midweek meal.	Stretch out from head to toe. Take a 30-minute POWER WALK to start your day. Add 10 minutes of weight lifting. Remember to start light.
thursday	Whole Grain Apple Muffins with Walnut Streusel.	Brown bag it! Take along a container of Peppery White Bean Salsa and a bag of Whole Wheat Pita Chips (pg. 189) to work to share with friends.	A dinner of Five-Spice Beef Wraps with Orange Ginger Dipping Sauce (pg. 280) will leave 'em smiling.	It's POWER WALK day. Spend 30 minutes walking. Add a few lunges to stretch out those legs.
friday	Gather the family for Apple Pie for Breakfast (pg. 267)—just kidding, of course!	Stay home for lunch. Build a super dish packed full of veggies. Summer Squash Salad with Baby Spinach, Roasted Tomatoes, and Parmesan Cheese (pg. 192) fits the bill.	Treat the family to Eggplant Boats Stuffed with Spicy Beef and Peas (pg. 271). Prepare Macadamia Nut Biscotti (pg. 193) with the kids for dessert tonight and snacks next week.	Start the day with a 40-minute POWER WALK with a pal that includes 10 minutes of jogging and 10 minutes of stretching!

For Week 33 Grocery Shopping List and Shopping Day Prep Tips visit www.GorgeousLifestyleGuide.com

gorgeous lifestyle guide week 34 — good to the bones, stress-free

Day	Breakfast	Lunch	Dinner	Revitalizing Activity
saturday	Bake up a batch of Whole Grain Apple Muffins and Walnut Streusel (pg. 177). Save extras for later in the week.	This is Shopping Day, so while you are running errands, stop and treat yourself to your favorite fresh deli sandwich piled high with fresh veggies.	Date night! Invite pals for Shrimp Scampi with Angel Hair Pasta (pg. 346), Summer Squash Salad with Baby Spinach, Roasted Tomatoes, and Parmesan Cheese (pg. 192), and Almond-Topped Ricotta Cheesecake for dessert (pg. 195).	Start the day with a 40-minute POWER WALK that includes 10 minutes of jogging! Today is Shopping Day! Hit the farmer's market.
sunday	Gather the group for a brunch of Bacon and Asparagus Quiche (pg. 342).	**Afternoon** Prepare Fresh Veggie Minestrone Soup with Chickpeas (pg. 356)—have a small cup for lunch and reserve the rest for later in the week.	Our comfort supper includes Really Good Turkey Burgers with Cheddar Cheese and Horseradish Sauce (pg. 354) and Peanut Butter Sandwich Cookies (pg. 194).	After supper, while the kids and Dad do the dishes, soak in a hot tub filled with Epsom salts and lavender oil.
monday	Warm up a Whole Grain Apple Muffin for a grab-and-go Monday breakfast.	Brown bag it! Choose whole grain bread to build a Spicy Flank Steak Sandwich with Roasted Pepper Blue Cheese Sauce (pg. 353).	Simple supper for a Monday night includes Baked Tilapia with Fresh Herbs (pg. 183) and leftover cheesecake from the weekend.	Take a 30-minute POWER WALK to start your day. Add 15 minutes of weight lifting. Schedule a Swedish massage. Buy an audiobook and put it in your car for rush-hour listening.
tuesday	Take an extra five minutes to build a better Grilled Peanut Butter and Banana Sandwich with Just a Touch of Honey (pg. 344).	Enjoy a bowl of Fresh Veggie Minestrone Soup with Chickpeas made earlier in the week.	A midweek veggie meal is re-invented with Rosemary Polenta with Spinach, Red Beans, and Goat Cheese (pg. 184), and Cocktail Nut Cookie Bars (pg. 196) for dessert.	Grab the entire family for an after-dinner walk around the neighborhood. Don't forget the dog!
wednesday	Grab a bowl of warm Oatmeal with Caramelized Fruit Topping (pg. 149) for a tummy-warming breakfast.	Invite your GORGEOUS gal pals to share Ginger-Marinated Tuna with Dill Lime Butter (pg. 347) and Key Lime Pound Cake (pg. 360).	Hearty Beef Stew (pg. 348) is a perfect midweek meal.	Stretch out from head to toe. Take a 30-minute POWER WALK to start your day. Add 10 minutes of weight lifting. Remember to start light.
thursday	Prepare an Open-Faced BLT Sandwich (pg. 340) for a quick and yummy breakfast.	Brown bag it! Take along a container of Peppery White Bean Salsa and a bag of Whole Wheat Pita Chips (pg. 189) to work to share with friends.	A dinner of Peppered Pork Pinwheels Stuffed with Swiss Chard, Sun-Dried Tomatoes, and Mozzarella (pg. 186) will leave 'em smiling.	It's POWER WALK day. Spend 30 minutes walking. Add a few lunges to stretch out those legs. Work off that frustration by spending 20 to 30 minutes in your garden.
friday	Sip Coconut Tropical Smoothies (pg. 148) for breakfast.	Stay home for lunch. Build a super dish packed full of veggies. Creamy Wild Mushroom Soup with Sherry and Fresh Thyme (pg. 357) fits the bill.	Treat the family to Parmesan Chicken Fingers with Green Cashew and Curry Dipping Sauce (pg. 181) and The Real Deal Fries with Ketchup of Course (pg. 358)!	Start the day with a 40-minute POWER WALK with a pal that includes 10 minutes of jogging and 10 minutes of stretching!

For Week 34 Grocery Shopping List and Shopping Day Prep Tips visit www.GorgeousLifestyleGuide.com

gorgeous lifestyle guide week 35 — you could be dancin', skin-savvy

	Breakfast	Lunch	Dinner	Revitalizing Activity
saturday	Bake up a batch of Whole Wheat Bran Muffins with Golden Raisins and Walnuts (pg. 207). Save extras for later in the week.	This is Shopping Day. While you are running errands, stop and treat yourself to your favorite deli sandwich with whole grain bread, fresh veggies, and lean meat.	Date night! Invite pals for Grilled Halibut with Salsa Verde (pg. 64), Stewed Tomatoes with Garlic and Black Beans (pg. 71) and Peach Gingerbread with Walnut Streusel (pg. 76).	Start the day with a 40-minute POWER WALK that includes 10 minutes of jogging! Today is Shopping Day! Hit the farmer's market.
sunday	Gather the group for Brunch Frittata with Red Potatoes and Kale (pg. 208).	**Afternoon** Prepare Sweet Pea Panzanella Salad (pg. 221). Have a small dish for lunch and reserve the rest for later in the week.	Sunday night supper fun includes Chicken Thighs with Sage and Caramelized Peaches (pg. 65) and Chilled Berry Sauce with Lime Sherbet and Coconut Garnish (pg. 225).	Stretch out those toes and soak in warm water after a long weekend. Me time! Luxuriate with a MINT FACIAL STEAM (pg. 78).
monday	Grab Whole Wheat Bran Muffin for the commute to work.	Brown bag it! Take along Sushi-Style Salmon Wraps (pg. 61) and share with your desk mate.	Prepare Better Veggie Chili (pg. 218) for an easy workweek supper.	Take a couple of minutes to visit the sporting goods store and update your athletic shoes. Remember to purchase a pair with just the support that you need to protect your tootsie toes.
tuesday	Fresh Fruit Salad with Citrus Basil Dressing (pg. 58) for a fun and fruity breakfast.	Butternut Squash Soup Flavored with Orange and Tarragon (pg. 70) can be prepared the night before and poured into a thermos for an on-the-run lunch.	Wild Ivory King Salmon Fillets with Macadamia Nut Crust (pg. 211) and Blueberry Shortbread Bars (pg. 223) make a super supper.	Get your kids together for a quick game of one-on-one. Give your dull skin a creamy shine with a MILKY CLEANSER (pg. 78).
wednesday	Blend up a batch of Juiced-Up Fruit-and-Herb Breakfast Drinks (Blueberry-Basil) (pg. 57).	Invite your GORGEOUS gal pals to share a lunch of Spinach Salad with Warm Chipotle Chili Vinaigrette Topped with Chicken Strips and Crisp Sweet Potato (pg. 66).	Hoisin Beef and Veggies (pg. 212) make for an easy supper.	Take a 30-minute POWER WALK to start your day. Add 15 minutes of weight lifting. Do a few more reps. Reward yourself with a pedicure appointment.
thursday	Whip up a batch of Double Berry Whole Wheat Pancakes (pg. 209) for the gang.	Brown bag it! Take along a container of salmon salad made from the leftovers from earlier in the week.	Feast on a menu of Sea Scallops with Blood Orange, Avocado, and Red Onion Salsa (pg. 215) and Peach Gingerbread with Walnut Streusel (pg. 76).	Remember your 30-minute POWER WALK. Add a few lunges to stretch out those legs and feet.
friday	Start the weekend with a great breakfast of Poached Eggs with Spinach and White Beans (pg. 210).	Home for lunch? Enjoy a Mediterranean Tuna Melt (pg. 62) for a TGIF lunch treat.	Treat the whole family to Veggie Night with Baked Potatoes Stuffed with Swiss Chard and Black Beans (pg. 217) and Roasted Veggie Stacks with Mozzarella (pg. 220).	Start the day with a 40-minute POWER WALK with a pal that includes 10 minutes of jogging and 10 minutes of stretching!

For Week 35 Grocery Shopping List and Shopping Day Prep Tips visit www.GorgeousLifestyleGuide.com

gorgeous lifestyle guide week 36, you could be dancin', hands-on glam

Day	Breakfast	Lunch	Dinner	Revitalizing Activity
saturday	Bake up a batch of Blueberry Buttermilk Coffee Cake Topped with Granola (pg. 236) Save extra pieces for later in the week.	This is Shopping Day. While you are running errands, stop and treat yourself to your favorite deli sandwich made with whole grain breads, fresh veggies, and lean meat.	Date night! Invite Pals for Snapper Veronique (pg. 244), Sautéed Red Cabbage with Drunken Raisins (pg. 251), and Tropical Strawberry Tiramisu (pg. 224).	Start the day with a 40-minute POWER WALK that includes 10 minutes of jogging! Today is Shopping Day! Hit the farmer's market.
sunday	Gather the group for Brunch Frittata with Red Potatoes and Kale (pg. 208).	**Afternoon** Prepare Sweet Pea Panzanella Salad (pg. 221). Have a small dish for lunch and reserve the rest for later in the week.	Sunday night supper fun includes Turkey Meatloaf Burgers 'with Sweet Potato Sticks (pg. 243) and Strike-It-Rich Chocolate Pudding with Chocolate Cookie Crumbles (pg. 252).	Stretch out those toes and soak in warm water after a long weekend. Give yourself a home spa manicure while you listen to your favorite new jazz cd.
monday	Grab a slice of Blueberry Buttermilk Coffee Cake Topped with Granola for the commute to work.	Brown bag it! Take along Roasted Asparagus Salad with Arugula, Radishes, and Lemon Vinaigrette (pg. 248).	Prepare Hoisin Beef and Veggies (pg. 212) for an easy workweek supper.	Take a couple of minutes to visit the sporting goods store and update your athletic shoes. Remember to purchase a pair with just the support that you need to protect your tootsie toes.
tuesday	Prepare Walnut-Stuffed Baked Apples with Maple Syrup (pg. 238).	Sweet Pea Panzanella Salad (made earlier in the week).	Chicken and Rice Meatball Hoagies (pg. 242) are easy and fun, especially when you add Blueberry Shortbread Bars (pg. 223) for dessert.	Hold hands with your special someone while you stroll through the neighborhood after supper.
wednesday	Bake Banana Bread Snack Cake (pg. 237) the night before for a simple grab-and-go breakfast.	Invite your GORGEOUS gal pals to share a lunch of Chilled Shrimp Salad with Red Grapes (pg. 241) and Pecan Graham Squares (pg. 226) for dessert.	Mojo Marinated Chicken Served over Black Beans (pg. 216) makes for a super supper.	Take a 30-minute POWER WALK to start your day. Add 15 minutes of weight lifting. Do a few more reps. Reward yourself with a pedicure appointment.
thursday	Granola Bars (pg. 239) are a super start during a busy week.	Brown bag it! Take along Asparagus Cheese Toasts (pg. 219) and heat them up at lunch time.	Feast on a menu of Sea Scallops with Blood Orange, Avocado, and Red Onion Salsa (pg. 215) and Chocoholic's Crutch (pg. 255).	Remember your 30-minute POWER WALK Add a few lunges to stretch out those legs and feet.
friday	Start the weekend with a great breakfast of Poached Eggs with Spinach and White Beans (pg. 210).	Home for lunch? Enjoy a lunch filled with veggie goodness. Roasted Veggie Stacks with Mozzarella (pg. 220) fits the bill.	Treat the whole family to Veggie Night with Baked Potatoes Stuffed with Swiss Chard and Black Beans (pg. 217) and leftover Pecan Graham Squares.	Start the day with a 40-minute POWER WALK with a pal that includes 10 minutes of jogging and 10 minutes of stretching!

For Week 36 Grocery Shopping List and Shopping Day Prep Tips visit www.GorgeousLifestyleGuide.com

gorgeous lifestyle guide week 37 — you could be dancin', sleepy time

Day	Breakfast	Lunch	Dinner	Revitalizing Activity
saturday	Bake up a batch of Orange Breakfast Muffins (pg. 305). Save extras for later in the week.	This is Shopping Day. While you are running errands, stop and treat yourself to your favorite deli sandwich made with whole grain bread, fresh veggies, and lean meat.	Date night! Invite pals for Charred Sirloin Steak with Mushroom and Red Wine Sauce (pg. 213) and Tropical Strawberry Tiramisu (pg. 224).	Start the day with a 40-minute POWER WALK that includes 10 minutes of jogging! Today is Shopping Day! Hit the farmer's market.
sunday	Gather the group for Sweet Potato Pancakes with Warm Raspberry Syrup (pg. 306).	**Afternoon:** Open Faced Eggplant, Tomato, and Cheddar Grilled Cheese (pg. 309) sandwiches are great for lunch and afternoon game watching.	Sunday night supper fun includes Stuffed Chicken Breasts with Mushrooms, Thyme, and Fontina Cheese (pg. 313) with Chilled Berry Sauce with Lime Sherbet and Coconut Garnish (pg. 225).	Stretch out those toes and soak in warm water after a long weekend. Get to bed early with a lavender sachet tucked under your pillow.
monday	Grab an Orange Breakfast Muffin for the commute to work.	Brown bag it! Take along a salad topped with leftover chicken from the night before.	Prepare Better Veggie Chili (pg. 218) for an easy workweek supper.	Take a couple of minutes to visit the sporting goods store and update your athletic shoes. Remember to purchase a pair with just the support that you need to protect your tootsie toes.
tuesday	Prepare Double-Berry Whole Wheat Pancakes (pg. 209) for the family and start the day off just fine.	Build a brown bag sandwich starring leftover Sirloin Steak on whole grain bread and pile high with fresh veggies.	Wild Ivory King Salmon Fillets with Macadamia Nut Crust (pg. 211) and Blueberry Shortbread Bars (pg. 223).	Get your kids together for a quick game of one-on-one. Place a blank piece of paper on your bedside table and quote your sleepy time mantra as you dose off.
wednesday	Blend up a batch of Fruit 'N Soy Milk Drinks (pg. 307).	Invite your GORGEOUS gal pals to share a lunch of Grilled Coconut Curry Shrimp with Soba Noodles (pg. 312) and Butterscotch Blondies (pg. 325).	Hoisin Beef and Veggies (pg. 212) make for a super supper.	Take a 30-minute POWER WALK to start your day. Add 15 minutes of weight lifting. Do a few more reps. Reward yourself with a pedicure appointment.
thursday	Breakfast Tomatoes with Smoked Salmon (pg. 308) are a fun way to start your day.	Grab your favorite work mate and visit the best salad bar for lunch. Choose citrus vinaigrette dressing and tons of fresh veggies.	Feast on a menu of Pecan-Crusted Chicken Fingers with Apricot Mustard Dipping Sauce (pg. 319).	Remember your 30-minute POWER WALK. Add a few lunges to stretch out those legs and feet.
friday	Start the weekend with a great breakfast of Poached Eggs with Spinach and White Beans (pg. 210).	Home for lunch? Enjoy Asparagus Cheese Toasts (pg. 219).	Treat the whole family to Linguini with Mussels and Snow Peas (pg. 318), Grilled Ratatouille Salad with Tomato Basil Vinaigrette (pg. 323) and Almond Cookies Two Ways (pg. 327).	Start the day with a 40-minute POWER WALK with a pal that includes 10 minutes of jogging and 10 minutes of stretching!

For Week 37 Grocery Shopping List and Shopping Day Prep Tips visit www.GorgeousLifestyleGuide.com

gorgeous lifestyle guide week 38 — you could be dancin', sexy glam

Day	Breakfast	Lunch	Dinner	Revitalizing Activity
saturday	Bake up a batch of Whole Wheat Bran Muffins with Golden Raisins and Walnuts (pg. 207). Save extras for later in the week.	This is Shopping Day. While you are running errands, stop and treat yourself to your favorite deli sandwich made with whole grain bread, fresh veggies, and lean meat.	Date night! Invite pals over for Roasted Beef Tenderloin Steaks Stuffed with Spinach and Gorgonzola with Béarnaise Sauce (pg. 384) and Lemon Vanilla Pudding with Mixed Berries (pg. 396).	Start the day with a 40-minute POWER WALK that includes 10 minutes of jogging! Today is Shopping Day! Hit the farmer's market.
sunday	**Breakfast:** Gather your honey for a special brunch of Creamy French-Style Eggs Garnished with Chopped Tomatoes and Chives (pg. 87).	**Afternoon:** Prepare a light lunch of Arugula Salad with Walnut-Crusted Goat Cheese (pg. 390).	**Dinner:** Sunday night supper fun includes Grilled Pork Chops with Cherry Ginger Chutney (pg. 389). and Chilled Berry Sauce with Lime Sherbet and Coconut Garnish (pg. 225).	**Revitalizing Activity:** Stretch out those toes and soak in warm water after a long weekend.
monday	Grab a Whole Wheat Bran Muffin for the commute to work.	Brown bag it! Choose whole grain bread to build a sandwich stuffed with veggies and leftover sliced steak from the weekend.	Prepare Better Veggie Chili (pg. 218) for an easy workweek supper.	Take a couple of minutes to visit the sporting goods store and update your athletic shoes. Remember to purchase a pair with just the support that you need to protect your tootsie toes.
tuesday	Prepare a batch of Cinnamon Chocolate-Chip Pancakes with Whipped Cream and Warm Maple Syrup (pg. 377)—all the better if it's a snow day!	Take along a container of Peel-and-Eat Jumbo Shrimp with Buffalo-Style Sauce (pg. 391; bring extra napkins!)	Wild Ivory King Salmon Fillets with Macadamia Nut Crust (pg. 211) and Blueberry Shortbread Bars (pg. 223).	Take a 30-minute POWER WALK to start your day. Add 15 minutes of weight lifting. After supper, grab his hand for an evening stroll around the neighborhood.
wednesday	Poached Eggs with Spinach and White Beans (pg. 210) makes a "egg-cellent" breakfast treat.	Invite your GORGEOUS gal pals to share a lunch of Grilled Lobster Tails with Parsley Butter Served over Creamy Hash (pg. 380) with leftover Blueberry Shortbread Bars.	Hoisin Beef and Veggies (pg. 212) make for a super supper.	Take a 30-minute POWER WALK to start your day. Add 15 minutes of weight lifting. Do a few more reps. Reward yourself with a pedicure appointment.
thursday	Warm up a leftover Whole Wheat Bran Muffin.	Brown bag it! Take along Olive, Onion, and Roasted Pepper Bruschetta (pg. 393) to share with coworkers.	Feast on a menu of Sea Scallops with Blood Orange, Avocado, and Red Onion Salsa (pg. 215) and Pecan Graham Squares (pg. 226).	Start the day with a 40-minute POWER WALK with your significant other that includes 10 minutes of jogging and 10 minutes of stretching!
friday	Start the weekend with a great breakfast of Baked Raspberry-Stuffed French Toast with Pecans and Maple Drizzle (pg. 379).	Home for lunch? Enjoy Asparagus Cheese Toasts (pg. 219) and an extra Pecan Graham Square from last night.	Treat the whole family to Butternut Squash Ravioli with Brown Butter, Sage, and Pine Nut Sauce (pg. 382) and Peanut Butter Chocolate Bars (pg. 394).	Start the day with a 40-minute POWER WALK with a pal that includes 10 minutes of jogging and 10 minutes of stretching!

For Week 38 Grocery Shopping List and Shopping Day Prep Tips visit www.GorgeousLifestyleGuide.com

gorgeous lifestyle guide week 39 — hands-on glam, good hair

Day	Breakfast	Lunch	Dinner	Revitalizing Activity
saturday	**Breakfast** Bake up a stunning Blueberry Buttermilk Coffee Cake Topped with Granola (pg. 236). Save extras for later in the week.	**Lunch** This is Shopping Day. While you are running errands, stop and treat yourself to a fresh veggie salad with your favorite (but light) dressing.	**Dinner** Date night! Invite pals for Roasted Asparagus Salad with Arugula, Radishes, and Lemon Vinaigrette (pg. 248), Lamb Chops with Coconut Skillet Sauce (pg. 92), and Strike-It-Rich Chocolate Pudding with Chocolate Crumbles (pg. 252).	**Revitalizing Activity** Start the day with a 40-minute POWER WALK that includes 10 minutes of jogging! Today is Shopping Day! Hit the farmer's market.
sunday	**Breakfast** Gather the group for Egg White Omelets with Bell Peppers and Turkey Sausage (pg. 88).	**Afternoon** Have a snacky lunch of Black Bean and Roasted Pepper Empanadas (pg. 250). Share extras with coworkers.	**Dinner** Prepare Jambalaya (pg. 245) for Sunday's supper and serve with Simple Zucchini Cake with Vanilla Glaze (pg. 254), reserving leftovers for later in the week.	**Revitalizing Activity** Me time!! Give yourself a home spa manicure while you listen to your favorite new jazz cd. Luxuriate with an OLIVE OIL MASK (pg. 110) for your hair. Buy a magazine and try out a new hairdo.
monday	**Breakfast** A batch of Pecan Bananadana Muffins (pg. 90) are quickly prepared and valuable later in the week.	**Lunch** Brown bag it! Make a batch of Creamy Cauliflower Soup with Arugula and Crispy Bacon Garnish (pg. 101). Take some to work and reserve the rest for later in the week.	**Dinner** Surprise!! Calf's Liver with Golden Onions (pg. 97) and Oatmeal Snack Cake (pg. 106) for dessert.	**Revitalizing Activity** Take a couple of minutes to visit the cosmetic counter and purchase a rich hand cream filled with collagen. Oh, and check out that bracelet in the glass counter.
tuesday	**Breakfast** Dash off to work with a slice of Blueberry Buttermilk Coffee Cake.	**Lunch** Make a batch of Turkey Meatloaf Burgers with Spicy Sweet Potato Sticks (pg. 243) and take them to the park for the other moms.	**Dinner** The kids (big and small) will dig into Chicken and Rice Meatball Hoagies (pg. 242).	**Revitalizing Activity** Hold hands with your special someone while you stroll through the neighborhood after supper. Let your fingers do the walking to make an appointment with a hip hairstylist.
wednesday	**Breakfast** Creamy French-Style Eggs Garnished with Chopped Tomatoes and Chives (pg. 87) is a super midweek meal.	**Lunch** Invite your GORGEOUS gal pals to share Paella with Chorizo, Asparagus, and Shellfish (pg. 98) for a fun lunch.	**Dinner** Enjoy a decadent supper of Poached Salmon in Infused Olive Oil with Horseradish Sauce (pg. 240) with leftover Simple Zucchini Cake slices.	**Revitalizing Activity** Take a 30-minute POWER WALK to start your day. Add 15 minutes of weight lifting. Do a few more reps than last week. Reward yourself with a manicure appointment.
thursday	**Breakfast** Whip up a batch of Granola Power Bars (pg. 239) for a real grab-and-go breakfast.	**Lunch** Brown bag it! Take along a container of veggie salad topped with slices of salmon leftovers from last evening.	**Dinner** A first course of leftover Creamy Cauliflower Soup with Arugula and Crispy Bacon Garnish followed by Mussels and Brussels in a White Wine Butter Sauce (pg. 94) makes for a cozy hand-holding supper.	**Revitalizing Activity** Walk this way—for 30 minutes. Add a few lunges to stretch out those legs and feet. Remember the sunscreen, especially on your hands.
friday	**Breakfast** Grab a Pecan Bananadana Muffin on your way out the door.	**Lunch** After your light midday restaurant meal, splurge on a cup of Chocoholic's Crutch (pg. 255).	**Dinner** Treat the whole family to Grilled Skirt Steak and Veggie Open-Faced Sandwiches (pg. 95) and Roasted Red Grape Parfaits with Orange and Maple-Flavored Ricotta Cheese (pg. 253).	**Revitalizing Activity** Start the day with a 40-minute POWER WALK with a pal that includes 10 minutes of jogging and 10 minutes of stretching!

For Week 39 Grocery Shopping List and Shopping Day Prep Tips visit www.GorgeousLifestyleGuide.com

gorgeous lifestyle guide week 40 — hands-on glam, tummy-pleasing

Day	Breakfast	Lunch	Dinner	Revitalizing Activity
saturday	Bake up a stunning Blueberry Buttermilk Coffee Cake Topped with Granola (pg. 236). Save extras for later in the week.	This is Shopping Day. While you are running errands, stop and treat yourself to a fresh veggie salad with your favorite (but light) dressing.	Date night! Invite pals for Roasted Asparagus Salad with Arugula, Radishes, and Lemon Vinaigrette (pg. 248), Snapper Fillets Smothered with Caramelized Onions (pg. 272), and Orange Cappuccino Parfaits (pg. 285).	Start the day with a 40-minute POWER WALK that includes 10 minutes of jogging! Today is Shopping Day! Hit the farmer's market.
sunday	Gather the group for Say "Ricotta Cheese" Pancakes with Very Berry Sauce (pg. 269).	**Afternoon** Have a snacky lunch of Black Bean and Roasted Pepper Empanadas (pg. 250). Share extras with coworkers.	Prepare Roasted Chipotle Salmon with Minted Couscous (pg. 279) for Sunday's supper and serve with Simple Zucchini Cake with Vanilla Glaze (pg. 254), reserving leftovers for later in the week.	Give yourself a home spa manicure. Turn on your Pilates DVD and get down with your inner core. Stretch out muscles and improve your squats. Work your way up to a perfect teaser.
monday	Start your work week with Apple Pie for Breakfast (pg. 267). Just kidding, of course!	Brown bag it! Build a better tuna sandwich by adding green pepper, celery, and onion to the salad. Choose whole grain bread and plenty of dark green lettuce with slices of tomato.	Surprise!! Serve Five-Spice Beef Wraps with Orange Ginger Dipping Sauce (pg. 280) and Poached Cherry Sundaes (pg. 254) for dessert.	Take a couple of minutes to visit the cosmetic counter and purchase a rich hand cream filled with collagen. Oh, and check out that bracelet in the glass counter.
tuesday	Dash off to work with a slice of Blueberry Buttermilk Coffee Cake.	Make a fresh veggie salad. Southwestern Chopped Salad with Toasted Peppers and Corn (pg. 284) fits the bill.	The kids (big and small) will dig into Chicken and Rice Meatball Hoagies (pg. 242).	Take a 30-minute WALK to start your day. Add 15 minutes of weight lifting. Do a few more reps than last week. Find a pal who wants to run a marathon and start training.
wednesday	Prepare Banana Bread Snack Cake (pg. 237), reserving extras for later in the week.	Invite your GORGEOUS gal pals to share Grilled Veggie Panini with Basil Pesto Sauce (pg. 274) with Chocoholic's Crutch (pg. 255) for dessert.	Enjoy a decadent supper of Poached Salmon in Infused Olive Oil with Horseradish Sauce (pg. 240) and leftover Simple Zucchini Cake slices for dessert.	Take a 30-minute POWER WALK to start your day. Add 15 minutes of weight lifting. Do a few more reps than last week. Reward yourself with a manicure appointment.
thursday	Enjoy Egg in a Frame with Basil Tomatoes (pg. 270) because the dish comes together in minutes.	Brown bag it! Take along a container of veggie salad topped with slices of salmon leftovers from last evening.	Sauteed Yellowtail Snapper with Braised Cabbage and Cheesy Mashed Potatoes (pg. 246) makes for a cozy hand-holding supper.	Walk this way—for 30 minutes. Add a few lunges to stretch out those legs and feet. Remember the sunscreen, especially on your hands.
friday	Grab a wedge of Banana Snack Cake on your way out the door.	A light luncheon includes Avocado and Grapefruit Salad (pg. 281).	Treat the whole family to Turkey Meatloaf Burgers with Sweet Potato Sticks (pg. 243) and Roasted Red Grape Parfaits with Orange and Maple-Flavored Ricotta Cheese (pg. 253).	Start the day with a 40-minute POWER WALK with a pal that includes 10 minutes of jogging and 10 minutes of stretching!

For Week 40 Grocery Shopping List and Shopping Day Prep Tips visit www.GorgeousLifestyleGuide.com

gorgeous lifestyle guide week 41 — hands-on glam, stress-free

Day	Breakfast	Lunch	Dinner	Revitalizing Activity
saturday	Bake up a stunning Blueberry Buttermilk Coffee Cake Topped with Granola (pg. 236). Save extras for later in the week.	This is Shopping Day. While you are running errands, stop and treat yourself to a fresh veggie salad with your favorite (but light) dressing.	Date night! Invite pals for Hunter's-Style Chicken Stew with Yellow Rice (pg. 352) and Key Lime Pound Cake (pg. 360) for dessert.	Start the day with a 40-minute POWER WALK that includes 10 minutes of jogging! Today is Shopping Day! Hit the farmer's market.
sunday	Gather the group for Bacon and Asparagus Quiche (pg. 342).	**Afternoon** Prepare a yummy pot of Creamy Wild Mushroom Soup with Sherry and Fresh Thyme (pg. 357).	Prepare Sunday's comfort supper of Old-Fashioned Turkeyloaf with Hidden Mushrooms (pg. 345) and serve with Simple Zucchini Cake with Vanilla Glaze (pg. 254), reserving leftovers for later in the week.	Take a 30-minute POWER WALK to start your day. Add 15 minutes of weight lifting. Schedule a Swedish massage. Buy an audiobook and put it in your car for rush-hour listening.
monday	Start the workweek off with a fun breakfast. Grilled Peanut Butter and Banana Sandwiches with Just a Touch of Honey (pg. 344) fill the bill.	Brown bag it! Build a better tuna sandwich by adding green pepper, celery, and onion to the salad. Choose whole grain bread and plenty of dark green lettuce with slices of tomato.	Surprise!! Serve Sliced Chicken Breast with Red Grape Sauce (pg. 247) and Sautéed Red Cabbage with Drunken Raisins (pg. 251). (Don't tell the kids!)	Take a couple of minutes to visit the cosmetic counter and purchase a rich hand cream filled with collagen. Oh, and check out that bracelet in the glass counter.
tuesday	Dash off to work with a slice of Blueberry Buttermilk Coffee Cake made earlier in the week.	Make a fresh veggie salad topped with slices of leftover chicken and your favorite citrus vinaigrette.	The kids (big and small) will dig into Really Good Turkey Burgers with Cheddar Cheese and Horseradish Sauce (pg. 354) and The Real Deal Fries (pg. 358) with Ketchup of Course.	Rest your muscles. Spend 20 minutes stretching. De-stress by preparing a batch of Maple Cake Doughnuts (pg. 361) to take to the office tomorrow morning. Eat one, share one!
wednesday	Prepare Banana Bread Snack Cake (pg. 237), reserving extras for later in the week.	Invite your GORGEOUS gal pals to share Spicy Flank Steak Sandwiches with Roasted Pepper Blue Cheese Sauce (pg. 353) for a fun lunch.	Enjoy a decadent supper of Poached Salmon in Infused Olive Oil with Horseradish Sauce (pg. 240) with leftover Simple Zucchini Cake slices.	Take a 30-minute POWER WALK to start your day. Add 15 minutes of weight lifting. Do a few more reps than last week. Reward yourself with a manicure appointment.
thursday	An Open-Faced BLT Breakfast Sandwich (pg. 340) is quick to make and fun to eat.	Brown bag it! Take along a container of leftover Creamy Wild Mushroom Soup with Sherry and Fresh Thyme from earlier in the week.	Shrimp Scampi with Angel Hair Pasta (pg. 346) makes for a cozy hand-holding supper. Serve with Chocolate Gingersnaps (pg. 362).	Walk this way—for 30 minutes. Add a few lunges to stretch out those legs and feet. Remember the sunscreen, especially on your hands.
friday	Grab a wedge of Banana Snack Cake on your way out the door.	Whip up Sweet Potato Soufflé (pg. 249) and invite your next door neighbor to lunch.	Treat the whole family to Hearty Beef Stew (pg. 348) and Roasted Red Grape Parfaits with Orange and Maple-Flavored Ricotta Cheese (pg. 253).	Start the day with a 40-minute POWER WALK with a pal that includes 10 minutes of jogging and 10 minutes of stretching!

For Week 41 Grocery Shopping List and Shopping Day Prep Tips visit www.GorgeousLifestyleGuide.com

gorgeous lifestyle guide week 42 — tummy-pleasing, skin-savvy

Day	Breakfast	Lunch	Dinner	Revitalizing Activity
saturday	Blend up a batch of Juiced-Up Fruit-and-Herb Breakfast Drinks (pg. 57) (Cantaloupe-Tarragon).	This is Shopping Day. While you are running errands, stop and treat yourself to your favorite deli sandwich made with whole grain bread, plenty of veggies, reduced-fat cheese, and lean meat.	Date night! Invite pals for Grilled Halibut with Salsa Verde (pg. 64), Grilled Veggie Skewers (pg. 283), and Poached Cherry Sundaes (pg. 288).	Start the day with a 40-minute POWER WALK that includes 15 minutes of jogging! Today is Shopping Day! Hit the farmer's market.
sunday	Gather the group for Say "Ricotta Cheese" Pancakes with Very Berry Sauce (pg. 269).	**Afternoon:** Have a simple lunch of roasted veggie soup made by blending leftover veggie skewers with homemade chicken broth.	Prepare a comfort food supper that includes Chicken Thighs with Sage and Caramelized Peaches (pg. 65) and Fresh Lime Cake with Warm Blueberry Sauce (pg. 286), saving extras for later in the week.	Turn on your Pilates DVD and get down with your inner core. Stretch out those muscles and improve your squats—work your way up to a perfect teaser.
monday	Prepare Egg in a Frame with Basil Tomatoes (pg. 270) for the gang to start off the week on the right foot.	Brown bag it! Take along a thermosful of Roasted Tomato Soup with Sea Bass Center (pg. 69).	Snapper Fillets Smothered with Caramelized Onions (pg. 272) and Sautéed Peas with Mint (pg. 282) make an easy weekday meal.	Sign up for an aerobics class with your best pal so that neither of you will skip out. Luxuriate with an OATMEAL PEEL (pg. 79). Visit the cosmetic counter for a makeover.
tuesday	Fruit and Yogurt Breakfast Parfaits with Granola Crunch (pg. 59) make morning time party time!	Enjoy Avocado and Grapefruit Salad (pg. 281) while reading the newest issue of your favorite magazine.	The kids will love Eggplant Boats Stuffed with Spicy Beef and Peas (pg. 271) with leftover slices of Fresh Lime Cake.	Rest your muscles and spend 20 minutes stretching out your tired parts, followed by a luxurious, scented bath.
wednesday	Time for Apple Pie for Breakfast (pg. 267), isn't it?	Invite your GORGEOUS gal pals to share a bowl of Butternut Squash Soup Flavored with Orange and Tarragon (pg. 70) and Oven-Roasted Fruit with Vanilla Yogurt Sorbet (pg. 77).	Spicy Tuna Dinner Salad with Balsamic Dressing (pg. 273) and Orange Cappuccino Parfaits (pg. 285) are yummy and simple to prepare.	Take a 30-minute POWER WALK to start your day. Add 15 minutes of weight lifting. Do a few more reps than last week. Find a pal who wants to run a marathon and start training.
thursday	Blend up your favorite Juiced-Up Fruit-and-Herb Breakfast Drinks (pg. 57) (Blueberry-Basil).	Brown bag it! Prepare Sushi-Style Salmon Wraps (pg. 61) and share extras with coworkers.	Prepare Baked Chicken Breasts with Artichoke and Sun-Dried Tomato Sauce (pg. 275) for an easy midweek supper.	Walk this way—for 30 minutes. Add a few lunges to stretch out those legs and butt. Add a few squats after your walk. Hold in your tummy during your workout to build muscles.
friday	Breakfast Burritos with Red Pepper Salsa (pg. 60) are a fun Friday breakfast.	Prepare Grilled Veggie Panini with Basil Pesto Sauce (pg. 274). Make one to share with your walking buddy.	Treat the whole family to Open-Faced Chicken Tacos (pg. 68). Add a bite of Tropical Buttermilk Panna Cotta with Strawberry Sauce (pg. 287) for dessert.	Start the day with a 40-minute POWER WALK with a pal that includes 10 minutes of jogging and 10 minutes of stretching! Me time! Apply a HONEY MASK (pg. 79).

For Week 42 Grocery Shopping List and Shopping Day Prep Tips visit www.GorgeousLifestyleGuide.com

gorgeous lifestyle guide week 43 — tummy-pleasing, sleepy time

Day	Breakfast	Lunch	Dinner	Revitalizing Activity
saturday	Bake up a batch of Orange Breakfast Muffins (pg. 305), reserving extras for later in the week.	This is Shopping Day. While you are running errands, stop and treat yourself to your favorite deli sandwich made with whole grain bread, plenty of veggies, reduced-fat cheese, and lean meat.	Date night! Invite pals for Broiled Tilapia Fillets with Arugula Aioli Sauce (pg. 315), Grilled Veggie Skewers (pg. 283), and Poached Cherry Sundaes (pg. 288).	Start the day with a 40-minute POWER WALK that includes 15 minutes of jogging! Today is Shopping Day! Hit the farmer's market.
sunday	Gather the group for Sweet Potato Pancakes with Warm Raspberry Syrup (pg. 306).	**Afternoon** Have a simple lunch of roasted veggie soup made by blending leftover veggie skewers with homemade chicken broth.	Sunday comfort supper includes Roast Turkey Breast with Cornbread-Cranberry Dressing and Madeira Mushroom Gravy (pg. 310) and Fresh Lime Cake with Warm Blueberry Sauce (pg. 286).	Turn on your Pilates DVD and get down with your inner core. Stretch out those muscles and improve your squats—work your way up to a perfect teaser.
monday	To start off the workweek, prepare Egg in a Frame with Basil Tomatoes (pg. 270) for the gang.	Brown bag it! Take along a light meal of Avocado and Grapefruit Salad (pg. 281).	Roasted Chipotle Salmon with Minted Couscous (pg. 279) and Sautéed Peas with Mint (pg. 282) make an easy weekday meal.	Sign up for an aerobics class with your best pal. Place a blank piece of paper on your bedside table and quote your sleepy time mantra as you dose off.
tuesday	Dash off to work with a Orange Breakfast Muffin from the batch made earlier.	Enjoy Southwestern Chopped Salad with Toasted Peppers and Corn (pg. 284) while reading the newest issue of your favorite magazine.	The kids will love Pecan-Crusted Chicken Fingers with Apricot Mustard Dipping Sauce (pg. 319) with slices of leftover Fresh Lime Cake.	Rest your muscles and spend 20 minutes stretching out your tired parts followed with a luxurious, scented bath.
wednesday	Whip up a batch of Fruit 'N Soy Milk Drinks (pg. 307) for a quick starter.	Invite your GORGEOUS gal pals to share Sautéed Cauliflower and Spinach Fettuccini Casserole (pg. 320) with Almond Cookies Two Ways (pg. 327).	Spicy Tuna Dinner Salad with Balsamic Dressing (pg. 273) and Orange Cappuccino Parfaits (pg. 285) are yummy and simple to prepare.	Take a 30-minute POWER WALK to start your day. Add 15 minutes of weight lifting. Do a few more reps than last week. Find a pal who wants to run a marathon and start training.
thursday	Breakfast Tomatoes with Smoked Salmon (pg. 308) are a fun start to your Thursday.	Brown bag it! Prepare fresh tuna salad with leftovers from last night's supper. Slip in an extra Almond Cookie.	Prepare Crab Cake Po' Boys (pg. 316) for an easy midweek supper.	Walk this way—for 30 minutes. Add a few lunges to stretch out those legs and butt. Add a few squats after your walk. Hold in your tummy during your workout to build muscles.
friday	Breakfast Tacos (pg. 268) are a fun Friday breakfast.	Prepare Grilled Veggie Panini with Basil Pesto Sauce (pg. 274). Make one to share with your walking buddy.	Treat the whole family to Rack of Lamb with Spinach and Breadcrumb Topping (pg. 311), Broccoli Mash (pg. 321), and Tropical Buttermilk Panna Cotta with Strawberry Sauce (pg. 287) for dessert.	Start the day with a 40-minute POWER WALK with a pal that includes 10 minutes of jogging and 10 minutes of stretching!

gorgeous lifestyle guide week 44 — sleepy time, good hair

	Breakfast	Lunch	Dinner	Revitalizing Activity
saturday	Bake up a batch of Orange Breakfast Muffins (pg. 305). Save extras for later in the week.	This is Shopping Day. While you are running errands, stop and treat yourself to your favorite fresh garden salad with whole grain bread on the side.	Date night! Invite pals for Rosemary Roasted Chicken Breasts with Smoky Almond Sauce (pg. 91), Broccoli Mash (pg. 321), and Simmering Blueberries with Cinnamon Dumplings (pg. 324).	Start the day with a 40-minute POWER WALK that includes 15 minutes of jogging! Today is Shopping Day!! Hit the farmer's market.
sunday	Gather the gang for Creamy French-Style Eggs Garnished with Chopped Tomatoes and Chives (pg. 87).	Afternoon: Have a simple lunch of Creamy Cauliflower Soup with Arugula and Crispy Bacon Garnish (pg. 101). Save extras for a quick lunch later in the week.	Serve a comfort meal of Roasted Pork Tenderloin with Swiss Chard (pg. 96) and Stuffed Zucchini, Yellow Squash, and Eggplant (pg. 322). Add Baked Pears in Brandy Sauce (pg. 104) for dessert.	Give your dull hair a COLOR LIFT (pg. 109). Don't forget to squeeze in your 30-minute POWER WALK. Relax with a soothing cup of decaffeinated tea and a hot, lavender-scented bath.
monday	Enjoy rich Fruit 'N Soy Milk Drinks (pg. 307) as a start to your workweek.	Brown bag it! Choose whole grain bread and lean meat or poultry to build your sandwich. Add dark green lettuce and sliced tomato.	Grilled Coconut Curry Shrimp with Soba Noodles (pg. 312) makes for a light and easy supper. Add leftover grilled veggies from earlier in the week.	Me time! Luxuriate with an OLIVE OIL HAIR MASK (pg. 110). Buy a magazine and try out a new hairdo. Get to bed early with a lavender sachet tucked under your pillow.
tuesday	Dash off to work with a warmed Orange Breakfast Muffin.	Prepare Open-Faced Eggplant, Tomato, and Cheddar Grilled Cheese (pg. 309). Make extras for your workout buddy.	Gather the family for a supper of Grilled Skirt Steak and Veggie Open-Faced Sandwich (pg. 95) and Sautéed Cauliflower and Spinach Fettuccini Casserole (pg. 320).	Rest your muscles and spend 20 minutes stretching out your tired parts, followed by a luxurious, scented bath.
wednesday	Enjoy a treat of Breakfast Tomatoes with Smoked Salmon (pg. 308).	Invite your GORGEOUS gal pals to share Mussels and Brussels in a White Wine Sauce (pg. 94) for lunch.	Simply prepared Broiled Tilapia Fillets with Arugula Aioli Sauce (pg. 315) come together so quickly, you will have time to bake a batch of Butterscotch Blondies (pg. 325) for dessert.	Take a 30-minute POWER WALK to start your day. Add 15 minutes of weight lifting. Schedule a Swedish massage.
thursday	Enjoy protein-rich Egg White Omelets with Bell Peppers and Turkey Sausage (pg. 89) for breakfast.	Brown bag it! Take along a fresh garden salad topped with flank steak slices from earlier in the week. Add a Butterscotch Blondie to the bag and another one for a pal.	Whip up Lamb Chops with Coconut Skillet Sauce (pg. 92) for a light meal on Thursday night. Prepare a batch of Almond Cookies Two Ways (pg. 327) and freeze half for next week.	Walk this way—for 30 minutes. Place a blank piece of paper on your bedside table and quote your sleepy time mantra as you dose off.
friday	Whip up a batch of Pecan Bananadana Muffins (pg. 90) and save extras for the weekend.	Prepare Grilled Veggie Panini with Basil Pesto Sauce (pg. 274). Make one to share with your walking buddy.	Treat the whole family to Pecan-Crusted Chicken Fingers with Apricot Mustard Dipping Sauce (pg. 319) and Simple Chocolate Mousse with Graham Cracker Crumbles (pg. 326).	Start the day with a 40-minute POWER WALK with a pal that includes 10 minutes of jogging and 10 minutes of stretching!

For Week 44 Grocery Shopping List and Shopping Day Prep Tips visit www.GorgeousLifestyleGuide.com

gorgeous lifestyle guide week 45 — sleepy time, stress-free

saturday	**Breakfast** Bake up a batch of Orange Breakfast Muffins (pg. 305). Save extras for later in the week.	**Lunch** This is Shopping Day. While you are running errands, stop and treat yourself to your favorite fresh garden salad with whole grain bread on the side.	**Dinner** Invite Pals for Butternut Squash and Swiss Chard Roll-Ups with Sun-Dried Tomato Basil Sauce (pg. 350), Broccoli Mash (pg. 321), and Simmering Blueberries with Cinnamon Dumplings (pg. 324).	**Revitalizing Activity** Start the day with a 40-minute POWER WALK that includes 15 minutes of jogging. Today is Shopping Day! Hit the farmer's market.
sunday	**Breakfast** Gather the group for Ham and Cheese Scramble (pg. 341).	**Afternoon** Have a simple lunch of Grilled Ratatouille Salad with Tomato Basil Vinaigrette (pg. 323). Save extra veggies for later in the week. They will make a great soup!	**Dinner** Serve a comfort meal of Shrimp Scampi with Angel Hair Pasta (pg. 346) and Stuffed Zucchini, Squash and Eggplant (pg. 322).	**Revitalizing Activity** After dinner relax with a warm and soothing cup of decaffeinated tea and a hot, lavender-scented bath.
monday	**Breakfast** Enjoy rich Fruit 'N Soy Milk Drinks (pg. 307) as a start to your workweek.	**Lunch** Splurge on a small dish of Pan-Sautéed Gnocchi with Sun-Dried Tomato and Sage (pg. 355).	**Dinner** Grilled Coconut Curry Shrimp with Soba Noodles (pg. 312) makes for a light and easy supper. Add leftover grilled veggies from earlier in the week.	**Revitalizing Activity** Get to bed early with a lavender sachet tucked under your pillow.
tuesday	**Breakfast** Dash off to work with a warmed Orange Breakfast Muffin.	**Lunch** Prepare Open-Faced Eggplant, Tomato, and Cheddar Grilled Cheese (pg. 309). Make extras for your workout buddy.	**Dinner** Gather the family for a supper of Spicy Flank Steak Sandwiches with Roasted Pepper Blue Cheese Sauce (pg. 353) and Sautéed Cauliflower and Spinach Fettuccini Casserole (pg. 320).	**Revitalizing Activity** Rest your muscles and spend 20 minutes stretching out your tired parts, followed by a luxurious, scented bath.
wednesday	**Breakfast** Enjoy a treat of Breakfast Tomatoes with Smoked Salmon (pg. 308).	**Lunch** Invite your GORGEOUS gal pals to share Crab Cake Po' Boys (pg. 316) for lunch.	**Dinner** Simply prepared Broiled Tilapia Fillets with Arugula Aioli Sauce (pg. 315) comes together so quickly you will have time to bake a batch of Butterscotch Blondies (pg. 325) for dessert.	**Revitalizing Activity** Take a 30-minute POWER WALK to start your day. Add 15 minutes of weight lifting. Schedule a Swedish massage.
thursday	**Breakfast** Enjoy an Open-Faced BLT Breakfast Sandwich (pg. 340) to start your day.	**Lunch** Brown bag it! Take along a fresh garden salad topped with steak slices from earlier in the week. Add a Butterscotch Blondie to the bag and another one for a pal.	**Dinner** Whip up Ginger-Marinated Tuna with Dill Lime Butter (pg. 347) for a light meal on Thursday night.	**Revitalizing Activity** Walk this way—for 30 minutes. Place a blank piece of paper on your bedside table and quote your sleepy time mantra as you dose off.
friday	**Breakfast** It's F-R-I-D-A-Y! Start the weekend with a treat of Grilled Peanut Butter and Banana Sandwich with Just a Touch of Honey (pg. 344).	**Lunch** Prepare Grilled Veggie Panini with Basil Pesto Sauce (pg. 274). Make one to share with your walking buddy.	**Dinner** Treat the whole family to Pecan-Crusted Chicken Fingers with Apricot Mustard Dipping Sauce (pg. 319) and Simple Chocolate Mousse with Graham Cracker Crumbles (pg. 326).	**Revitalizing Activity** Start the day with a 40-minute POWER WALK with a pal that includes 10 minutes of jogging and 10 minutes of stretching!

For Week 45 Grocery Shopping List and Shopping Day Prep Tips visit www.GorgeousLifestyleGuide.com

gorgeous lifestyle guide week 46 — stress-free, skin-savvy

Day	Breakfast	Lunch	Dinner	Revitalizing Activity
saturday	Just for fun, make the gang Grilled Peanut Butter and Banana Sandwiches with Just a Touch of Honey (pg. 344) for breakfast.	This is Shopping Day. While you run your errands, stop and treat yourself to your favorite garden fresh salad and whole grain roll.	Date night. Invite pals for an easy menu of Creamy Wild Mushroom Soup with Sherry and Fresh Thyme (pg. 357), Grilled Halibut with Salsa Verde (pg. 64), and Key Lime Pound Cake (pg. 360).	Start the day with a 40-minute POWER WALK that includes 15 minutes of jogging! Today is Shopping Day!! Hit the farmer's market.
sunday	Gather the group for Bacon and Asparagus Quiche (pg. 342) for brunch.	**Afternoon** Have a simple lunch of leftover Creamy Wild Mushroom Soup from last night's supper.	Serve Hearty Beef Stew (pg. 348) and Pretty in Peach (pg. 363) for dessert to start the week off just fine.	Me time! Apply a HONEY MASK (pg. 79). Don't forget that 30-minute POWER WALK. After dinner, relax with a warm and soothing cup of tea and a hot, lavender-scented bath.
monday	Juiced-Up Fruit-and-Herb Drinks (pg. 57) (like Blueberry-Basil) make an easy and nourishing breakfast.	Brown bag it! Choose whole grain bread and fresh veggies to build your favorite Mediterranean Tuna Melt (pg. 62) and take it on the road, alongside a slice of leftover Key Lime Pound Cake.	Ginger-Marinated Tuna with Dill Lime Butter (pg. 347) makes for a simple midweek super.	Me time! Luxuriate with an OATMEAL PEEL (pg. 79). Visit the cosmetic counter for a makeover. Work off that frustration by spending 20 to 30 minutes in your garden.
tuesday	Dash off to work after enjoying Breakfast Burritos with Red Pepper Salsa (pg. 60).	Prepare a huge pot of Fresh Minestrone Soup with Chickpeas (pg. 356). Have a bowl for lunch and reserve leftovers for later in the week.	Chicken Thighs with Sage and Caramelized Peaches (pg. 65) are totally comforting for a midweek supper.	Rest your muscles. Spend 20 minutes stretching. De-stress by preparing a batch of Maple Cake Doughnuts (pg. 36) to take to the office tomorrow morning. Eat one, share the rest!
wednesday	Fresh Fruit Salad with Citrus Basil Dressing (pg. 58) makes a FUN and fruity starter!	Invite your GORGEOUS gal pals for Spinach Salad with Warm Chipotle Chili Vinaigrette Topped with Chicken Strips and Crisp Sweet Potato (pg. 66). It's to die for.	Butternut Squash and Swiss Chard Roll-Ups with Sun-Dried Tomato Basil Sauce (pg. 350) are easily prepared and soothing to eat.	Take a 30-minute POWER WALK to start your day. Add 15 minutes of weight lifting. Schedule a Swedish massage. Buy an audiobook and put it in your car for rush-hour listening.
thursday	You will just love Ham and Cheese Scramble (pg. 341) for breakfast.	Brown bag it! Take along a childhood favorite of Open-Faced Chicken Tacos (pg. 68).	Hunter's-Style Stew with Yellow Rice (pg. 352) can be prepared in your slow cooker and served to a hungry crowd.	Remember to hold in your stomach on your 30-minute POWER WALK. Afterward, enjoy a cup of soothing tea.
friday	There's always time for Fruit and Yogurt Breakfast Parfaits with Granola Crunch (pg. 59).	Enjoy Spicy Flank Steak Sandwich with Roasted Pepper Blue Cheese Sauce (pg. 353) shared with the other moms at the park.	Treat the whole family to Really Good Turkey Burgers with Cheddar Cheese and Horseradish Sauce (pg. 354) and The Real Deal Fries with Ketchup of Course (pg. 358).	Start the day with a 40-minute POWER WALK with a pal that includes 10 minutes of jogging and 10 minutes of stretching!

For Week 46 Grocery Shopping List and Shopping Day Prep Tips visit www.GorgeousLifestyleGuide.com

gorgeous lifestyle guide week 47 — stress-free, sexy glam

	Breakfast	Lunch	Dinner	Revitalizing Activity
saturday	Just for fun, make the gang Grilled Peanut Butter and Banana Sandwiches with Just a Touch of Honey (pg. 344) for breakfast.	This is Shopping Day. While you run your errands, stop and treat yourself to your favorite garden fresh salad and whole grain roll.	Date night. Invite pals for an easy menu of Creamy Wild Mushroom Soup with Sherry and Fresh Thyme (pg. 357), Saltimbocca (pg. 386), and Key Lime Pound Cake (pg. 360).	Start the day with a 40-minute POWER WALK that includes 15 minutes of jogging! Today is Shopping Day! Hit the farmer's market.
sunday	Enjoy the morning after by serving Very Sexy Scrambled Eggs with Caviar and Peppered Strawberries (pg. 376) for brunch.	**Afternoon** Have a simple lunch of leftover Creamy Wild Mushroom Soup from last night's supper.	Serve Chicken Wings with Mole Sauce (pg. 387) and Pretty in Peach (pg. 363) dessert to start the week off just fine.	Take a 30-minute POWER WALK to start your day. After supper, grab his hand for an evening stroll around the neighborhood. Then enjoy a lavender-scented bath.
monday	Fruit 'N Soy Milk Drinks (pg. 307) make an easy and nourishing breakfast.	Brown bag it! Choose whole grain bread and fresh veggies to build your favorite deli sandwich and take it on the road, alongside a slice of Saturday's Key Lime Pound Cake.	Ginger-Marinated Tuna with Lime Butter (pg. 347) makes for a simple midweek supper.	Work off that frustration by spending 20 to 30 minutes in your garden. Grab your partner and enter the "Love Gym." Work on your Pilates moves.
tuesday	Dash off to work with an Open-Faced BLT Sandwich (pg. 340).	Prepare a huge pot of Fresh Veggie Minestrone Soup with Chickpeas (pg. 356). Have a bowl for lunch and reserve leftovers for later in the week.	Grilled Pork Chops with Cherry Ginger Chutney (pg. 389) make for a yummy midweek supper.	Rest your muscles. Spend 20 minutes stretching. De-stress by preparing a batch of Maple Cake Doughnuts (pg. 361) to take to the office tomorrow morning. Eat one, share the rest!
wednesday	Whip up a batch of Cinnamon Chocolate-Chip Pancakes with Whipped Cream and Warm Maple Syrup (pg. 377).	Invite your GORGEOUS gal pals for Grilled Lobster Tails with Parsley Butter Served over Creamy Hash (pg. 380). It's to die for.	Duck Breasts with Pinot Noir Red Grape Sauce (pg. 388) is easily prepared and soothing to eat.	Take a 30-minute POWER WALK to start your day. Add 15 minutes of weight lifting. Schedule a Swedish massage. Buy an audiobook and put it in your car for rush-hour listening.
thursday	You will just love Ham and Cheese Scramble (pg. 341) for breakfast.	Brown bag it! Take along a container of Peel and Eat Shrimp with Buffalo-Style Sauce (pg. 391). Share with your deskmate. Bring extra napkins!	Hunter's Style Stew with Yellow Rice (pg. 352) can be prepared in your slow cooker and served to a hungry crowd.	Remember to hold in your stomach on your 30-minute POWER WALK. Afterward, enjoy a cup of soothing tea.
friday	There's always time for Baked Raspberry-Stuffed French Toast with Pecans and Maple Syrup (pg. 379).	Enjoy Spicy Flank Steak Sandwich with Roasted Pepper Blue Cheese Sauce (pg. 353) shared with the other moms at the park.	Treat the whole family to Really Good Turkey Burgers with Cheddar Cheese and Horseradish Sauce (pg. 354) and The Real Deal French Fries with Ketchup of Course (pg. 358).	Start the day with a 40-minute POWER WALK with a pal that includes 10 minutes of jogging and 10 minutes of stretching!

For Week 47 Grocery Shopping List and Shopping Day Prep Tips visit www.GorgeousLifestyleGuide.com

gorgeous lifestyle guide week 48 — sleepy time, eye-catching

Day	Breakfast	Lunch	Dinner	Revitalizing Activity
saturday	Bake up a batch of Orange Breakfast Muffins (pg. 305). Save extras for later in the week.	This is Shopping Day. While you are running errands, stop and treat yourself to your favorite fresh garden salad with whole grain bread on the side.	Date night! Invite pals for Grilled New York Strip Steaks with Garlic Herb Oil (pg. 125), Broccoli Mash (pg. 321) and Chocolate Ricotta-Filled Crepes (pg. 136).	Start the day with a 40-minute POWER WALK that includes 15 minutes of jogging! Today is Shopping Day! Hit the farmer's market.
sunday	Gather the group for Scrambled Eggs with Red Grape and Avocado Salsa (pg. 118).	**Afternoon** Have a simple lunch of Grilled Ratatouille Salad with Tomato Basil Vinaigrette (pg. 323). Save extra veggies for later in the week. They will make a great soup!	Serve a comfort meal of Chicken Papricash Over Egg Noodles (pg. 122) and Stuffed Zucchini, Yellow Squash, and Eggplant (pg. 322).	After dinner relax with a warm and soothing cup of decaffeinated tea and a hot, lavender-scented bath.
monday	Enjoy rich Fruit 'N Soy Milk Drinks (pg. 307) as a start to your workweek.	Brown bag it! Choose whole grain bread to go with your Roasted Veggie-Stuffed Tomatoes (pg. 131).	Stir Fry Chicken and Broccoli with Chopped Peanuts (pg. 123) makes for a light and easy supper. Add leftover grilled veggies from earlier in the week.	Lighten dark circles and smooth puffiness with raw ingredients like potatoes and egg whites. Get to bed early with a lavender sachet tucked under your pillow.
tuesday	Dash off to work with a warmed Orange Breakfast Muffin.	Prepare Open-Faced Eggplant, Tomato, and Cheddar Grilled Cheese (pg. 309). Make extras for your workout buddy.	Gather the family for a supper of Pork Medallions with Asparagus and Sweet Potatoes (pg. 127) and Sautéed Cauliflower and Spinach Fettuccini Casserole (pg. 320).	Rest your muscles and spend 20 minutes stretching out your tired parts, followed by a luxurious, scented bath.
wednesday	Enjoy a treat of Breakfast Tomatoes with Smoked Salmon (pg. 308).	Invite your GORGEOUS gal pals to share Italian-Style Strata (pg. 126) and Orange-Glazed Yogurt Cake (pg. 134) for lunch.	Simply prepared Broiled Tilapia Fillets with Arugula Aioli Sauce (pg. 315) comes together so quickly, you will have time to bake a batch of Butterscotch Blondies (pg. 325) for dessert.	See clearly. Identify something beautiful in your environment and appreciate the sight. Pull out the digital camera and create a picture to frame for your desk.
thursday	Melon Bowls with Strawberry Ginger Sauce (pg. 120) are perfect for a fast starter.	Brown bag it! Take along a fresh garden salad topped with your favorite lean poultry. Add a Butterscotch Blondie to the bag and another one for a pal.	Whip up linguini with Roasted Vegetable Burritos with Chipotle Chili Sauce (pg. 121) for a light meal on Thursday night. Serve leftover Orange-Glazed Yogurt Cake for dessert.	Walk this way—for 30 minutes. Place a blank piece of paper on your bedside table and quote your sleepy time mantra as you dose off.
friday	Poached Eggs in Spicy Tomato Sauce (pg. 119) are a perfect way to start your day.	Prepare Grilled Veggie Panini with Basil Pesto Sauce (pg. 274). Make one to share with your walking buddy.	Treat the whole family to Pecan-Crusted Chicken Fingers with Apricot Mustard Dipping Sauce (pg. 319) and Simple Chocolate Mousse with Graham Cracker Crumbles (pg. 326).	Start the day with a 40-minute POWER WALK with a pal that includes 10 minutes of jogging and 10 minutes of stretching!

For Week 48 Grocery Shopping List and Shopping Day Prep Tips visit www.GorgeousLifestyleGuide.com

gorgeous lifestyle guide week 49 — stress-free, smile pretty

	Breakfast	Lunch	Dinner	Revitalizing Activity
saturday	Just for fun, make the gang Grilled Peanut Butter and Banana Sandwiches with Just a Touch of Honey (pg. 344) for breakfast.	This is Shopping Day. While you run your errands, stop and treat yourself to your favorite garden fresh salad and whole grain roll.	Date night! Invite pals for Creamy Wild Mushroom Soup with Sherry and Fresh Thyme (pg. 357), Lemon Veal with Sautéed Spinach, Pine Nuts and Goat Cheese (pg. 158), and Key Lime Pound Cake. (pg. 360)	Start the day with a 40-minute POWER WALK that includes 15 minutes of jogging! Today is Shopping Day! Hit the farmer's market.
sunday	Gather the group for Spicy Roasted Veggie and Shrimp Salsa with Fried Egg and Warm Cheese Sauce (pg. 146) for brunch.	**Afternoon** Have a simple lunch of leftover Creamy Wild Mushroom Soup with Sherry and Fresh Thyme from last night's supper.	Serve Sunday night comfort supper that includes Seared Jumbo Scallops with Herbed Butter Sauce (pg. 152) and Mango-Walnut Crumble (pg. 165).	After dinner, relax with a warm and soothing cup of tea and a hot, lavender-scented bath.
monday	Fruit 'N Soy Milk Drinks (pg. 307) make an easy and nourishing breakfast.	Brown bag it! Choose whole grain bread and fresh veggies to build your favorite deli sandwich and take it on the road, alongside a slice of Saturday's Key Lime Pound Cake.	Ginger-Marinated Tuna with Dill Lime Butter (pg. 347) makes for a simple midweek supper.	Work off that frustration by spending 20 to 30 minutes in your garden. Make an appointment with the cosmetic counter to check out the new seasonal lipstick colors.
tuesday	Dash off to work with Coconut Tropical Smoothies (pg. 148).	Prepare a huge pot of Fresh Veggie Minestrone Soup with Chickpeas (pg. 356). Have a bowl for lunch and reserve leftovers for later in the week.	Double-Cheese and Sausage Calzone with Marinara Dipping Sauce (pg. 153) makes for a fun midweek supper.	Rest your muscles. Spend 20 minutes stretching. De-stress by preparing a batch of Maple Cake Doughnuts (pg. 361) to take to the office tomorrow morning. Remember—eat one, share the rest!
wednesday	Prepare Breakfast Panini with Chicken Sausage (pg. 178) and share half with your special someone.	Invite your GORGEOUS gal pals for Buffalo Chicken Cobb Salad with Buttermilk Dressing (pg. 150) and Emergency Key Lime Pie (pg. 166) for dessert. Yum!	Butternut Squash and Swiss Chard Roll-Ups with Sun-Dried Tomato Basil Sauce (pg. 350) are easily prepared and soothing to eat.	Take a 30-minute POWER WALK to start your day. Add 15 minutes of weight lifting. Schedule a Swedish massage. Buy an audiobook and put it in your car for rush-hour listening.
thursday	You will just love Ham and Cheese Scramble (pg. 341) for breakfast.	Brown bag it! Take along a sandwich reminiscent of a childhood favorite. Turkey with Caramelized Onion and Smoked Gouda Panini (pg. 151) is perfect.	Hunter's-Style Stew with Yellow Rice (pg. 352) can be prepared in your slow cooker and served to a hungry crowd.	Smile at everyone you meet today and see how many smile back at you. Smile while cars pass you on your 30-minute POWER WALK.
friday	There's always time for Fruit 'N Soy Milk Drinks (pg. 307).	Enjoy Spicy Flank Steak Sandwich with Roasted Pepper Blue Cheese Sauce (pg. 353) shared with the other moms at the park.	Treat the whole family to Really Good Turkey Burgers with Cheddar Cheese and Horseradish Sauce (pg. 354) and The Real Deal Fries with Ketchup of Course (pg. 358).	Start the day with a 40-minute POWER WALK with a pal that includes 10 minutes of jogging and 10 minutes of stretching!

For Week 49 Grocery Shopping List and Shopping Day Prep Tips visit www.GorgeousLifestyleGuide.com

gorgeous lifestyle guide week 50 — sexy glam, smile pretty

	Breakfast	Lunch	Dinner	Revitalizing Activity
saturday	Start off your sexy weekend with Cinnamon Chocolate-Chip Pancakes with Whipped Cream and Warm Maple Syrup (pg. 377).	This is Shopping Day. While you are running your errands, stop and enjoy your favorite deli sandwich filled with fresh veggies, lean meat, and reduced-fat cheese.	Couples supper club menu: Baked Oysters with Pancetta Topping (pg. 392), Seared Jumbo Scallops with Herbed Butter Sauce (pg. 152), and Basil-Roasted Strawberry Cheesecake with Rich Chocolate Crust (pg. 397).	Start the day with a 40-minute POWER WALK that includes 15 minutes of jogging! Today is Shopping Day! Hit the farmer's market and the specialty wine shop.
sunday	Enjoy a Luxurious Brunch of Very Sexy Scrambled Eggs with Caviar and Peppered Strawberries (pg. 376). Yum!	**Afternoon** Plan a workout for two—prepare a batch of Orgasmic Braised Ribs with Chili and Chocolate (pg. 381).	Serve Orgasmic Braised Ribs with Arugula Salad with Walnut-Crusted Goat Cheese (pg. 390) and a small sliver of last night's cheesecake.	After your 30-minute POWER WALK, curl up with a good book and a cup of non-teeth staining herbal tea and a hot, revitalizing bath.
monday	Perfect for a quick pick-me-up, choose Oatmeal with Caramelized Fruit Topping (pg. 149).	Brown bag it! Build a take-along Shrimp Salad with Mango and Cucumber (pg. 159).	Monday . . . Monday's dinner is purrrfect when it stars Crisp Roasted Chicken with Penne Pasta (pg. 154).	Grab your partner and enter the "Love Gym." Work on your Pilates moves. Smile at everyone you meet today and see how many smile back at you.
tuesday	Whip up Coconut Tropical Smoothies (pg. 148).	Lighten up with Avocado and Grapefruit Salad (pg. 281) for a quick lunch.	Saltimbocca (pg. 386) is a dish that comes together quickly in order to "spice up" that weekday night meal.	Rest your muscles and spend 20 minutes stretching. De-stress further by preparing a batch of Peanut Butter Chocolate Bars (pg. 394) to take to the office tomorrow morning.
wednesday	Fresh Papaya and Grapefruit with Yogurt and Mint (pg. 147) is a special start to your day.	Invite your GORGEOUS gal pals for a luscious lunch of Turkey with Caramelized Onions and Smoked Gouda Panini (pg. 151).	Reconnect as you graze on Chicken with Bel Paese, Prosciutto, and Capers with White Wine Pan Sauce (pg. 156).	Take a 30-minute POWER WALK to start your day. Add 15 minutes of weight lifting. After supper, grab his hand for an evening stroll around the neighborhood.
thursday	Start the day off with a hearty breakfast of Egg, Sausage, and Spinach Skillets (pg. 378). (You might have to call in late for work!)	Brown bag it! Take along a fresh veggie salad topped with chicken that you couldn't finish last evening.	Take advantage of your slow cooker when you prepare Chicken Wings with Mole Sauce (pg. 387) and eat at your leisure.	Walk this way—for 30 minutes followed by a cup of soothing tea and perhaps a neck and shoulder massage from your honey.
friday	Baked Raspberry-Stuffed French Toast with Pecans and Maple Drizzle (pg. 379) is an excellent way to kick off your Friday.	Enjoy a light lunch of Olive, Onion, and Roasted Pepper Bruschetta (pg. 393).	Dinner for two stars Grilled Lobster Tails with Parsley Butter Served over Creamy Hash (pg. 380). Does it get any better than this?	Start the day with a 40-minute POWER WALK with a your significant other that includes 10 minutes of jogging and 10 minutes of stretching!

For Week 50 Grocery Shopping List and Shopping Day Prep Tips visit www.GorgeousLifestyleGuide.com

gorgeous lifestyle guide week 51 — sexy glam, good hair

Day	Breakfast	Lunch	Dinner	Revitalizing Activity
saturday	Start off your sexy weekend with Cinnamon Chocolate-Chip Pancakes with Whipped Cream and Warm Maple Syrup (pg. 377).	This is Shopping Day. While you are running your errands, stop and enjoy your favorite deli sandwich filled with fresh veggies, lean meat, and reduced-fat cheese.	Couples supper club menu: Baked Oysters with Pancetta Topping (pg. 392), Paella with Chorizo, Asparagus, and Shellfish (pg. 98), and Basil-Roasted Strawberry Cheesecake with Rich Chocolate Crust (pg. 397).	Start the day with a 40-minute POWER WALK that includes 15 minutes of jogging! Today is Shopping Day! Hit the farmer's market and the specialty wine shop.
sunday	Enjoy a luxurious brunch of Very Sexy Scrambled Eggs with Caviar and Peppered Strawberries (pg. 376). Yum!	**Afternoon** Enjoy a light lunch of Arugula Salad with Walnut-Crusted Goat Cheese (pg. 390).	Sunday night supper for two is divine when it includes Grilled Pork Chops with Cherry Ginger Chutney (pg. 389).	After dinner relax with a warm and soothing cup of tea and a hot, revitalizing bath. Later that night treat your hair to a FRUIT MASK (pg. 109).
monday	For a quick pick-me-up choose Fruit 'N Soy Milk Drinks (pg. 307) for breakfast.	Brown bag it! Take along a thermos of Creamy Cauliflower Soup with Arugula and Crispy Bacon Garnish (pg. 101).	Monday . . . Monday's dinner is purrrfect when it stars a Grilled Skirt Steak and Veggie Open-Faced Sandwich (pg. 95).	Grab your partner and enter the "Love Gym." Work on your Pilates moves. Me time! Luxuriate with an OLIVE OIL MASK (pg. 110) for your hair. Buy a magazine and try out a new hairdo.
tuesday	Whip up a batch of Raspberry Oatmeal Muffins with Macadamia Nut Butter (pg. 89) and save extras for snacks during the week.	Lighten up with Avocado and Grapefruit Salad (pg. 281) for a quick lunch.	Lamb Chops with Coconut Skillet Sauce (pg. 92) is a dish that comes together quickly in order to "spice up" that weekday night meal.	Rest your muscles and spend 20 minutes stretching. De-stress further by preparing a batch of Peanut Butter Chocolate Bars (pg. 394) to take to the office tomorrow morning.
wednesday	Egg White Omelets with Bell Peppers and Turkey Sausage (pg. 88) are filled with lean protein.	Invite your GORGEOUS gal pals for a luscious lunch of Lobster in an Orange Curry Butter Sauce (pg. 93) with Sautéed Bananas with Sweet Mascarpone and Walnut Crunch (pg. 107).	Reconnect as you graze over Peel-and-Eat Jumbo Shrimp with Buffalo-Style Sauce (pg. 391).	Take a 30-minute POWER WALK to start your day. Add 15 minutes of weight lifting. After supper, grab his hand for an evening stroll around the neighborhood.
thursday	Start the day off with a hearty breakfast of Eggs, Sausage, and Spinach Skillets (pg. 378). (You might have to call in late for work!)	Brown bag it! Take along spicy shrimp salad using up the shrimp that you couldn't finish last evening.	Take advantage of your slow cooker when you prepare Chicken Wings with Mole Sauce (pg. 387) and eat at your leisure.	Walk this way—for 30 minutes followed by a cup of soothing tea and perhaps a neck and shoulder massage from your honey.
friday	Baked Raspberry-Stuffed French Toast with Pecans and Maple Drizzle (pg. 379) is an excellent way to start the weekend.	Enjoy a light lunch of Olive, Onion, and Roasted Pepper Bruschetta (pg. 393).	Dinner stars Rosemary Roasted Chicken Breasts with Smoky Almond Sauce (pg. 91), Toasted Corn with Sautéed Spinach & Cherry Tomatoes (pg. 103), and Baked Pears in Brandy Sauce (pg. 104).	Start the day with a 40-minute POWER WALK with your significant other that includes 10 minutes of jogging and 10 minutes of stretching!

For Week 51 Grocery Shopping List and Shopping Day Prep Tips visit www.GorgeousLifestyleGuide.com

gorgeous lifestyle guide week 52 — sexy glam, eye-catching

Day	Breakfast	Lunch	Dinner	Revitalizing Activity
saturday	Start off your sexy weekend with Cinnamon Chocolate-Chip Pancakes with Whipped Cream and Warm Maple Syrup (pg. 377).	This is Shopping Day. While you are running your errands, stop and enjoy your favorite deli sandwich filled with fresh veggies, lean meat, and reduced-fat cheese.	Couples supper club menu: Baked Oysters with Pancetta Topping (pg. 392), Pork Medallions with Asparagus and Sweet Potatoes (pg. 127), and Basil-Roasted Strawberry Cheesecake (pg. 397).	Start the day with a 40-minute POWER WALK that includes 15 minutes of jogging! Today is Shopping Day! Hit the farmer's market and the specialty wine shop.
sunday	Enjoy a Luxurious Brunch of Very Sexy Scrambled Eggs with Caviar and Peppered Strawberries (pg. 376). Yum!	**Afternoon:** Prepare a fresh veggie salad for two and top with leftovers from last evening's party. Diced pork and asparagus are great salad toppers.	Sexy Saltimbocca (pg. 386) comes together quickly and has just enough plate appeal to make you feel like a gourmet chef. Serve with a side of Sweet Balsamic Onions (pg. 129).	After dinner relax with a soothing cup of tea and a hot, revitalizing bath. Lighten dark circles and smooth puffiness with raw ingredients like potatoes and egg whites.
monday	Perfect for a quick pick-me-up, choose Melon Bowls with Strawberry Ginger Sauce (pg. 120) for breakfast.	Brown bag it! Build a take-along a lunch of Roasted Veggie-Stuffed Tomatoes (pg. 131).	Monday . . . Monday's dinner is purrrfect when it stars Chicken Paprikash Served over Egg Noodles (pg. 122).	Work on your Pilates moves. Make frozen eye pads. Relax with eyes closed for 15 minutes. Did your remember your 30-minute POWER WALK?
tuesday	Scrambled Eggs with Red Grape and Avocado Salsa (pg. 118) are a yummy start to your day.	Lighten up with Avocado and Grapefruit Salad (pg. 281)for a quick lunch.	Mushroom and Spinach-Filled Frittata (pg. 128) is a dish that comes together quickly in order to "spice up" that weeknight meal.	Rest your muscles and spend 20 minutes stretching. De-stress further by preparing a batch of Peanut Butter Chocolate Bars (pg. 394) to take to the office tomorrow morning.
wednesday	Grab a Granola Bar from that stash in your freezer.	Invite your GORGEOUS gal pals for a luscious lunch of Roasted Vegetable Burritos with Chipotle Chili Sauce (pg. 121) and Pear and Strawberry Crisp (pg. 133) to cool down their spicy palates.	Reconnect with your family as you graze over Peel-and-Eat Jumbo Shrimp with Buffalo-Style Sauce (pg. 391).	Take a 30-minute POWER WALK to start your day. Add 15 minutes of weight lifting. After supper, grab his hand for an evening stroll around the neighborhood.
thursday	Start the day off with a hearty breakfast of Eggs, Sausage, and Spinach Skillets (pg. 378). (You might have to call in late for work!)	Brown bag it! Take along Arugula Salad with Walnut Crusted Goat Cheese (pg. 390) for a fun lunch.	Take advantage of your veggie side when you prepare Spaghetti Squash Carbonara and Olive, Onion, and Roasted Pepper Bruschetta (pg. 393) for a nibbly supper.	Walk this way—for 30 minutes followed by a cup of soothing tea and perhaps a neck and shoulder massage from your honey.
friday	Baked Raspberry-Stuffed French Toast with Pecans and Maple Drizzle (pg. 379) gets Friday off to an excellent start.	Enjoy a light lunch of Italian-Style Strata (pg. 126). Save extras for the other carpool moms.	Dinner for two stars Grilled New York Strip Steaks with Garlic Herb Oil (pg. 125). Does it get any better than this?	Start the day with a 40-minute POWER WALK with your significant other that includes 10 minutes of jogging and 10 minutes of stretching!

For Week 52 Grocery Shopping List and Shopping Day Prep Tips visit www.GorgeousLifestyleGuide.com

NUTRITIONAL APPENDIX

Start Your Day

Apple Pie for Breakfast
Tummies—page 267
Per serving: 376 calories;
14 grams fat; 14 grams protein;
50 grams carbohydrates;
7 grams fiber

Bacon and Asparagus Quiche
Stress—page 342
Per serving: 414 calories;
32 grams fat; 15 grams protein;
17 grams carbohydrates;
0 grams fiber

Baked Raspberry-Stuffed French Toast with Pecans and Maple Drizzle
Sexy—page 379
Per serving: 340 calories;
8 grams fat; 10 grams protein;
59 grams carbohydrates;
2 grams fiber

Banana Bread Snack Cake
Hands—page 237
Per serving: 186 calories;
6 grams fat; 4 grams protein;
31 grams carbohydrates;
3 grams fiber

Blueberry Buttermilk Coffee Cake Topped with Granola
Hands— page 236
Per serving: 159 calories;
6 grams fat; 4 grams protein;
25 grams carbohydrates;
3 grams fiber

Breakfast Burritos with Red Pepper Salsa
Skin—page 60
Per serving: 536 calories;
23 grams fat; 26 grams protein;
55 grams carbohydrates;
6 grams fiber

Breakfast Panini with Chicken Sausage
Bones—page 178
Per serving: 541 calories;
41 grams fat; 22 grams protein;
21 grams carbohydrates;
3 grams fiber

Breakfast Tacos
Tummies—page 268
Per serving: 130 calories;
3 grams fat; 10 grams protein;
16 grams carbohydrates;
2 grams fiber

Breakfast Tomatoes with Smoked Salmon
Sleep—page 308
Per serving: 89 calories;
3 grams fat; 8 grams protein;
9 grams carbohydrates;
2 grams fiber

Broiled Grapefruit with Honey Mascarpone Cream
Eyes—page 117
Per serving: 248 calories;
14 grams fat; 3 grams protein;
29 grams carbohydrates;
2 grams fiber

Brunch Frittata with Red Potatoes and Kale
Feet—page 208
Per serving: 563 calories;
37 grams fat; 31 grams protein;
25 grams carbohydrates;
2 grams fiber

Cinnamon Chocolate-Chip Pancakes with Whipped Cream and Warm Maple Syrup
Sexy—page 377
Per serving: 517 calories;
21 grams fat; 14 grams protein;
71 grams carbohydrates;
2 grams fiber

Creamy French-Style Eggs Garnished with Chopped Tomatoes and Chives
Hair—page 87
Per serving: 291 calories;
16 grams fat; 15 grams protein;
21 grams carbohydrates;
3 grams fiber

Coconut Tropical Smoothies
Smile—page 148
Per serving: 306 calories;
4 grams fat; 7 grams protein;
64 grams carbohydrates;
3 grams fiber

Double-Berry Whole Wheat Pancakes
Feet—page 209
Per serving: 389 calories;
15 grams fat; 13 grams protein;
53 grams carbohydrates;
7 grams fiber

Egg in a Frame with Basil Tomatoes
Tummies—page 270
Per serving: 256 calories;
13 grams fat; 11 grams protein;
26 grams carbohydrates;
5 grams fiber

Egg White Omelets with Bell Peppers and Turkey Sausage
Hair—page 88
Per serving: 358 calories;
19 grams fat; 38 grams protein;
7 grams carbohydrates;
1 gram fiber

Eggs Benedict with Swiss Chard and Whole Grain English Muffins
Bones—page 175
Per serving: 423 calories;
35 grams fat; 12 grams protein;
17 grams carbohydrates;
3 grams fiber

Egg, Sausage, and Spinach Skillets
Sexy—page 378
Per serving: 696 calories;
52 grams fat; 27 grams protein;
8 grams carbohydrates;
2 grams fiber

Fresh Fruit Salad with Citrus Basil Dressing
Skin—page 58
Per serving: 135 calories;
1 gram fat; 2 grams protein;
34 grams carbohydrates;
4 grams fiber

Fresh Papaya and Grapefruit with Yogurt and Mint
Smile—page 147
Per serving: 162 calories;
2 grams fat; 7 grams protein;
32 grams carbohydrates;
3 grams fiber

Fruit 'N Soy Milk Drinks
Sleep—page 307
Per serving: 151 calories;
3 grams fat; 4 grams protein;
30 grams carbohydrates;
5 grams fiber

Fruit and Yogurt Breakfast Parfaits with Granola Crunch
Skin—page 59
Per serving: 308 calories;
10 grams fat; 10 grams protein;
48 grams carbohydrates;
8 grams fiber

Granola Power Bars
Hands—page 239
Per serving: 274 calories;
17 grams fat; 4 grams protein;
28 grams carbohydrates;
3 grams fiber

Grilled Peanut Butter and Banana Sandwiches with Just a Touch of Honey
Stress—page 344
Per serving: 290 calories;
6 grams fat; 7 grams protein;
57 grams carbohydrates;
6 grams fiber

Ham and Cheese Scramble
Stress—page 341
Per serving: 397 calories;
29 grams fat; 29 grams protein;
3 grams carbohydrates;
0 grams fiber

Juiced-Up Fruit-and-Herb Breakfast Drinks
Skin—page 57
Per serving: 222 calories;
2 grams fat; 6 grams protein;
47 grams carbohydrates;
3 grams fiber

Melon Bowls with Strawberry Ginger Sauce
Eyes—page 120
Per serving: 73 calories;
1 gram fat; 1 gram protein;
18 grams carbohydrates;
2 grams fiber

Oatmeal with Caramelized Fruit Topping
Smile—page 149
Per serving: 454 calories;
16 grams fat; 9 grams protein;
73 grams carbohydrates;
9 grams fiber

Open-Faced BLT Breakfast Sandwich
Stress—page 340
Per serving: 324 calories;
17 grams fat; 23 grams protein;
22 grams carbohydrates;
5 grams fiber

Orange Breakfast Muffins
Sleep—page 305
Per serving: 92 calories;
3 grams fat; 1 gram protein;
17 grams carbohydrates;
0 grams fiber

Pecan Bananadana Muffins
Hair—page 90
Per serving: 165 calories;
5 grams fat; 3 grams protein;
28 grams carbohydrates;
1 gram fiber

Poached Eggs in Spicy Tomato Sauce
Eyes—page 119
Per serving: 351 calories;
23 grams fat; 20 grams protein;
16 grams carbohydrates;
3 grams fiber

Poached Eggs with Spinach and White Beans
Feet—page 210
Per serving: 410 calories;
19 grams fat; 27 grams protein;
34 grams carbohydrates;
9 grams fiber

Raspberry Oatmeal Muffins with Macadamia Nut Butter

Hair—page 89
Per serving: 247 calories;
15 grams fat; 5 grams protein;
26 grams carbohydrates;
3 grams fiber

Say "Ricotta Cheese" Pancakes with Very Berry Sauce

Tummies—page 269
Per serving: 623 calories;
19 grams fat; 16 grams protein;
125 grams carbohydrates;
11 grams fiber

Scrambled Eggs with Red Grape and Avocado Salsa

Eyes—page 118
Per serving: 270 calories;
18 grams fat; 13 grams protein;
15 grams carbohydrates;
2 grams fiber

Spicy Roasted Veggie and Shrimp Salsa with Fried Egg and Warm Cheese Sauce

Smile—page 146
Per serving: 419 calories;
22 grams fat; 36 grams protein;
19 grams carbohydrates;
4 grams fiber

Sweet Potato and Country Ham Frittata

Bones—page 176
Per serving: 321 calories;
20 grams fat; 19 grams protein;
16 grams carbohydrates;
2 grams fiber

Sweet Potato Pancakes with Warm Raspberry Syrup

Sleep—page 306
Per serving: 429 calories;
8 grams fat; 8 grams protein;
84 grams carbohydrates;
10 grams fiber

Very Sexy Scrambled Eggs with Caviar and Peppered Strawberries

Sexy—page 376
Per serving: 401 calories;
29 grams fat; 16 grams protein;
19 grams carbohydrates;
2 grams fiber

Walnut-Stuffed Baked Apples with Maple Syrup

Hands—page 238
Per serving: 152 calories;
6 grams fat; 3 grams protein;
22 grams carbohydrates;
2 grams fiber

Whole Grain Apple Muffins with Walnut Streusel

Bones—page 177
Per serving: 186 calories;
6 grams fat; 4 grams protein;
31 grams carbohydrates;
2 grams fiber

Whole Wheat Bran Muffins with Golden Raisins and Walnuts

Feet—page 207
Per serving: 228 calories;
10 grams fat; 6 grams protein;
32 grams carbohydrates;
2 grams fiber

•••••Main Plates•••••

Baked Chicken Breasts with Artichoke and Sun-Dried Tomato Sauce

Tummies—page 275
Per serving: 583 calories;
38 grams fat; 42 grams protein;
21 grams carbohydrates;
5 grams fiber

Baked Potatoes Stuffed with Swiss Chard and Black Beans

Feet—page 217
Per serving: 565 calories;
9 grams fat; 31 grams protein;

96 grams carbohydrates;
23 grams fiber

Baked Tilapia with Fresh Herbs
Bones—page 183
Per serving: 179 calories;
5 grams fat; 28 grams protein;
3 grams carbohydrates;
0 grams fiber

Better Veggie Chili
Feet—page 218
Per serving: 388 calories;
6 grams fat; 20 grams protein;
68 grams carbohydrates;
23 grams fiber

Broiled Tilapia Fillets with Arugula Aioli Sauce
Sleep—page 315
Per serving: 307 calories;
16 grams fat; 31 grams protein;
7 grams carbohydrates;
0 grams fiber

Buffalo Chicken Cobb Salad with Buttermilk Dressing
Smile—page 150
Per serving: 840 calories;
64 grams fat; 55 grams protein;
17 grams carbohydrates;
4 grams fiber

Butternut Squash and Swiss Chard Roll-Ups with Sun-Dried Tomato Basil Sauce
Stress—page 350
Per serving: 697 calories;
29 grams fat; 31 grams protein;
79 grams carbohydrates;
10 grams fiber

Butternut Squash Ravioli with Brown Butter, Sage, and Pine Nut Sauce
Sexy—page 382
Per serving: 798 calories;
54 grams fat; 26 grams protein;
56 grams carbohydrates;
6 grams fiber

Calf's Liver with Golden Onions
Hair—page 97
Per serving: 532 calories;
35 grams fat; 32 grams protein;
22 grams carbohydrates;
1 gram fiber

Charred Sirloin Steak with Mushroom and Red Wine Sauce
Feet—Page 213
Per serving: 430 calories;
31 grams fat; 24 grams protein;
11 grams carbohydrates;
2 grams fiber

Chicken and Rice Meatball Hoagies
Hands—page 242
Per serving: 542 calories;
21 grams fat; 30 grams protein;
64 grams carbohydrates;
10 grams fiber

Chicken Paprikash Served over Egg Noodles
Eyes—page 122
Per serving: 607 calories;
21 grams fat; 39 grams protein;
66 grams carbohydrates;
5 grams fiber

Chicken Portobello with Linguini in Butter Sauce
Tummies—page 276
Per serving: 461 calories;
27 grams fat; 33 grams protein;
14 grams carbohydrates;
4 grams fiber

Chicken Thighs with Sage and Caramelized Peaches
Skin—page 65
Per serving: 368 calories;
24 grams fat; 24 grams protein;
34 grams carbohydrates;
1 gram fiber

Chicken Wings with Mole Sauce
Sexy—page 387
Per serving: 547 calories;
36 grams fat; 31 grams protein;
29 grams carbohydrates;
7 grams fiber

Chicken with Bel Paese, Prosciutto, and Capers with White Wine Pan Sauce
Smile—page 156
Per serving: 374 calories;
25 grams fat; 21 grams protein;
7 grams carbohydrates;
0 gram fiber

Chilled Shrimp Salad with Red Grapes
Hands—page 241
Per serving: 180 calories;
4 grams fat; 24 grams protein;
12 grams carbohydrates;
1 gram fiber

Crab Cake Po' Boys
Sleep—page 316
Per serving: 555 calories;
31 grams fat; 22 grams protein;
49 grams carbohydrates;
4 grams fiber

Crispy Roasted Chicken with penne Pasta
Smile—page 154
Per serving: 623 calories;
31 grams fat; 36 grams protein;
47 grams carbohydrates;
4 grams fiber

Double-Cheese and Sausage Calzones with Marinara Dipping Sauce
Smile—page 153
Per serving: 733 calories;
44 grams fat; 29 grams protein;
55 grams carbohydrates;
4 gram fiber

Duck Breasts with Pinot Noir Red Grape Sauce
Sexy—page 388
Per serving: 293 calories;
13 grams fat; 13 grams protein;
29 grams carbohydrates;
2 grams fiber

Eggplant Boats Stuffed with Spicy Beef and Peas
Tummies—page 271
Per serving: 524 calories;
35 grams fat; 28 grams protein;
24 grams carbohydrates;
8 grams fiber

Five-Spice Beef Wraps with Orange Ginger Dipping Sauce
Tummies—page 280
Per serving: 424 calories;
22 grams fat; 28 grams protein;
25 grams carbohydrates;
4 grams fiber

Ginger-Marinated Tuna with Dill Lime Butter
Stress—page 347
Per serving: 526 calories;
26 grams fat; 54 grams protein;
18 grams carbohydrates;
1 gram fiber

Green Gazpacho Soup with Navy Bean Garnish
Bones—page 188
Per serving: 687 calories;
18 grams fat; 35 grams protein;
104 grams carbohydrates;
35 grams fiber

Grilled Coconut Curry Shrimp with Soba Noodles
Sleep—page 312
Per serving: 478 calories;
9 grams fat; 44 grams protein;
58 grams carbohydrates;
4 grams fiber

Grilled Halibut with Salsa Verde
Skin—page 64
Per serving: 789 calories;
58 grams fat; 52 grams protein;
17 grams carbohydrates;
7 grams fiber

Grilled Lamb Chops with White Bean Salad

Bones—page 182
Per serving: 688 calories;
23 grams fat; 53 grams protein;
69 grams carbohydrates;
27 grams fiber

Grilled Lobster Tails with Parsley Butter Served Over Creamy Hash

Sexy—page 380
Per serving: 760 calories;
25 grams fat; 53 grams protein;
83 grams carbohydrates;
15 grams fiber

Grilled New York Strip Steaks with Garlic Herb Oil

Eyes—page 125
Per serving: 754 calories;
67 grams fat; 33 grams protein;
4 grams carbohydrates;
1 gram fiber

Grilled Pork Chops with Cherry Ginger Chutney

Sexy—page 389
Per serving: 425 calories;
9 grams fat; 30 grams protein;
59 grams carbohydrates;
4 grams fiber

Grilled Skirt Steak and Veggie Open-Faced Sandwich

Hair—page 95
Per serving: 758 calories;
32 grams fat; 38 grams protein;
82 grams carbohydrates;
9 grams fiber

Grilled Swordfish Steaks with Spicy Papaya Relish and Herbed Compound Butter

Smile—page 157
Per serving: 501 calories;
33 grams fat; 35 grams protein;
19 grams carbohydrates;
1 gram fiber

Grilled Veggie Panini with Basil Pesto Sauce

Tummies—page 274
Per serving: 729 calories;
33 grams fat; 27 grams protein;
87 grams carbohydrates;
11 grams fiber

Hearty Beef Stew

Stress—page 348
Per serving: 581 calories;
33 grams fat; 33 grams protein;
27 grams carbohydrates;
4 grams fiber

Hoisin Beef and Veggies

Feet—page 212
Per serving: 664 calories;
29 grams fat; 29 grams protein;
72 grams carbohydrates;
8 grams fiber

Hunter's-Style Chicken Stew with Yellow Rice

Stress—page 352
Per serving: 725 calories;
40 grams fat; 43 grams protein;
42 grams carbohydrates;
4 grams fiber

Italian-Style Strata

Eyes—page 126
Per serving: 522 calories;
21 grams fat; 36 grams protein;
49 grams carbohydrates;
7 grams fiber

Jambalaya

Hands—page 245
Per serving: 871 calories;
53 grams fat; 58 grams protein;
37 grams carbohydrates;
3 grams fiber

Lamb Chops with Coconut Skillet Sauce

Hair—page 92
Per serving: 242 calories;
23 grams fat; 6 grams protein;
5 grams carbohydrates;
2 grams fiber

Lemon Veal with Sautéed Spinach, Pine Nuts, and Goat Cheese
Smile—page 158
Per serving: 419 calories;
29 grams fat; 30 grams protein;
11 grams carbohydrates;
2 grams fiber

Linguini with Mussels and Snow Peas
Sleep—page 318
Per serving: 400 calories;
12 grams fat; 25 grams protein;
41 grams carbohydrates;
3 grams fiber

Lobster in an Orange Curry Butter Sauce
Hair—page 93
Per serving: 529 calories;
25 grams fat; 47 grams protein;
27 grams carbohydrates;
2 grams fiber

Mediterranean Tuna Melt
Skin—page 62
Per serving: 675 calories;
13 grams fat; 46 grams protein;
94 grams carbohydrates;
25 grams fiber

Mojo Marinated Chicken Served over Black Beans
Feet—page 216
Per serving: 764 calories;
22 grams fat; 63 grams protein;
79 grams carbohydrates;
18 grams fiber

Mushroom and Spinach–Filled Frittata
Eyes—page 128
Per serving: 387 calories;
17 grams fat; 17 grams protein;
48 grams carbohydrates;
8 grams fiber

Mussels with Brussels in a White Wine Butter Sauce
Hair—page 94
Per serving: 246 calories;
12 grams fat; 15 grams protein;
11 grams carbohydrates;
1 gram fiber

Mustard-Garlic Roasted Chicken Served with Arugula and Artichoke Salad
Bones—page 179
Per serving: 572 calories;
43 grams fat; 36 grams protein;
11 grams carbohydrates;
4 grams fiber

Old-Fashioned Turkeyloaf with Hidden Mushrooms
Stress—page 345
Per serving: 451 calories;
21 grams fat; 42 grams protein;
21 grams carbohydrates;
3 grams fiber

Open-Faced Eggplant, Tomato, and Cheddar Grilled Cheese
Sleep—page 309
Per serving: 378 calories;
15 grams fat; 16 grams protein;
45 grams carbohydrates;
4 grams fiber

Open-Faced Chicken Tacos
Skin—page 68
Per serving: 644 calories;
32 grams fat; 38 grams protein;
50 grams carbohydrates;
5 grams fiber

Orgasmic Braised Ribs with Chili and Chocolate
Sexy—page 381
Per serving: 727 calories;
31 grams fat; 19 grams protein;
22 grams carbohydrates;
5 grams fiber

Overstuffed Beefsteak Tomatoes with Tortellini Salad
Feet—page 214
Per serving: 740 calories;
48 grams fat; 33 grams protein;
46 grams carbohydrates;
4 grams fiber

Paella with Chorizo, Asparagus, and Shellfish

Hair—page 98
Per serving: 675 calories;
26 grams fat; 54 grams protein;
53 grams carbohydrates;
5 grams fiber

Pancetta-Wrapped Turkey Medallions with Broccoli Rabe, Peppers, and Onions

Tummies—page 278
Per serving: 436 calories;
19 grams fat; 42 grams protein;
8 grams carbohydrates;
3 grams fiber

Parmesan Chicken Fingers with Green Cashew and Curry Dipping Sauce

Bones—page 181
Per serving: 561 calories;
31 grams fat; 23 grams protein;
54 grams carbohydrates;
4 grams fiber

Pecan-Crusted Chicken Fingers with Apricot Mustard Dipping Sauce

Sleep—page 319
Per serving: 521 calories;
32 grams fat; 42 grams protein;
17 grams carbohydrates;
3 grams fiber

Peppered Pork Pinwheels Stuffed with Swiss Chard, Sun-Dried Tomatoes, and Mozzarella

Bones—page 186
Per serving: 278 calories;
20 gram fat; 17 grams protein;
9 grams carbohydrates;
2 grams fiber

Poached Salmon in Infused Olive Oil with Horseradish Sauce

Hands—page 240
Per serving: 790 calories;
77 grams fat; 23 grams protein;
4 grams carbohydrates;
1 gram fiber

Pork Medallions with Asparagus and Sweet Potatoes

Eyes—page 127
Per serving: 440 calories;
29 grams fat; 23 grams protein;
18 grams carbohydrates;
3 grams fiber

Rack of Lamb with Spinach and Breadcrumb Topping

Sleep—page 311
Per serving: 605 calories;
46 grams fat; 32 grams protein;
15 grams carbohydrates;
1 gram fiber

Really Good Turkey Burgers with Cheddar Cheese and Horseradish Sauce

Stress—page 354
Per serving: 789 calories;
59 grams fat; 45 grams protein;
23 grams carbohydrates;
2 grams fiber

Roast Turkey Breast with Cornbread-Cranberry Dressing and Madeira Mushroom Gravy

Sleep—page 310
Per serving: 802 calories;
38 grams fat; 69 grams protein;
38 grams carbohydrates;
4 grams fiber

Roasted Beef Tenderloin Steaks Stuffed with Spinach and Gorgonzola with Béarnaise Sauce

Sexy—page 384
Per serving: 1018 calories;
91 grams fat; 40 grams protein;
6 grams carbohydrates;
1 gram fiber

Roasted Chipotle Salmon with Minted Couscous

Tummies—page 279
Per serving: 600 calories;
17 grams fat; 63 grams protein;
46 grams carbohydrates;
3 grams fiber

Roasted Pork Tenderloin with Swiss Chard

Hair—page 96
Per serving: 148 calories;
7 grams fat; 15 grams protein;
5 grams carbohydrates;
1 gram fiber

Roasted Tomato Basil Soup with Sea Bass Center

Skin—page 69
Per serving: 551 calories;
27 grams fat; 35 grams protein;
55 grams carbohydrates;
22 grams fiber

Roasted Veggie Burritos with Chipotle Chili Tomato Sauce

Eyes—page 121
Per serving: 418 calories;
22 grams fat; 17 grams protein;
47 grams carbohydrates;
11 grams fiber

Rosemary Polenta with Spinach, Red Beans, and Goat Cheese

Bones—page 184
Per serving: 855 calories;
38 grams fat; 37 grams protein;
95 grams carbohydrates;
27 grams fiber

Rosemary Roasted Chicken Breasts with Smoky Almond Sauce

Hair—page 91
Per serving: 319 calories;
25 grams fat; 15 grams protein;
11 grams carbohydrates;
2 grams fiber

Saltimbocca

Sexy—page 386
Per serving: 372 calories;
23 grams fat; 30 grams protein;
1 gram carbohydrates;
0 grams fiber

Sautéed Yellowtail Snapper with Braised Cabbage and Cheesy Mashed Potatoes

Hands—page 246
Per serving: 725 calories;
32 grams fat; 89 grams protein;
18 grams carbohydrates;
5 grams fiber

Sea Scallops with Blood Orange, Avocado, and Red Onion Salsa

Feet—page 215
Per serving: 304 calories;
19 gram fat; 21 grams protein;
14 grams carbohydrates;
3 grams fiber

Seared Jumbo Scallops with Herbed Butter Sauce

Smile—page 152
Per serving: 473 calories;
31 grams fat; 31 grams protein;
9 grams carbohydrates;
1 gram fiber

Shrimp Scampi with Angel Hair Pasta

Stress—page 346
Per serving: 451 calories;
17 grams fat; 34 grams protein;
39 grams carbohydrates;
3 grams fiber

Sliced Chicken Breast with Red Grape Sauce

Hands—page 247
Per serving: 496 calories;
24 grams fat; 39 grams protein;
29 grams carbohydrates;
1 gram fiber

Snapper Fillets Smothered with Caramelized Onions

Tummies—page 272
Per serving: 298 calories;
7 grams fat; 47 grams protein;
10 grams carbohydrates;
1 gram fiber

Snapper Veronique

Hands—page 244
Per serving: 398 calories;
14 grams fat; 49 grams protein;
13 grams carbohydrates;
1 gram fiber

Spaghetti Squash Carbonara
Eyes—page 124
Per serving: 576 calories;
33 grams fat; 34 grams protein;
41 grams carbohydrates;
0 grams fiber

Spicy Flank Steak Sandwich with Roasted Pepper Blue Cheese Sauce
Stress—page 353
Per serving: 692 calories;
49 grams fat; 40 grams protein;
25 grams carbohydrates;
3 grams fiber

Spicy Tuna Dinner Salad with Balsamic Dressing
Tummies—page 273
Per serving: 672 calories;
34 grams fat; 37 grams protein;
58 grams carbohydrates;
14 grams fiber

Spinach Salad with Warm Chipotle Chili Vinaigrette Topped with Chicken Strips and Crisp Sweet Potato
Skin—page 66
Per serving: 595 calories;
46 grams fat; 19 grams protein;
34 grams carbohydrates;
10 grams fiber

Stir-Fry Chicken and Broccoli with Chopped Peanuts
Eyes—page 123
Per serving: 545 calories;
30 grams fat; 29 grams protein;
39 grams carbohydrates;
4 grams fiber

Stuffed Chicken Breast with Mushrooms, Thyme and Fontina Cheese
Sleep—page 313
Per serving: 467 calories;
31 grams fat; 42 grams protein;
3 grams carbohydrates;
1 gram fiber

Sushi-Style Salmon Wraps
Skin—page 61
Per serving: 684 calories;
14 grams fat; 26 grams protein;
113 grams carbohydrates;
6 grams fiber

Sweet Potato Apple Salad with Honey, Ginger and Mustard Dressing
Skin—page 63
Per serving: 403 calories;
22 grams fat; 7 grams protein;
52 grams carbohydrates;
5 grams fiber

Turkey Meatloaf Burgers with Spicy Sweet Potato Sticks
Hands—page 243
Per serving: 595 calories;
23 grams fat; 38 grams protein;
58 grams carbohydrates;
5 grams fiber

Turkey with Caramelized Onion and Smoked Gouda Panini Sandwiches
Smile—page 151
Per serving: 661 calories;
38 grams fat; 37 grams protein;
45 grams carbohydrates;
7 grams fiber

Whole Wheat Spaghetti with Grilled Turkey, Broccoli Rabe, Red Peppers, and Peas
Bones—page 180
Per serving: 775 calories;
22 grams fat; 53 grams protein;
96 grams carbohydrates;
16 grams fiber

Wild Ivory King Salmon Fillets with Macadamia Nut Crust
Feet—page 211
Per serving: 626 calories;
41 grams fat; 59 grams protein;
5 grams carbohydrates;
3 grams fiber

•••• On the Side ••••

Artichoke and Asiago Crostini
Smile—page 162
Per serving: 298 calories;
16 grams fat; 9 grams protein;
31 grams carbohydrates;
3 grams fiber

Arugula Salad with Walnut-Crusted Goat Cheese
Sexy—page 390
Per serving: 1103 calories;
107 grams fat; 33 grams protein;
6 grams carbohydrates;
2 grams fiber

Asparagus Cheese Toasts
Feet—Page 219
Per serving: 361 calories;
20 grams fat; 20 grams protein;
26 grams carbohydrates;
4 grams fiber

Avocado and Grapefruit Salad
Tummies—page 281
Per serving: 157 calories;
11 grams fat; 2 grams protein;
15 grams carbohydrates;
3 grams fiber

Baked Oysters with Pancetta Topping
Sexy—page 392
Per serving: 210 calories;
11 grams fat; 11 grams protein;
16 grams carbohydrates;
1 gram fiber

Black Bean and Roasted Pepper Empanadas
Hands—page 250
Per serving: 198 calories;
5 grams fat; 12 grams protein;
28 grams carbohydrates;
6 grams fiber

Blue Cheese Dip with All Kinds of Dippers
Smile—page 161
Per serving: 108 calories;
10 grams fat; 4 grams protein;
1 gram carbohydrates;
0 grams fiber

Broccoli Mash
Sleep—page 321
Per serving: 232 calories;
17 grams fat; 5 grams protein;
16 grams carbohydrates;
2 grams fiber

Buttermilk Rolls with Sweet Onion Filling
Eyes—page 130
Per serving: 196 calories;
10 grams fat; 4 grams protein;
23 grams carbohydrates;
0 grams fiber

Butternut Squash Soup Flavored with Orange and Tarragon
Skin—page 70
Per serving: 168 calories;
5 grams fat; 7 grams protein;
17 grams carbohydrates;
2 grams fiber

Creamy Cauliflower Soup with Arugula and Crispy Bacon Garnish
Hair—page 101
Per serving: 435 calories;
25 grams fat; 18 grams protein;
28 grams carbohydrates;
4 grams fiber

Creamy Wild Mushroom Soup with Sherry and Fresh Thyme
Stress—page 357
Per serving: 526 calories;
27 grams fat; 13 grams protein;
63 grams carbohydrates;
11 grams fiber

Fresh Veggie Minestrone Soup with Chickpeas
Stress—page 356
Per serving: 148 calories;
3 grams fat; 7 grams protein;
25 grams carbohydrates;
8 grams fiber

Fried Plantains

Hair—page 100
Per serving: 211 calories;
14 grams fat; 1 gram protein;
24 grams carbohydrates;
2 grams fiber

Grilled Ratatouille Salad with Tomato Basil Vinaigrette

Sleep—page 323
Per serving: 365 calories;
28 grams fat; 6 grams protein;
28 grams carbohydrates;
10 grams fiber

Grilled Vegetable Skewers

Tummies—page 283
Per serving: 111 calories;
4 grams fat; 3 grams protein;
18 grams carbohydrates;
3 grams fiber

Lentils with Wild Rice and Mushrooms

Bones—page 190
Per serving: 315 calories;
7 grams fat; 21 grams protein;
43 grams carbohydrates;
13 grams fiber

Louisiana-Style Red Beans

Hair—page 102
Per serving: 581 calories;
20 grams fat; 27 grams protein;
74 grams carbohydrates;
15 grams fiber

Olive, Onion, and Roasted Pepper Bruschetta

Sexy—page 393
Per serving: 613 calories;
39 grams fat; 9 grams protein;
56 grams carbohydrates;
5 grams fiber

Pan-Sautéed Gnocchi with Sun-Dried Tomato and Sage

Stress—page 355
Per serving: 313 calories;
14 grams fat; 14 grams protein;
35 grams carbohydrates;
2 grams fiber

Peel-and-Eat Jumbo Shrimp with Buffalo-Style Sauce

Sexy—page 391
Per serving: 461 calories;
28 grams fat; 47 grams protein;
4 grams carbohydrates;
0 grams fiber

Peppery White Bean Salsa with Whole Wheat Pita Chips

Bones—page 189
Per serving: 520 calories;
17 grams fat; 22 grams protein;
72 grams carbohydrates;
11 grams fiber

Roasted Asparagus Salad with Arugula, Radishes, and Lemon Vinaigrette

Hands—page 248
Per serving: 217 calories;
22 grams fat; 2 grams protein;
6 grams carbohydrates;
2 grams fiber

Roasted Veggie Stacks with Mozzarella

Feet—page 220
Per serving: 129 calories;
6 grams fat; 8 grams protein;
15 grams carbohydrates;
5 grams fiber

Roasted Veggie-Stuffed Tomatoes

Eyes—page 131
Per serving: 205 calories;
12 grams fat; 10 grams protein;
19 grams carbohydrates;
5 grams fiber

Rosemary Roasted Carrot Sticks

Skin—page 72
Per serving: 115 calories;
7 grams fat; 1 gram protein;
13 grams carbohydrates;
4 grams fiber

Sautéed Cauliflower and Spinach Fettuccini Casserole

Sleep—page 320
Per serving: 588 calories;
32 grams fat; 29 grams protein;
49 grams carbohydrates;
6 grams fiber

Sautéed Peas with Mint

Tummies—page 282
Per serving: 118 calories;
7 grams fat; 4 grams protein;
11 grams carbohydrates;
4 grams fiber

Sautéed Red Cabbage with Drunken Raisins

Hands—page 251
Per serving: 86 calories;
0 grams fat; 2 grams protein;
18 grams carbohydrates;
3 grams fiber

Shrimp Salad with Mango and Cucumber

Smile—page 159
Per serving: 700 calories;
65 grams fat; 25 grams protein;
12 grams carbohydrates;
1 gram fiber

Slowly Stewed Collard Greens

Feet—page 222
Per serving: 198 calories;
12 grams fat; 13 grams protein;
10 grams carbohydrates;
3 grams fiber

Southwestern Chopped Salad with Toasted Peppers and Corn

Tummies—page 284
Per serving: 755 calories;
27 grams fat; 28 grams protein;
110 grams carbohydrates;
22 grams fiber

Stewed Tomatoes with Garlic and Black Beans

Skin—page 71
Per serving: 318 calories;
4 grams fat; 18 grams protein;
56 grams carbohydrates;
14 grams fiber

Stuffed Sweet Potatoes with Spinach and Corn

Skin—page 73
Per serving: 321 calories;
8 grams fat; 7 grams protein;
59 grams carbohydrates;
9 grams fiber

Stuffed Zucchini, Yellow Squash, and Eggplant

Sleep—page 322
Per serving: 56 calories;
2 grams fat; 3 grams protein;
7 grams carbohydrates;
2 grams fiber

Summer Squash Salad with Baby Spinach, Roasted Tomatoes, and Parmesan Cheese

Bones—page 192
Per serving: 303 calories;
26 grams fat; 7 grams protein;
16 grams carbohydrates;
7 grams fiber

Sweet Balsamic Onions

Eyes—page 129
Per serving: 72 calories;
4 grams fat; 1 gram protein;
10 grams carbohydrates;
2 grams fiber

Sweet Pea Panzanella Salad

Feet—page 221
Per serving: 277 calories;
18 grams fat; 8 grams protein;
23 grams carbohydrates;
5 grams fiber

Sweet Potato Soufflé

Hands—page 249
Per serving: 233 calories;
9 grams fat; 6 grams protein;
32 grams carbohydrates;
3 grams fiber

Swiss Cheese Wafers
Smile—page 160
Per serving: 115 calories;
9 grams fat; 4 grams protein;
5 grams carbohydrates;
0 grams fiber

The Real Deal Fries with Ketchup of Course!
Stress—page 358
Per serving: 499 calories;
18 grams fat; 10 grams protein;
81 grams carbohydrates;
11 grams fiber

Toasted Corn with Sautéed Spinach and Cherry Tomatoes
Hair—page 103
Per serving: 86 calories;
4 grams fat; 4 grams protein;
11 grams carbohydrates;
4 grams fiber

Unfried Fried Onions
Eyes—page 132
Per serving: 181 calories;
14 grams fat; 2 grams protein;
14 grams carbohydrates;
3 grams fiber

Watercress Salad with Raspberry Vinaigrette and Blood Orange
Bones—page 191
Per serving: 298 calories;
27 gram fat; 2 grams protein;
14 grams carbohydrates;
3 grams fiber

•••• Snacks & Sweets ••••

Almond Cookies Two Ways
Sleep—page 327
Per serving: 191 calories;
10 grams fat; 3 grams protein;
24 grams carbohydrates;
1 gram fiber

Almond-Topped Ricotta Cheesecake
Bones—page 195
Per serving: 186 calories;
10 gram fat; 10 grams protein;
14 grams carbohydrates;
1 gram fiber

Baked Pears in Brandy Sauce
Hair—page 104
Per serving: 346 calories;
8 grams fat; 1 gram protein;
56 grams carbohydrates;
4 grams fiber

Banana Flaxseed Bread with Warm Strawberry Sauce
Skin—page 75
Per serving: 446 calories;
11 grams fat; 7 grams protein;
84 grams carbohydrates;
5 grams fiber

Basil-Roasted Strawberry Cheesecake with Rich Chocolate Crust
Sexy—page 397
Per serving: 882 calories;
67 grams fat; 14 grams protein;
61 grams carbohydrates;
3 grams fiber

Blueberry Shortbread Bars
Feet—page 223
Per serving: 171 calories;
8 grams fat; 2 grams protein;
24 grams carbohydrates;
1 gram fiber

Butterscotch Blondies
Sleep—page 325
Per serving: 241 calories;
11 grams fat; 3 grams protein;
33 grams carbohydrates;
0 grams fiber

Chilled Berry Sauce with Lime Sherbet and Coconut Garnish
Feet—page 225
Per serving: 78 calories;
1 gram fat; 1 gram protein;
19 grams carbohydrates;
6 grams fiber

Chocoholic's Crutch
Hands—page 255
Per serving: 379 calories;
33 grams fat; 10 grams protein;
25 grams carbohydrates;
7 grams fiber

Chocolate Gingersnaps
Stress—page 362
Per serving: 122 calories;
6 grams fat; 1 gram protein;
17 grams carbohydrates;
0 grams fiber

Chocolate Ricotta-Filled Crepes
Eyes—page 136
Per serving: 221 calories;
6 grams fat; 10 grams protein;
32 grams carbohydrates;
1 gram fiber

Cocktail Nut Cookie Bars
Bones—page 196
Per serving: 312 calories;
20 grams fat; 4 grams protein;
36 grams carbohydrates;
3 grams fiber

Cranberry Wedding Cookies
Eyes—page 135
Per serving: 145 calories;
12 grams fat; 2 grams protein;
9 grams carbohydrates;
1 gram fiber

Emergency Key Lime Pie
Smile—page 166
Per serving: 413 calories;
22 grams fat; 72 grams protein;
50 grams carbohydrates;
1 gram fiber

Fresh Lime Cake with Warm Blueberry Sauce
Tummies—page 286
Per serving: 308 calories;
14 grams fat; 4 grams protein;
43 grams carbohydrates;
1 gram fiber

Individual Brownie Cakes Loaded with Chocolate Chunks and Walnuts Served with Ice Cream and Hot Fudge Sauce
Sexy—page 395
Per serving: 592 calories;
39 grams fat; 8 grams protein;
61 grams carbohydrates;
3 grams fiber

Key Lime Pound Cake
Stress—page 360
Per serving: 286 calories;
12 grams fat; 3 grams protein;
42 grams carbohydrates;
0 grams fiber

Lemon Vanilla Pudding With Mixed Berries
Sexy—page 396
Per serving: 355 calories;
8 grams fat; 8 grams protein;
67 grams carbohydrates;
3 grams fiber

Macadamia Nut Biscotti Dipped in Chocolate and Coconut
Bones—page 193
Per serving: 150 calories;
9 grams fat; 2 grams protein;
17 grams carbohydrates;
1 gram fiber

Mango-Walnut Crumble
Smile—page 165
Per serving: 239 calories;
13 grams fat; 3 grams protein;
31 grams carbohydrates;
2 grams fiber

Maple Cake Doughnuts
Stress—page 361
Per serving: 253 calories;
7 grams fat; 5 grams protein;
44 grams carbohydrates;
0 grams fiber

New York–Style Cheesecake
Smile—page 164
Per serving: 231 calories;
11 grams fat; 7 grams protein;

27 grams carbohydrates;
0 grams fiber

Oatmeal Snack Cake
Hair—page 106
Per serving: 346 calories;
13 grams fat; 5 grams protein;
54 grams carbohydrates;
1 gram fiber

Orange and Tarragon–Infused Crème Brûlées with Sliced Bananas
Smile—page 163
Per serving: 386 calories;
18 grams fat; 10 grams protein;
49 grams carbohydrates;
2 grams fiber

Orange Cappuccino Parfaits
Tummies—page 285
Per serving: 208 calories;
3 grams fat; 16 grams protein;
28 grams carbohydrates;
0 grams fiber

Orange-Glazed Yogurt Cake
Eyes—page 134
Per serving: 247 calories;
10 grams fat; 4 grams protein;
35 grams carbohydrates;
0 grams fiber

Oven-Roasted Fruit with Vanilla Yogurt Sorbet
Skin—page 77
Per serving: 206 calories;
4 grams fat; 5 grams protein;
40 grams carbohydrates;
4 grams fiber

Peach Gingerbread with Walnut Streusel
Skin—page 76
Per serving: 284 calories;
10 grams fat; 6 grams protein;
43 grams carbohydrates;
2 grams fiber

Peanut Butter Chocolate Bars
Sexy—page 394
Per serving: 391 calories;
26 grams fat; 9 grams protein;
36 grams carbohydrates;
2 grams fiber

Peanut Butter Sandwich Cookies
Bones—page 194
Per serving: 291 calories;
25 gram fat; 4 grams protein;
14 grams carbohydrates;
1 gram fiber

Pear and Strawberry Crisp
Eyes—page 133
Per serving: 280 calories;
10 grams fat; 4 grams protein;
49 grams carbohydrates;
5 grams fiber

Pecan Graham Squares
Feet—page 226
Per serving: 187 calories;
10 grams fat; 3 grams protein;
22 grams carbohydrates;
1 gram fiber

Poached Cherry Sundaes
Tummies—page 288
Per serving: 162 calories;
9 grams fat; 1 gram protein;
36 grams carbohydrates;
2 grams fiber

Pretty in Peach
Stress—page 363
Per serving: 478 calories;
18 grams fat; 6 grams protein;
76 grams carbohydrates;
4 grams fiber

Rhubarb and Strawberry Frozen Yogurt with Fresh Mint
Hair—page 105
Per serving: 169 calories;
1 gram fat; 4 grams protein;
37 grams carbohydrates;
3 grams fiber

Roasted Figs with Sweetened Orange Sauce
Skin—page 74
Per serving: 86 calories;
0 grams fat; 1 gram protein;
22 grams carbohydrates;
3 grams fiber

Roasted Red Grape Parfaits with Orange and Maple-Flavored Ricotta Cheese
Hands—page 253
Per serving: 301 calories;
13 grams fat; 14 grams protein;
33 grams carbohydrates;
1 gram fiber

Sautéed Bananas with Sweet Mascarpone and Walnut Crunch
Hair—page 107
Per serving: 527 calories;
35 grams fat; 10 grams protein;
52 grams carbohydrates;
4 grams fiber

Simmering Blueberries with Cinnamon Dumplings
Sleep—page 324
Per serving: 209 calories;
1 gram fat; 3 grams protein;
49 grams carbohydrates;
2 grams fiber

Simple Chocolate Mousse with Graham Cracker Crumbles
Sleep—page 326
Per serving: 353 calories;
15 grams fat; 6 grams protein;
56 grams carbohydrates;
3 grams fiber

Simple Zucchini Cake with Vanilla Glaze
Hands—page 254
Per serving: 202 calories;
7 grams fat; 4 grams protein;
31 grams carbohydrates;
0 grams fiber

Strike-It-Rich Chocolate Pudding with Chocolate Cookie Crumbles
Hands—page 252
Per serving: 453 calories;
22 grams fat; 9 grams protein;
58 grams carbohydrates;
2 grams fiber

Tropical Buttermilk Panna Cotta with Strawberry Sauce
Tummies—page 287
Per serving: 238 calories;
4 grams fat; 5 grams protein;
48 grams carbohydrates;
2 grams fiber

Tropical Strawberry Tiramisu
Feet—page 224
Per serving: 355 calories;
26 grams fat; 3 grams protein;
28 grams carbohydrates;
1 gram fiber

RECIPE INDEX

• D–E •

• F •

• G •

• H •

• I–L •

• M •

• n–o •

• P •

Your GORGEOUS Lifestyle Made Easy

By now you realize that being *gorgeous* is all about living life to the fullest. To make this easy for you, we've created a website that will help you organize your week! Hair a little dull? Mood a little cranky? The lifestyle plans in this book are designed to let you focus on those areas that you feel need a little extra attention. You needn't follow them from week to week. Pick one or two that look interesting and get started by going to *www.GorgeousLifestyleGuide.com*. Click on the week that you have chosen. You will find a shopping list for all of the meals that you want to prepare. You will also find organizing shopping day tips for food prep that allows for simple meals during your busy week.

Don't stop there. While you are visiting *www.GorgeousLifestyleGuide.com* check out the latest Gorgeous Home Spa Secrets and news from Jorj's Glam Kitchen. Feel free to Ask Dr. Moon and get answers to your gorgeous questions. We'll even throw in a couple of relaxation and exercise tips to help you balance your life. And for those of you who are joining our Gorgeous Gal Pal Lunch Club, we'll offer special themes and menus so that you and your friends will enjoy the path to *Gorgeous* even more! Now, what can be easier than this?

Drop by and check us out, and you are well on your way to a *gorgeous* you!